Rapid
Medicine

Second Edition

Amir H. Sam
Hammersmith Hospital
Imperial College London
UK

James T.H. Teo
National Hospital for Neurology and Neurosurgery, London
UK

WILEY-BLACKWELL
A John Wiley & Sons, Ltd., Publication

This edition first published 2010, © 2003, 2010 by Amir H Sam and James T H Teo.

Blackwell Publishing was acquired by John Wiley & Sons in February 2007. Blackwells publishing program has been merged with Wileys global Scientific, Technical and Medical business to form Wiley-Blackwell.

Registered office: John Wiley & Sons Ltd, The Atrium, Southern Gate, Chichester, West Sussex, PO19 8SQ, UK

Editorial offices: 9600 Garsington Road, Oxford, OX4 2DQ, UK
                     The Atrium, Southern Gate, Chichester, West Sussex, PO19 8SQ, UK
                     111 River Street, Hoboken, NJ 07030-5774, USA

For details of our global editorial offices, for customer services and for information about how to apply for permission to reuse the copyright material in this book please see our website at www.wiley.com/wiley-blackwell

The right of the author to be identified as the author of this work has been asserted in accordance with the Copyright, Designs and Patents Act 1988.

Wiley also publishes its books in a variety of electronic formats. Some content that appears in print may not be available in electronic books.

Designations used by companies to distinguish their products are often claimed as trademarks. All brand names and product names used in this book are trade names, service marks, trademarks or registered trademarks of their respective owners. The publisher is not associated with any product or vendor mentioned in this book. This publication is designed to provide accurate and authoritative information in regard to the subject matter covered. It is sold on the understanding that the publisher is not engaged in rendering professional services. If professional advice or other expert assistance is required, the services of a competent professional should be sought.

Library of Congress Cataloging-in-Publication Data

Sam, Amir H.
   Rapid medicine / Amir H. Sam, James T.H. Teo. – 2nd ed.
        p. ; cm. – (Rapid series)
   Rev. ed. of: Rapid medicine / Amir H. Sam ... [et al.]. 2003.
   Includes index.
   ISBN 978-1-4051-8323-9
   1. Internal medicine–Handbooks, manuals, etc. I. Teo, James T. H. II. Rapid medicine. III. Title. IV. Series:
Rapid series.
   [DNLM: 1. Clinical Medicine–Handbooks. 2. Signs and Symptoms–Handbooks. WB 39 S187ra 2010]
   RC55.R37 2010
   616–dc22

                                                                                       2010015319

ISBN: 9781405183239

A catalogue record for this book is available from the British Library.

Set in 7.5pt/9.5pt Frutiger-Light by Thomson Digital, Noida, India

Printed and bound in Malaysia by Vivar Printing Sdn Bhd

1   2010

Contents

Preface

In the conception of this book, we envisioned a text encompassing core medical conditions in an easily accessible format. *Rapid Medicine* covers over 200 diseases in a structured manner. For each condition we have summarised the Definition, Aetiology, Epidemiology, History, Examination, Investigations, Management, Complications and Prognosis. We hope that this will provide a useful pocketbook on the wards and in preparation for exams.

In clinical practice however, patients present with symptoms and signs rather than confirmed diagnoses. It is therefore essential to supplement the knowledge of various diseases with an understanding of the differential diagnoses of clinical presentations. The second edition of *Rapid Medicine* has been configured with this learning strategy in mind. This new edition contains a separate section on the differential diagnoses for a range of symptoms, signs and laboratory test results, reflecting the way in which most of your patients will present to you during your study and clinical practice.

This edition also contains an additional section named 'Shorter Topics'. Here we have included a number of important conditions that medical students need to know about, but perhaps not in as much detail. We hope that you enjoy this book and use it to consolidate your ward-based learning.

Amir H. Sam
James T.H. Teo

List of abbreviations

ABG	arterial blood gas
ABPA	allergic bronchopulmonary aspergillosis
ACAG	acute closed-angle glaucoma
ACE	angiotensin-converting enzyme
ACh	acetylecholine
ACTH	adrenocorticotrophic hormone
ADH	antidiuretic hormone
AF	atrial fibrillation
AFP	alpha feto-protein
AIDS	acquired immune deficiency syndrome
ALP	alkaline phosphatase
ALA	δ-aminolaevulinic acid
ALL	acute lymphoblastic leukaemia
ALS	amyotrophic lateral sclerosis
ALT	alanine transaminase
AML	acute myeloblastic leukaemia
ANA	anti-nuclear antibody
ANCA	anti-neutrophil cytoplasm antibody
APP	amyloid precursor protein
APTT	activated partial thromboplastin time
ARDS	acute respiratory distress syndrome
ARF	acute renal failure
5-ASA	5-aminosalicyclic acid
ASD	atrioseptal defect
ASM	anti-smooth muscle antibody
AST	aspartate aminotransferase
ATN	acute tubular necrosis
AV	atrioventricular
AXR	abdominal X-ray
BCC	basal cell carcinoma
BCG	Bacille Calmette–Guérin
BiPAP	biphasic positive airway pressure
BMI	body mass index
BP	blood pressure
CABG	coronary artery bypass graft
CAH	congenital adrenal hyperplasia
c-ANCA	cytoplasmic anti-neutrophil cytoplasmic antibodies
CAPD	continuous ambulatory peritoneal dialysis
CEA	carcinoembyonic antigen
CHD	coronary heart disease
CK	creatine kinase
CLL	chronic lymphocytic leukaemia
CM	cardiomyopathy
CML	chronic myelocytic leukaemia
CMML	chronic myelomonocytic leukaemia
CMV	cytomegalovirus
CNS	central nervous system
COAD	chronic obstructive airway disease
COMT	catechol-O-methyltransferase
COPD	chronic obstructive pulmonary disease

CPAP	continuous positive airway pressure
CPR	cardiopulmonary resuscitation
CREST	syndrome of calcinosis, Raynaud's, oesophageal dysmotility, sclerodactyly and telangiectasia
CRF	corticotrophin-releasing factor/chronic renal failure
CRH	cortisol-releasing hormone
CRP	C-reactive protein
CSF	cerebrospinal fluid
CSS	Churg–Strauss syndrome
CT	computerized tomography
CTP	carboxyterminal propeptide
CVA	cerebrovascular accident
CVP	central venous pressure
CVS	chorionic villus sampling/cardiovascular system
CXR	chest X-ray
DCM	dilated cardiomyopathy
DDAVP	desmopressin
DHEA	dehydroepiandrosterone
DHEAS	dehydroepiandrosterone sulphate
DIC	disseminated intravascular coagulation
DIDMOAD	syndrome of diabetes insipidus, diabetes mellitus, optic atrophy and deafness
DIP	desquamative interstitial pneumonia/distal interphalangeal
DKA	diabetic ketoacidosis
DMD	duchenne muscular dystrophy
DNA	deoxyribonucleic acid
DOPA	dihydroxyphenylalanine
DPTA	diethylenetriamine penta-acetate
DVT	deep vein thrombosis
EBV	Epstein–Barr virus
ECG	electrocardiogram
EDTA	ethylenediaminetetra-acetate
EEG	electroencephalogram
ELISA	enzyme-linked immunoabsorbent assay
EMD	electrical–mechanical dissociation
EMG	electromyogram
ENT	ear, nose and throat
ERCP	endoscopic retrograde cholangio-pancreatography
ESR	erythrocyte sedimentation rate
ETT	exercise tolerance test
FAB	French–American–British classification
FBC	full blood count
FEV_1	forced expiratory volume in 1 s
FFP	fresh frozen plasma
FSH	follicle-stimulating hormone
FVC	forced vital capacity
GABA	gamma-aminobutyric acid
GAD	glutamic acid decarboxylase
GBM	glomerular basement membrane
GCA	giant cell arteritis
GCS	glasgow Coma Scale
GFR	glomerular filtration rate
GGT	γ-glutamyl transferase
GH	growth hormone

GHRH	growth-hormone-releasing hormone
GI	gastrointestinal
GnRH	gonadotrophin-releasing hormone
G6PD	glucose-6-phosphate dehydrogenase
GTT	glucose tolerance test
HAART	highly active antiiretroviral treatment
HACEK	haemophilus, actinobacillus, cardiobacterium, eikenella, kingella
HAV	hepatitis A
Hb	haemoglobin
HBIG	hepatitis B immunoglobulin
HBV	hepatitis B virus
HCC	hepatocellular carcinoma
hCG	human chorionic gonadotrophin
HCM	hypertrophic cardiomyopathy
HCV	hepatitis C virus
HDL	high-density lipoprotein
HDV	hepatitis D virus
HEV	hepatitis E
5-HIAA	5-hydroxyindole acetic acid
HIDA	hepatoiminodiacetic acid
HIV	human immunodeficiency virus
HLA	human leukocyte antigen
HNF	hepatocyte nuclear factor
HONK	hyperosmolar non-ketotic
HSP	Henoch–Schönlein purpura
HSV	herpes simplex virus
HTLV	human T-cell lymphoma virus
HUS	haemolytic–uraemic syndrome
IBD	inflammatory bowel disease
IBS	irritable bowel syndrome
ICP	intracranial pressure
ICT	immunochromato- graphic test
IDDM	insulin-dependent diabetes mellitus
Ig	immunoglobulin
IGF-	insulin-like growth factor
IHD	ischaemic heart disease
IL	interleukin
IM	intramuscular
INR	international normalized ratio
IOP	intraocular pressure
IPPV	intermittent positive pressure ventilation
ITP	immune thrombocytopenic purpura
ITU	intensive therapy unit
IV	intravenous
IVIG	intravenous infusions of immunoglobulin
IVU	intravenous urogram
JVP	jugular venous pressure
KD	Kawasaki's disease
KUB	abdominal radiograph of kidneys, ureter and bladder
LBBB	left bundle branch block
LDH	lactate dehydrogenase
LDL	low-density lipoprotein
LFT	liver function test
LH	luteinizing hormone/laparoscopic hysterectomy

LKM	liver/kidney microsomal (antibodies)
LMN	lower motor neurone
LMW	low molecular weight
MAO	monoamine oxidase
MCH	mean cell haemoglobin
MCP	metacarpal-phalangeal
MCV	mean cell volume
MEC	mixed essential cryoglobulinaemia
MEN	multiple endocrine neoplasia
MI	myocardial infarct
MIBG	meta-iodobenzyguanidine
MODS	multiple organ dysfunction syndrome
MODY	maturity-onset diabetes of the young
MP	microscopic polyangiitis
MPGN	membranoproliferative glomerulonephritis
MRCP	magnetic resonance cholangio-pancreography
MPTP	1-methyl-4-phenyl-1,2,3,6-tetrahydro- pyridine
MRI	magnetic resonance imaging
MS	multiple sclerosis
MSE	mental state examination
MSU	midstream urine
MTP	metatarsophalangeal
NAC	*N*-acetylcysteine
NAPQI	*N*-acetyl-*p*-benzoquinoneimine
NASH	non-alcoholic streatohepatitis
NIDDM	non-insulin-dependent diabetes mellitus
NK	natural killer
NSAIDs	non-steroidal anti-inflammatory drugs
NSIP	non-specific interstitial pneumonia
OGD	oesaphago-gastro-duodenoscopy
OTC	over-the-counter
PAF	platelet-activating factor
PAN	polyarteritis nodosa
pANCA	perinuclear antineutrophil cytoplasmic antibodies
PAS	periodic acid–Schiff
PBG	porphobilinogen
PCOS	polycystic ovarian syndrome
PCP	*Pneumocystis carinii* pneumonia
PCR	polymerase chain reaction
PCS	primary sclerosing cholangitis
PCV	packed cell volume
PCWP	pulmonary capillary wedge pressure
PEEP	positive end expiratory pressure
PEFR	peak expiratory flow rate
PEG	percutaneous endoscopic gastronomy
PET	positron emission tomography
PIP	peripheral-interphalangeal
PKD	polycystic kidney disease
PKDL	post kala azar dermal leishmaniasis
PMR	polymyalgia rheumatica
POAG	primary open-angle glaucoma
POEMS	syndrome of polyneuropathy, endocrinopathy, monoclonal gammopathy and skin pigmentation
PPAR	peroxisome proliferator-activated receptor

PPD	purified protein derivative of tuberculin
PR	per rectum
PSC	primary sclerosing cholangitis
PT	prothrombin time
PTH	parathyroid hormone
PUVA	psoralen and ultraviolet A therapy
QBC	quantitative buffy coat test
RA	refractory anaemia
RAEB	refractory anaemia with excess blasts
RAEB-t	RAEB in transformation
RAO	retinal artery occlusion
RAPD	relative afferent pupillary defect
RARS	refractory anaemia with ring sideroblasts
RAST	radio-allergosorbent test
RBBB	right bundle branch block
RBC	red blood cell
RCM	restrictive cardiomyopathy
REAL	Revised American and European Lymphoma classification
RP	relapsing polychondritis
RNA	ribonucleic acid
RTA	renal tubular acidosis
RUQ	right upper quadrant
RVO	retinal vein occlusion
SAA	serum amyloid A
SAP	serum amyloid P
SAPHO	syndrome of synovitis, acne, palmoplantar pustulosis, hyperostosis, osteitis
SBP	spontaneous bacterial peritonitis
SC	subcutaneous
SCC	squamous cell carcinoma
SHBG	sex-hormone-binding globulin
SIADH	syndrome of inappropriate ADH
SIRS	systemic inflammatory response syndrome
SLE	systemic lupus erythematosus
SMA	smooth muscle antibody
SPECT	single photon emission computerized tomography
SXR	skull X-ray
$t_{1/2}$	half-life
T_3	tri-iodothyronine
T_4	thyroxine
TA	Takayasu's disease
TB	tuberculosis
t.d.s.	three times per day
TEN	toxic epidermal necrolysis
TFT	thyroid function test
TIA	transient ischaemic attack
TIBC	total iron-binding capacity
TIPS	transjugular intrahepatic portosystemic shunt
TLCO	carbon monoxide transfer factor
TNF	tumour necrosis factor
tPA	tissue plasminogen activator
TPN	total parenteral nutrition
TRAP	tartrate-resistant acid phosphatase
TRH	thyroid-releasing hormone
TSH	thyroid-stimulating hormone

TTP	thrombotic thrombocytopenic purpura
UC	ulcerative colitis
U&E	urea and electrolytes
UIP	usual interstitial pneumonia
UMN	upper motor neurone
UTI	urinary tract infection
UV	ultraviolet
VCA	viral capsid antigen
VDRL	venereal disease research laboratory
VF	ventricular fibrillation
VLDL	very low-density lipoprotein
VQ	ventilation: perfusion ratio
VSD	ventriculoseptal defect
VT	ventricular tachycardia
vWF	von Willebrand's factor
VZV	varicella zoster virus
VZIG	varicella zoster immunoglobulin
WCC	white cell count
WG	Wegener's granulomatosis
WHO	World Health Organization

List of symbols

<	less than
>	greater than
/	or
↑	increased
↓	decreased
♀	female
♂	male

Medical Conditions

Aortic dissection

DEFINITION   A condition where a tear in the aortic intima allows blood to surge into the aortic wall, causing a split between the inner and outer tunica media, and creating a false lumen.

AETIOLOGY   Degenerative changes in the smooth muscle of the aortic media are the predisposing event. Common causes and predisposing factors are:
* hypertension;
* aortic atherosclerosis;
* connective tissue disease (e.g. SLE, Marfan's, Ehlers–Danlos);
* congenital cardiac abnormalities (e.g. aortic coarctation);
* aortitis (e.g. Takayasu's aortitis, tertiary syphilis);
* iatrogenic (e.g. during angiography or angioplasty);
* trauma;
* crack cocaine.

Stanford classification divides dissection into:

* *type A* with ascending aorta tear (most common);
* *type B* with descending aorta tear distal to the left subclavian artery.

Expansion of the false aneurysm may obstruct the subclavian, carotid, coeliac and renal arteries.

EPIDEMIOLOGY   Most common in ♂ between 40 and 60 years.

HISTORY   Sudden central 'tearing' pain, may radiate to the back (may mimic an MI). Aortic dissection can lead to occlusion of the aorta and its branches:

Carotid obstruction: Hemiparesis, dysphasia, blackout.
Coronary artery obstruction: Chest pain (angina or MI).
Subclavian obstruction: Ataxia, loss of consciousness.
Anterior spinal artery: Paraplegia.
Coeliac obstruction: Severe abdominal pain (ischaemic bowel).
Renal artery obstruction: Anuria, renal failure.

EXAMINATION   Murmur on the back below left scapula, descending to abdomen.
Blood pressure (BP): Hypertension (BP discrepancy between arms of >20 mmHg), wide pulse pressure. If hypotensive may signify tamponade, check for pulsus paradoxus.
Aortic insufficiency: Collapsing pulse, early diastolic murmur over aortic area.
Unequal arm pulses.
There may be a palpable abdominal mass.

INVESTIGATIONS
Bloods: FBC, cross-match 10 units of blood, U&E (renal function), clotting.
CXR: Widened mediastinum, localized bulge in the aortic arch.
ECG: Often normal. Signs of left ventricular hypertrophy or inferior MI if dissection compromises the ostia of the right coronary artery.
CT-thorax: False lumen of dissection can be visualized.
Echocardiography: Transoesophageal is highly specific.
Cardiac catheterization and aortography.

MANAGEMENT
Acute: If suspected, CT-thorax should be performed urgently concurrent to resuscitation. Resuscitate and restore blood volume with blood products. Monitor pulse and BP in both arms, central venous pressure monitoring, urinary catheter. Best managed in ITU setting.

Aortic dissection (continued)

Type A dissection: Treated surgically. Emergency surgery because of the risk of cardiac tamponade. Affected aorta is replaced by a tube graft. Aortic valve may also be replaced.

Type B dissection: Can be treated medically, surgically or by endovascular stenting. Control BP and prevent further dissection with IV nitroprusside and/or IV labetalol (use calcium channel blocker if β-blocker contraindicated). Surgical repair may be appropriate for patients with intractable or recurrent pain, aortic expansion, end-organ ischemia or progression of dissection, and has similar outcome rates. Endovascular repair is a newer technique using endovascular stents and is available in some centres, although evidence of benefit is still lacking (ADSORB trial results pending).

COMPLICATIONS   Aortic rupture, cardiac tamponade, pulmonary oedema, MI, syncope, cerebrovascular, renal, mesenteric or spinal ischaemia.

PROGNOSIS   Untreated mortality: 30% at 24 h, 75% at 2 weeks.
Operative mortality of 5–10%. A further 10% have neurological sequelae.
Prognosis for type B better than type A.

Aortic regurgitation

DEFINITION   Reflux of blood from aorta into left ventricle (LV) during diastole. Aortic regurgitation (AR) is also called aortic insufficiency.

AETIOLOGY
Aortic valve leaflet abnormalities or damage: Bicuspid aortic valve, infective endocarditis, rheumatic fever, trauma.
Aortic root/ascending aorta dilation: Systemic hypertension, aortic dissection, aortitis (e.g. syphilis, Takayasu's arteritis), arthritides (rheumatoid arthritis, seronegative arthritides), Marfan's syndrome, pseudoxanthoma elasticum, Ehlers–Danlos syndrome, osteogenesis imperfecta.
Reflux of blood into the LV during diastole results in left ventricular dilation and ↑ end-diastolic volume and ↑ stroke volume. The combination of ↑ stroke volume and low end-diastolic pressure in the aorta may explain the collapsing pulse and the wide pulse pressure. In acute AR, the LV cannot adapt to the rapid increase in end-diastolic volume caused by regurgitant blood.

EPIDEMIOLOGY   Chronic AR often begins in the late 50s, documented most frequently in patients >80 years.

HISTORY   Chronic AR: initially asymptomatic. Later, symptoms of heart failure: exertional dyspnoea, orthopnoea, fatigue. Occasionally angina.
Severe acute AR: sudden cardiovascular collapse.
Symptoms related to the aetiology, e.g. chest or back pain in patients with aortic dissection.

EXAMINATION   Collapsing 'water-hammer' pulse and wide pulse pressure. Thrusting and heaving (volume-loaded) displaced apex beat.
Early diastolic murmur at lower left sternal edge, better heard with the patient sitting forward with the breath held in expiration. An ejection systolic murmur is often heard because of ↑ flow across the valve.
Austin Flint mid-diastolic murmur: Over the apex, from turbulent reflux hitting anterior cusp of the mitral valve and causing a physiological mitral stenosis.
Rare signs associated with a hyperdynamic pulse:
  Quincke's sign: Visible pulsations on nail-bed.
  de Musset's sign: Head nodding in time with pulse.
  Becker's sign: Visible pulsations of the pupils and retinal arteries.
  Müller's sign: Visible pulsation of the uvula.
  Corrigan's sign: Visible pulsations in neck.
  Traube's sign: 'Pistol shot' (systolic and diastolic sounds) heard on auscultation of the femoral arteries.
  Duroziez's sign: A systolic and diastolic bruit heard on partial compression of femoral artery with a stethoscope.
  Rosenbach's sign: Systolic pulsations of the liver.
  Gerhard's sign: Systolic pulsations of the spleen.
  Hill's sign: Popliteal cuff systolic pressure exceeding brachial pressure by >60 mmHg.

INVESTIGATIONS
CXR: Cardiomegaly. Dilation of the ascending aorta. Signs of pulmonary oedema may be seen with left heart failure.
ECG: May show signs of left ventricular hypertrophy (deep S wave in V_{1-2}, tall R wave in V_{5-6}, inverted T waves in I, aVL, V_{5-6} and left-axis deviation).

Aortic regurgitation (continued)

Echocardiogram: 2D echo and M-mode may indicate the underlying cause (e.g. aortic root dilation, bicuspid aortic valve) or the effects of AR (left ventricular dilation/dysfunction and fluttering of the anterior mitral valve leaflet). Doppler echocardiography for detecting AR and assessing severity. Periodic (annual) follow-up echocardiogram for serial measurements of LV size and function.

Cardiac catheterization with angiography: If there is uncertainty about the functional state of the ventricle or the presence of coronary artery disease.

MANAGEMENT

Aortic valve replacement: In patients with symptoms of ventricular decompensation, or LV dysfunction: ejection fraction <50%, LV enlargement (end-systolic dimension >55 mm; end-diastolic dimension >75 mm).

Vasodilators (ACE inhibitor or nifedipine): In patients with LV systolic dysfunction (left ventricular ejection fraction (LVEF) <50%), or progressive LV dilatation. Vasodilators ↓ systemic vascular resistance and the afterload, i.e. the burden on the volume-loaded LV. Treat the complications (e.g. heart failure).

COMPLICATIONS   Left ventricular failure and pulmonary oedema.

PROGNOSIS   Chronic AR is often well tolerated for many years without symptoms.

Prognosis depends on the underlying aetiology. Acute AR caused by aortic dissection or infective endocarditis is fatal if not treated urgently.

Aortic stenosis

DEFINITION   Narrowing of the left ventricular outflow at the level of the aortic valve.

AETIOLOGY
1. Stenosis secondary to rheumatic heart disease (commonest worldwide);
2. calcification of a congenital bicuspid aortic valve;
3. calcification/degeneration of a tricuspid aortic valve in the elderly.

EPIDEMIOLOGY   Prevalence in ~3% of 75-year-olds. ♂ > ♀. Those with bicuspid aortic valve may present earlier (as young adults).

HISTORY   May be asymptomatic initially.
Angina (because of ↑ oxygen demand of the hypertrophied ventricles).
Syncope or dizziness on exercise.
Symptoms of heart failure (e.g. dyspnoea).

EXAMINATION
BP: Narrow pulse pressure.
Pulse: Slow-rising.
Palpation: Thrill in the aortic area (if severe). Forceful sustained thrusting undisplaced apex beat.
Auscultation: Harsh ejection systolic murmur at aortic area, radiating to the carotid artery and apex. Second heart sound (A2 component) may be softened or absent (because of calcification). A bicuspid valve may produce an ejection click.
Distinguish from aortic sclerosis[1] and hypertrophic obstructive cardiomyopathy (HOCM).[2]

INVESTIGATIONS
ECG: Signs of left ventricular hypertrophy (deep S wave in V_{1-2}, tall R wave in V_{5-6}, inverted T waves in I, aVL, V_{5-6} and left-axis deviation), LBBB.
CXR: Post-stenotic enlargement of the ascending aorta, calcification of aortic valve.
Echocardiogram: Visualizes structural changes of the valves and level of stenosis (valvar, supravalvar or subvalvar). Estimation of aortic valve area and pressure gradient across the valve in systole and left ventricular function may be assessed.
Cardiac angiography: Allows differentiation from other causes of angina, and to assess for concomitant coronary artery disease (50% of patients with severe aortic stenosis have significant coronary artery disease).

MANAGEMENT   General principle is surgical management unless contraindicated.
Surgical: Valve replacement is recommended if valve pressure difference is >50 mmHg in a symptomatic patient. If unfit for surgery, balloon dilation (valvoplasty) may be performed but this is considered to be a palliative procedure due to high rate of complications (e.g. MI, myocardial perforation, severe AR).
Medical: Manage left ventricular failure (see Cardiac failure); ACE inhibitors and vasodilators should be used very cautiously in aortic stenosis. Antibiotic prophylaxis against infective endocarditis.

---

[1] Aortic sclerosis is senile degeneration with no left ventricular outflow tract obstruction. The pulse character is normal, a thrill is not palpable and the ejection systolic murmur radiates only faintly. The S_2 heart sound is normal.

[2] HOCM: see Cardiomyopathy.

Aortic stenosis (continued)

COMPLICATIONS   Arrhythmias, Stokes–Adams attacks, MI, left ventricular failure and sudden death.

PROGNOSIS   Survival differs according to symptoms. In symptomatic patients with severe aortic stenosis causing left ventricular failure, average survival 50% at 18 months without surgery. Average survival with angina 5 years; syncope 3 years; dyspnoea 2 years.

Atrial fibrillation

DEFINITION   Characterized by rapid, chaotic and ineffective atrial electrical conduction. Often subdivided into: 'permanent', 'persistent' and 'paroxysmal'.

AETIOLOGY   There may be no identifiable cause ('lone' atrial fibrillation (AF)). Secondary causes lead to abnormal atrial electrical pathways that result in AF.

Systemic causes: Thyrotoxicosis, hypertension, pneumonia, alcohol.

Heart: Mitral valve disease, ischaemic heart disease, rheumatic heart disease, cardiomyopathy, pericarditis, sick sinus syndrome,[1] atrial myxoma.

Lung: Bronchial carcinoma, pulmonary embolism.

EPIDEMIOLOGY   Very common in the elderly ($\sim$5% of those >65 years). May be paroxysmal.

HISTORY   Often asymptomatic. Some patients experience palpitations or syncope. Symptoms of the cause of the AF.

EXAMINATION   Irregularly irregular pulse, difference in apical beat and radial pulse. Look for thyroid disease and valvular heart disease.

INVESTIGATIONS

ECG: Uneven baseline (fibrillations) with absent P waves, irregular QRS complexes. If there is a saw-tooth baseline, consider if there is atrial flutter.[2]

Blood: Cardiac enzymes, TFT, lipid profile, U&E, Mg^{2+}, Ca^{2+} (risk of digoxin toxicity ↑ with hypokalaemia, hypomagnesaemia or hypercalcaemia).

Echocardiogram: To assess for mitral valve disease, left atrial dilation, left ventricular dysfunction or structural abnormalities.

MANAGEMENT   Treat any reversible cause (e.g. thyrotoxicosis, chest infection). Specific treatment strategy focuses on:

(1) **Rhythm control**[3]:

If the AF is >48 h from onset, anticoagulate (at least 3–4 weeks) before attempting cardioversion.

DC cardioversion: Synchronized DC shock (2 × 100 J, 1 × 200 J).

Chemical cardioversion: Flecainide (contraindicated if there is history of ischaemic heart disease) or amiodarone.

Prophylaxis against AF: Sotalol, amiodarone or flecainide. Also consider providing 'pill-in-the-pocket' strategy for suitable patients.

(2) **Rate control**[3]

Chronic 'permanent' AF: Ventricular rate control with digoxin, verapamil and/or β-blockers. Aim for rate of $\sim$90/min..

---

[1]Sick sinus (or tachy–brady) syndrome: caused by ischaemia, infarction or fibrosis of the sinus node, presenting with bradycardia (caused by intermittent failure of sinus node depolarization), with ↑ P–P intervals (>2 s) and intermittent tachycardia (caused by ↑ ectopic pacemaker activity). Treated with pacemaker insertion for symptomatic bradycardia, anti-arrhythmics for tachycardia and anticoagulation to reduce risk of thromboembolism.

[2]Atrial flutter is characterized by atrial rate of 300 min^{-1} and ventricular rate of 150 min^{-1} (2:1 heart block as atrioventricular (AV) node conducts every second beat). ECG shows a regular 'saw-tooth' baseline (rate $\sim$300 min^{-1}). Can be reversed by vagal manoeuvres, IV adenosine (with cardiac monitoring) or chemical cardioversion.

[3]The AFFIRM trial showed that rhythm control offers no survival advantage over rate control.

Atrial fibrillation (continued)

(3) **Stroke risk stratification**:

Low-risk patients can be managed with aspirin, and high-risk patients require anticoagulation with warfarin. Risk factors indicating high risk are previous thromboembolic event, age $\geq$75 years with hypertension, diabetes or vascular disease, and/or clinical evidence of valve disease, heart failure or impaired left ventricular function.

COMPLICATIONS   Thromboembolism (e.g. embolic stroke ~4% risk per year, ↑ risk with left atrial enlargement or left ventricular dysfunction). Worsens any existing heart failure.

PROGNOSIS   Chronic AF in a diseased heart does not usually return to sinus rhythm.

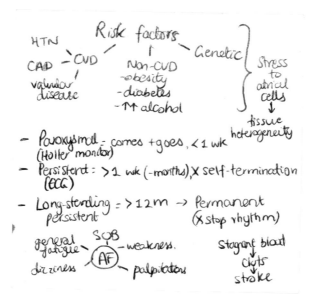

Cardiac Arrest[1]

DEFINITION   Acute cessation of cardiac function.

AETIOLOGY   Classical reversible causes of cardiac arrest are the four H's and four T's:

Hypoxia	Tamponade
Hypothermia	Tension pneumothorax
Hypovolaemia	Thromboembolism
Hypo- or hyperkalaemia	Toxins and other metabolic disorders (drugs, therapeutic agents, sepsis)

EPIDEMIOLOGY   N/A.

HISTORY   Management precedes or is concurrent to history (e.g. from witnesses).

EXAMINATION   Unconscious, patient is not breathing, absent carotid pulses.

INVESTIGATIONS
Cardiac monitor: Classification of the rhythm directs management (see below).
Bloods: ABG, U&E, FBC, cross-match, clotting, toxicology screen, glucose.

MANAGEMENT
Safety: Approach any arrest scene with caution as the cause of the arrest may still pose
   a threat. Defibrillators and oxygen are hazards. Help should be summoned as soon as
   possible.
Basic life support[1]:
1. If the arrest is witnessed and monitored, consider giving a precordial thump if no
   defibrillator immediately available.
2. Clear and maintain *airway* with head tilt (if no spinal injury), jaw thrust and chin lift.
3. Assess *breathing* by look, listen and feel.
   If not breathing, give two effective breaths immediately.
4. Assess *circulation* at carotid pulse for 10 s.
   If absent, give 30 chest compressions at rate of $\sim 100\,min^{-1}$. Continue cycles of 30
   compressions for every two breaths.
5. Proceed to advanced life support as soon as possible.

Advanced life support[1]:
1. Attach cardiac monitor and defibrillator.
2. Assess the rhythm:
   (A) If pulseless ventricular tachycardia (VT)[2] or ventricular fibrillation (VF)[3] ('shockable
   rhythm'):
   - Defibrillate once: 150–360 J biphasic, 360 J monophasic. (Ensure no one is touching
     patient or bed when defibrillating.)
   - Resume CPR immediately for 2 min, and then return to 2.
   - Administer adrenaline (1 mg IV) after second defibrillation and again every 3–5 min.
   - If 'shockable rhythm' persists after third shock, administer amiodarone 300 mg IV bolus
     (or lidocaine).

---

[1] Refer to latest UK Resuscitation Council guidelines.

[2] *VT*: >3 successive ventricular extrasystoles (broad QRS complexes: >120 ms) at a rate of >120 min^{-1}.
Patients at high risk of recurrent VT should be considered for implantable defibrillator which has been
shown to be more effective than amiodarone.

[3] *VF*: Irregular, rapid ventricular activation with no cardiac output.

Cardiac Arrest (continued)

(B) If pulseless electrical activity (PEA) or asystole:
- CPR for 2 min, and then return to 2.
- Administer adrenaline (1 mg IV) every 3–5 min.
- Atropine (3 mg IV, once only) if asystole or PEA with rate $<60\,min^{-1}$.

(C) During CPR:
- Check electrodes, paddle positions and contacts.
- Secure airway (e.g. attempt endotracheal intubation, high-flow oxygen). Once airway secure, give continuous compressions and breaths.
- Consider magnesium, bicarbonate, external pacing.
- Stop CPR and check pulse only if change in rhythm or signs of life.

Treatment of reversible causes:
Hypothermia: Warm slowly.
Hypo- or hyperkalaemia: Correction of electrolytes.
Hypovolaemia: IV colloids, crystalloids or blood products.
Tamponade: Pericardiocentesis under xiphisternum up and leftwards.
Tension pneumothorax: Needle into second intercostal space, mid-clavicular line.
Thromboembolism: (*see* Pulmonary embolism, Myocardial infarction).
Toxins: (*see* drug formulary for antidotes).

COMPLICATIONS   Irreversible hypoxic brain damage, death.

PROGNOSIS   Resuscitation is less successful in the arrests that occur outside hospital. Duration of inadequate effective cardiac output is associated with poor prognosis.

Cardiac failure

DEFINITION   Inability of the cardiac output to meet the body's demands despite normal venous pressures.

AETIOLOGY:
Low output (↓ cardiac output):
Left heart failure: Ischaemic heart disease, hypertension, cardiomyopathy, aortic valve disease, mitral regurgitation.
Right heart failure: Secondary to left heart failure, infarction, cardiomyopathy, pulmonary hypertension/embolus/valve disease, chronic lung disease, tricuspid regurgitation, constrictive pericarditis/pericardial tamponade.
Biventricular failure: Arrhythmia, cardiomyopathy (dilated or restrictive), myocarditis, drug toxicity.
High output (↑ demand): Anaemia, beriberi, pregnancy, Paget's disease, hyperthyroidism, arteriovenous malformation.

EPIDEMIOLOGY   10% of > 65-year-olds.
Left: Tachycardia, tachypnoea, displaced apex beat, bilateral basal crackles, third heart sound ('gallop' rhythm: rapid ventricular filling), pansystolic murmur (functional mitral regurgitation).
Acute LVF: Tachypnoea, cyanosis, tachycardia, peripheral shutdown, pulsus alternans, gallop rhythm, wheeze 'cardiac asthma', fine crackles throughout the lung.
Right: ↑ JVP, hepatomegaly, ascites, ankle/sacral pitting, oedema, signs of functional tricuspid regurgitation (*see* Tricuspid regurgitation).

HISTORY
Left (symptoms caused by pulmonary congestion): Dyspnoea (New York Heart Association classification):
1. no dyspnoea;
2. dyspnoea on ordinary activities;
3. dyspnoea on less than ordinary activities;
4. dyspnoea at rest.
Orthopnoea, paroxysmal nocturnal dyspnoea, fatigue.
Acute LVF: Dyspnoea, wheeze, cough and pink frothy sputum.
Right: Swollen ankles, fatigue, ↑ weight (resulting from oedema), ↓ exercise tolerance, anorexia, nausea.

INVESTIGATIONS
Blood: FBC, U&Es, LFTs, CRP, glucose, lipids, TFTs.
In acute LVF: ABG, troponin, brain natriuretic peptide (BNP). ↑ Plasma BNP suggests the diagnosis of cardiac failure. A low plasma BNP rules out cardiac failure (90% sensitivity).
CXR (in acute LVF): Cardiomegaly (heart >50 % of thoracic width), prominent upper lobe vessels, pleural effusion, interstitial oedema ('Kerley B lines'), perihilar shadowing ('bat's wings'), fluid in the fissures.
ECG: May be normal. May have ischaemic changes, arrhythmia, left ventricular hypertrophy (seen in hypertension).
Echocardiogram: To assess ventricular contraction. If left ventricular ejection fraction (LVEF) <40%: systolic dysfunction. Diastolic dysfunction: ↓ compliance leading to a restrictive filling defect.
Swan–Ganz catheter: Allows measurements of right atrial, right ventricular, pulmonary artery, pulmonary wedge and left ventricular end-diastolic pressures.

MANAGEMENT
Acute LVF: *Cardiogenic shock*: Severe cardiac failure with low BP requires the use of inotropes (e.g. dopamine, dobutamine) and should be managed in ITU.

Cardiac failure (continued)

Pulmonary oedema: Sit up patient, 60–100% O_2 and consider CPAP. Other first-line therapies are diamorphine (venodilator and anxiolytic effect), GTN infusion ($\downarrow$ preload), IV furosemide if fluid overloaded (venodilator and later diuretic effect). Monitor BP, respiratory rate, sat. O_2, urine output, ECG. Treat the cause, e.g. myocardial infarction, arrhythmia.

Chronic LVF: Treat the cause, e.g. hypertension. Treat exacerbating factors, e.g. anaemia. The following drug therapies are evidence-based.[1]

ACE-inhibitors (e.g. enalapril, perindopril, ramipril): Inhibit intracardiac renin-angiotensin system which may contribute to myocardial hypertrophy and remodelling. ACE inhibitors slow progression of the heart failure and improve survival.

β-Blockers (bisprolol or carvedilol): Block the effects of chronically activated sympathetic system, slow progression of the heart failure and improve survival. The benefits of ACE inhibitors and β-blockers are additive.

Loop diuretics (e.g. furosemide) and dietary salt restriction to correct fluid overload.

Aldosterone antagonists (spironolactone or, if not tolerated, eplerenone) improve survival in patients with NYHA class III/IV symptoms and on standard therapy. Monitor K^+ (may cause hyperkalaemia). May be used to assist in the management of diuretic-induced hypokalaemia.

Angiotensin receptor blockers (ARB) (e.g. candesartan): May be added in patients with persistent symptoms despite ACE inhibitors and β-blockers. Monitor K^+ (may cause hyperkalaemia).

Hydralazine and a nitrate: May be added in patients (particularly in Afro-Caribbeans) with persistent symptoms despite therapy with an ACE inhibitor and β-blocker.

Digoxin: Positive inotrope, $\downarrow$ hospitalization, but does not improve survival.

n-3 polyunsaturated fatty acids: Provide a small beneficial advantage in terms of mortality.

Cardiac resynchronization therapy (CRT): Biventricular pacing improves symptoms and survival in patients with LVEF $\leq$ 35%, cardiac dyssynchrony (QRS > 120 msec) and moderate to severe symptoms despite optimal medical therapy. Most patients who meet these criteria are also candidates for an implantable *cardiac* defibrillator (ICD) and receive a combined device.

Avoid drugs that can adversely affect patients with heart failure due to systolic dysfunction, e.g. NSAIDs, non-dihydropyridine calcium channel blockers (i.e. diltiazem and verapamil).

COMPLICATIONS   Respiratory failure, cardiogenic shock, death.

PROGNOSIS   Fifty per cent of patients with severe heart failure die within 2 years.

---

[1]Important trials include: CIBIS-II and US-Carvedilol (role of β-blockers); SOLVD and CONSENSUS (role of ACE-inhibitors); DIG study (role of digoxin); CHARM-Added trial (value of adding an ARB to appropriate doses of an ACE inhibitor); RALES trial (benefit of spironolactone in severe heart failure); CARE-HF, COMPANION and MIRACLE trial (benefits of CRT); GISSI-HF trial (benefit of n-3 polyunsaturated fatty acids).

Cardiomyopathy

DEFINITION   Primary disease of the myocardium. Cardiomyopathy may be dilated, hypertrophic or restrictive.

AETIOLOGY   The majority are idiopathic.

Dilated: Post-viral myocarditis, alcohol, drugs (e.g. doxorubicin, cocaine), familial (~25% of idiopathic cases, usually autosomal dominant), thyrotoxicosis, haemochromatosis, peripartum.

Hypertrophic: Up to 50% of cases are genetic (autosomal dominant) with mutations in β-myosin, troponin T or α-tropomyosin (components of the contractile apparatus).

Restrictive: Amyloidosis, sarcoidosis, haemochromatosis.

EPIDEMIOLOGY   Prevalence of dilated cardiomyopathy and hypertrophic cardiomyopathy is ~0.05–0.20%. Restrictive cardiomyopathy is rare.

HISTORY

Dilated: Symptoms of heart failure, arrhythmias, thromboembolism, family history of sudden death.

Hypertrophic: Usually none. Syncope, angina, arrhythmias, family history of sudden death.

Restrictive: Dyspnoea, fatigue, arrhythmias, ankle or abdominal swelling.

Enquire about family history of sudden death.

EXAMINATION

Dilated: ↑ JVP, displaced apex beat, functional mitral and tricuspid regurgitations, third heart sound.

Hypertrophic: Jerky carotid pulse, double apex beat, ejection systolic murmur.

Restrictive: ↑ JVP (Kussmaul's sign: further ↑ on inspiration), palpable apex beat, third heart sound, ascites, ankle oedema, hepatomegaly.

INVESTIGATIONS

CXR: May show cardiomegaly, and signs of heart failure.

ECG:

All types: Non-specific ST changes, conduction defects, arrhythmias

Hypertrophic: Left-axis deviation, signs of left ventricular hypertrophy (*see* Aortic stenosis), Q waves in inferior and lateral leads.

Restrictive: Low voltage complexes.

Echocardiography:

Dilated: Dilated ventricles with 'global' hypokinesia.

Hypertrophic: Ventricular hypertrophy (disproportionate septal involvement)

Restrictive: Non-dilated non-hypertrophied ventricles. Atrial enlargement, preserved systolic function, diastolic dysfunction, granular or 'sparkling' appearance of myocardium in amyloidosis.

Cardiac catheterization: May be necessary for measurement of pressures.

Endomyocardial biopsy: May be helpful in restrictive cardiomyopathy.

Pedigree or genetic analysis: Rarely necessary.

MANAGEMENT

Dilated: Treat heart failure and arrhythmias. Consider implantable cardiac defibrillators (ICD) for recurrent VTs.

Hypertrophic: Treat arrhythmias with drugs, ICD for survivors of sudden death, reduce outflow tract gradients, pacemaker, surgery (e.g. septal myomectomy, septal ablation with ethanol). Screen family members with ECG or echocardiography.

Restrictive: No specific treatment. Manage the underlying cause.

Cardiac transplantation: May be considered in end-stage heart failure in all cardiomyopathy types.

Cardiomyopathy (continued)

COMPLICATIONS   Heart failure, arrhythmias (atrial and ventricular).
Dilated and hypertrophic cardiomyopathy: Sudden death and embolism.
Hypertrophic: Infective endocarditis.

PROGNOSIS
Dilated: Depends on the aetiology, New York Heart Association functional class and ejection fraction.
Hypertrophic: Ventricular tachyarrhythmias are the major cause of sudden death.
Restrictive: Poor prognosis, many die within the first year after diagnosis.

Heart block

DEFINITION   Impairment of the atrioventricular (AV) node impulse conduction, as represented by the interval between P wave and QRS complex.

First-degree AV block: Prolonged conduction through the AV node.

Second-degree AV block: Mobitz type I (Wenckebach): Progressive prolongation of AV node conduction culminating in one atrial impulse failing to be conducted through the AV node. The cycle then begins again.

Mobitz type II: Intermittent or regular failure of conduction through AV node. Also defined by the number of normal conductions per failed or abnormal one (e.g. 2 : 1 or 3 : 1).

Third-degree (complete) AV block: No relationship between atrial and ventricular contraction. Failure of conduction through the AV node leads to a ventricular contraction generated by a focus of depolarization within the ventricle (ventricular escape).

AETIOLOGY
MI or ischaemic heart disease (most common cause).
Infection (e.g. rheumatic fever, infective endocarditis).
Drugs (e.g. digoxin, β-blockers, Ca^{2+} channel antagonists).
Metabolic (e.g. hyperkalaemia, cholestatic jaundice, hypothermia).
Infiltration of conducting system (e.g. sarcoidosis, cardiac neoplasms, amyloidosis).
Degeneration of the conducting system.

EPIDEMIOLOGY   Majority of the 250 000 pacemakers implanted annually are for heart block.

HISTORY
First degree: Asymptomatic.
Wenckebach: Usually asymptomatic.
Mobitz type II and third-degree block: May cause Stokes–Adams attacks (syncope caused by ventricular asystole). Other presentations include dizziness, palpitations, chest pain and heart failure.

EXAMINATION   Often normal. Examine for signs of the cause.
Complete heart block: Slow large volume pulse; JVP may show 'cannon waves'.
Mobitz type II and third-degree block: Signs of a reduced cardiac output (e.g. hypotension, heart failure).

INVESTIGATIONS
ECG (consider ambulatory Holter or 24 h):

Type of heart block	ECG appearances
First degree	Prolonged PR interval (>0.2 s)
Mobitz type I (Wenckebach)	Progressively prolonged PR interval, culminating in a P wave that is not followed by a QRS. The pattern then begins again
Mobitz type II	Intermittently a P wave is not followed by a QRS. There may be a regular pattern of P waves not followed by a QRS (e.g. two P waves per QRS, indicating 2 : 1 block)
Third degree (complete)	No relationship between P waves and QRS complexes. If QRS initiated by focus in the bundle of His, the QRS is narrow. QRS initiated more distally are wide and slow rate (∼30 beats/min)

Look for other signs of cause, e.g. ischaemia.
CXR: Cardiac enlargement, pulmonary oedema.
Blood: TFT, digoxin level, cardiac enzymes, troponin.
Echocardiogram: Wall motion abnormalities, aortic valve disease, vegetations.

Heart block (continued)

MANAGEMENT

Chronic block: Permanent pacemaker (PPM) insertion is recommended in patients with third-degree heart block, advanced Mobitz type II and symptomatic Mobitz type I.

Acute block (e.g. secondary to anterior MI): If associated with clinical deterioration, IV atropine and consider temporary (external) pacemaker.

COMPLICATIONS   Asystole. Cardiac arrest. Heart failure. Complications of any pacemaker inserted.

PROGNOSIS   Mobitz type II and third-degree block usually indicate serious underlying cardiac disease.

Hypertension

DEFINITION   Defined as systolic BP >140 mmHg and/or diastolic BP >85 mmHg measured on three separate occasions. Malignant hypertension is defined as BP $\geq 200/130$ mmHg.

AETIOLOGY
Primary:
- Essential or idiopathic hypertension (Commonest, >90% of cases).

Secondary:
- *Renal*: Renal artery stenosis, chronic glomerulonephritis, chronic pyelonephritis, polycystic kidney disease, chronic renal failure.
- *Endocrine*: Diabetes mellitus, hyperthyroidism, Cushing's syndrome, Conn's syndrome, hyperparathyroidism, phaeochromocytoma, congenital adrenal hyperplasia, acromegaly.
- *Cardiovascular*: Aortic coarctation, ↑ intravascular volume.
- *Drugs*: Sympathomimetics, corticosteroids, oral contraceptive pill.
- *Pregnancy*: Pre-eclampsia.

EPIDEMIOLOGY   Very common. 10–20% of adults in the Western world.

HISTORY
Often asymptomatic.
Symptoms of complications (*see* Complications).
Symptoms of the cause.
Accelerated or malignant hypertension: Scotomas (visual field loss), blurred vision, headache, seizures, nausea, vomiting, acute heart failure.

EXAMINATION   Measure on two to three different occasions before diagnosing hypertension and record lowest reading.
There may be loud second heart sound, fourth heart sound.
Examine for causes, e.g. radiofemoral delay (aortic coarctation), renal artery bruit (renal artery stenosis). Examine for end-organ damage, e.g. fundoscopy for retinopathy.
Keith–Wagner classification of retinopathy:
  (I)   'silver wiring';
  (II)   as above, plus arteriovenous nipping;
  (III) as above, plus flame haemorrhages and cotton wool exudates;
  (IV)   as above, plus papilloedema.

PATHOLOGY/PATHOGENESIS   Fibrotic intimal thickening of the arteries, reduplication of elastic lamina and smooth muscle hypertrophy. Arteriolar wall layers replaced by pink hyaline material with luminal narrowing (hyaline arteriosclerosis).

INVESTIGATIONS
Blood: U&E, glucose, lipids.
Urine dipstick: Blood and protein.
ECG: May show signs of left ventricular hypertrophy (deep S wave in V_{1-2}, tall R wave in V_{5-6}, inverted T waves in I, aVL, V_{5-6}, left-axis deviation) or ischaemia.
Ambulatory BP monitoring (BP measured throughout the day): Excludes 'white coat' hypertension, allows monitoring of treatment response, assesses preservation of nocturnal dip.
Others: Especially in patients <35 years or other suspected secondary cases (see relevant topics).

MANAGEMENT   Assessment and modification of other cardiovascular risk factors.
Conservative: Stop smoking, lose weight, ↓ alcohol, reduce dietary Na^+.

Hypertension (continued)

Investigate for secondary causes: Worthwhile in young patients, malignant hypertension or poor response to treatment.

Medical[1]: Treatment recommended for systolic BP $\geq$ 160 mmHg and/or diastolic BP $\geq$ 100 mmHg, or if evidence of end-organ damage. Other hypertension patients may still require treatment depending on other cardiac risk factors. Multiple drug therapies often necessary.

- *Thiazide diuretics (e.g. bendrofluamethiazide)*: Recommended first line, especially in >55-year-olds or black patients.
- *ACE inhibitors (e.g. ramipril) or angiotensin-II antagonist (e.g. losartan)*: First line in <55-year-olds, diabetic patients, heart failure or left ventricular dysfunction.
- *Ca^{2+} channel antagonists (e.g. amlodipine)*: Recommended first line, especially in >60-year-olds or black patients.
- *β-Blockers (e.g. atenolol)*: Not preferred initial therapy, but may be considered in younger patients. Avoid combining with thiazide diuretic to reduce patient risk of developing diabetes. May increase risk of heart failure.
- *α-Blockers (e.g. doxazosin)*: Fourth-line agent. May be useful for patients with prostatism.

Target BP:
- $\leq$140/85 mmHg (non-diabetic);
- $\leq$130/80 mmHg (diabetes without proteinuria);
- $\leq$125/75 mmHg (diabetes with proteinuria).

Severe hypertension (diastolic BP > 140 mmHg): Atenolol or nifedipine.

Acute malignant hypertension: IV β-blocker, labetolol or hydralazine sodium nitroprusside. Avoid very rapid lowering which can cause cerebral infarction.

COMPLICATIONS   Heart failure, coronary artery disease and MI, CVA, peripheral vascular disease, emboli, retinopathy, renal failure, hypertensive encephalopathy, posterior reversible encephalopathy syndrome (PRES), malignant hypertension.

PROGNOSIS   Good, if BP controlled. Uncontrolled hypertension linked with increased mortality (6× stroke risk and 3× cardiac death risk). Treatment reduces incidence of renal damage, stroke and heart failure.

[1]See NICE guidelines 2006 (available at http://www.nice.org.uk/nicemedia/pdf/CG034NICEguideline.pdf).

Ischaemic heart disease

DEFINITION   Characterized by ↓ blood supply (ischaemia) to the heart muscle resulting in chest pain (angina pectoris). May present as 'stable angina' or 'acute coronary syndrome' (ACS).

ACS can be further subdivided into unstable angina (no cardiac injury), non-ST-elevation myocardial infarction (NSTEMI) or ST-elevation MI (STEMI, transmural infarction). MI refers to cardiac muscle necrosis resulting from ischaemia.

AETIOLOGY   Angina pectoris occurs when myocardial oxygen demand exceeds oxygen supply. The most common cause is atherosclerosis. Other causes of coronary artery narrowing such as spasm (e.g. from cocaine), arteritis and emboli are rare.

MI is caused by sudden occlusion of a coronary artery due to rupture of an atheromatous plaque and thrombus formation.

Atherosclerosis: Endothelial injury is followed by migration of monocytes into subendothelial space and differentiation into macrophages. Macrophages accumulate LDL lipids insudated in the subendothelium and become foam cells. They release growth factors, which stimulate smooth muscle proliferation, production of collagen and proteoglycans. This leads to the formation of an atheromatous plaque.

ASSOCIATIONS/RISK FACTORS   Male, diabetes mellitus, family history, hypertension, hyperlipidaemia, smoking, previous history.

EPIDEMIOLOGY   Common, prevalence is >2%. More common in males. Annual incidence of MI in the United Kingdom is ~5 in 1000.

HISTORY

ACS: Chest pain or discomfort of acute onset. Central heavy tight 'gripping' pain that radiates to arms (usually left), neck, jaw or epigastrium. Occurring at rest, ↑ severity and frequency of previously stable angina.

May be associated with breathlessness, sweating, nausea and vomiting.

May be silent in elderly or in patients with diabetes.

Stable angina: Brought on by exertion and relieved by rest.

EXAMINATION

Stable angina: Look for signs of risk factors.

ACS: May have no clinical signs. Pale, sweating, restless, low-grade pyrexia. Check both radial pulses for aortic dissectio.

Arrhythmias, disturbances of BP. New heart murmurs (e.g. pansystolic murmur of mitral regurgitation from papillary muscle rupture or ventricular septal defect).

Signs of complications, i.e. acute heart failure, cardiogenic shock (hypotension, cold peripheries, oliguria).

INVESTIGATIONS

Blood: FBC, U&Es, CRP, glucose, lipid profile, cardiac enzymes: CK-MB and troponin-T or I[1] (sensitive marker of cardiac injury, ↑ after 12 h), amylase (pancreatitis may mimic MI), TFTs. AST and LDH ↑ after 24 and 48 h, respectively; occasionally used only to make retrospective diagnosis.

ECG:

Unstable angina or NSTEMI: May show ST depression, T-wave inversion (Q waves in these patients may indicate old MIs).

ST-elevation (Q-wave) MI: Hyperacute T waves, ST elevation (>1 mm in limb leads, >2 mm in chest leads), new-onset LBBB. Later: T inversion (hours) and Q waves (days).

---

[1]Causes of ↑ troponin other than acute thrombotic coronary artery occlusion include sepsis, tachycardia, myocarditis/pericarditis, pulmonary embolism, cardiac failure, renal failure, stroke and cardiac contusion.

Ischaemic heart disease (continued)

Location of infarct	Changes in leads
Inferior wall	II, III, aVF
Anterior wall	Septum (V_1–V_2), apex (V_3–V_4), anterolateral wall (V_5–V_6)
Lateral wall	I, aVL
Posterior infarct	Tall R wave and ST depression in V_1–V_3

CXR: To look for signs of heart failure. Useful to look for differentials (e.g. aortic dissection).

Exercise ECG testing (treadmill test)[2]: To determine prognosis and management.

Indications: In patients with troponin-negative ACS, or stable angina with an intermediate or high pretest probability of coronary heart disease (based on the characteristics of their chest pain, cardiac risk factors, age and gender). Patients should not be on digoxin (associated with a false-positive result).

Positive test: Defined as $\geq$ 1 mm horizontal or downsloping ST-segment depression measured at 80 ms after the end of the QRS complex (sensitivity: 60% and specificity: 90%).

Failed test: Failure to achieve at least 85% of the predicted maximal heart rate (220 – age) and otherwise negative (i.e. absence of chest discomfort or ECG findings). β-Blockers ↓ the maximal heart rate that is achieved and may be stopped prior to the test.

Resting ECG abnormalities (e.g. preexcitation syndrome, >1mm of ST depression, LBBB or paced ventricular rhythm) interfere with interpretation.

Radionuclide myocardial perfusion imaging (rMPI): Uses Tc-99m sestamibi or tetrofosmin. Can be performed under stress (exercise or pharmacological) or at rest. Stress testing would show low uptake in ischaemic myocardium. Rest testing can be used in patient with ACS, no previous MI but non-diagnostic troponin and ECGs.

Echocardiogram: Measure LVEF (early measurements may be misleading because of myocardial stunning). Exercise (or dobutamine stress) echocardiography may detect inducible wall motion abnormalities.

Pharmacologic stress testing: For patients who cannot exercise or if the exercise test is inconclusive. Pharmacological agents such as dipyridamole, adenosine or dobutamine can be used to induce a tachycardia. Various imaging modalities (e.g. rMPI, echocardiography) can be used to detect ischaemic myocardium. Dipyridamole and adenosine are contraindicated in AV block and reactive airway disease.

Cardiac catheterization/angiography: In ACS with positive troponin or TIMI score 5–7, or if high risk on stress testing (using Duke treadmill score based on exercise time, maximum ST-segment deviation and exercise angina).

Coronary calcium scoring using specialized CT (if available): may have a role in outpatients with atypical chest pain or in acute chest pain that is not clearly due to ischaemia (absence of CAC excludes obstructive coronary artery disease).

MANAGEMENT
Stable angina:
- *Minimize cardiac risk factors*: Control BP, hyperlipidaemia and diabetes. Provide advice on smoking, exercise, weight loss and low-fat diet. All patients should receive aspirin (75 mg/day) unless contraindicated.

---

[2]Contraindications to exercise ECG testing: severe aortic stenosis, uncontrolled arrhythmia, hypertension or heart failure. Stop if breathlessness or chest pain occurs, patient feels faint, arrhythmia, development of left bundle branch block, ST-segment elevation or depression >2 mm, fall in BP, BP > 230 mmHg, or if 90% maximal heart rate for age is achieved.

- *Immediate symptom relief*: GTN as a spray or sublingually.
- *Long-term treatment*: β-Blockers, e.g. atenolol, unless contraindicated (contraindications include acute heart failure, cardiogenic shock, bradycardia, heart block, asthma), calcium channel blockers (e.g. verapamil, diltiazem), nitrates (e.g. isosorbide dinitrate). Dual therapy may be indicated if monotherapy is ineffective.
- *Percutaneous coronary intervention (PCI)*: For localized areas of stenosis, in patients with angina not controlled despite maximal tolerable medical therapy. Restenosis rate is ∼25% at 6 months but drug-eluting coronary stents ↓ restenosis rates (release an anti-restenotic drug, e.g. sirolimus or paclitaxel).
- *Coronary artery bypass graft (CABG)*: For more severe cases (three-vessel disease). The rates of MI and overall survival are generally similar between PCI and CABG.

Unstable angina/NSTEMI[3]:
- Admit to coronary care unit (CCU), oxygen, IV access, monitor vital signs and serial ECG.
- Analgesia: GTN (initially sublingual, IV infusion if persistent chest pain), morphine sulphate/diamorphine, antiemetic (metoclopramide).
- Aspirin (loading): 300 mg chewed. Maintenance: 75 mg, indefinite.
- Clopidogrel (loading): 300 mg. Maintenance: 75 mg for at least 1 year if troponin positive or high risk.
- Low-molecular-weight heparin (e.g. enoxaparin or dalteparin).
- β-Blocker (e.g. metoprolol) if not contraindicated.
- Glucose–insulin infusion if blood glucose >11 mmol/L.
- Consider glycoprotein (GP) IIb/IIIa inhibitors, e.g. tirofiban (initiated on presentation and continued for 48–72 h or until PCI) in patients:
  - undergoing PCI; *or*
  - at high risk for further cardiac events (troponin positive, TIMI risk score ≥4, continuing ischaemia or other high-risk features).
- If little improvement, consider urgent angiography ± revascularization.

STEMI:
- Admit to CCU, oxygen, IV access, monitor vital signs and serial ECG.
- Analgesia: GTN (initially sublingual, IV infusion if persistent chest pain), morphine sulphate/diamorphine, antiemetic (metoclopramide)
- Aspirin (loading): 300 mg chewed. Maintenance: 75 mg, indefinite.
- Clopidogrel (loading): 600 mg if patient going to primary PCI, 300 mg if undergoing thrombolysis and ≤75 years of age, 75 mg if undergoing thrombolysis and >75 years of age. Maintenance: 75 mg, for at least 1 year.
- β-Blocker (e.g. metoprolol) if not contraindicated.
- If undergoing primary PCI: IV heparin (plus GP IIb/IIIa inhibitor) or bivalirudin (an antithrombin). If undergoing thrombolysis with recombinant tissue plasminogen activator (rtPA): IV heparin.
- Glucose–insulin infusion if blood glucose >11 mmol/L.

[3]Evidence-based medicine for management of ACS:
- ISIS-1: beta-blockers.
- ISIS-2: aspirin and streptokinase.
- ISIS-4: ACE inhibitors.
- PROVE IT trial: initial high dose statin therapy.
- DIGAMI: initial insulin–glucose infusion and insulin for 3 months in all diabetic patients.
- CURE: combined clopidogrel and aspirin in NSTEMI.
- CLARITY: combined clopidogrel, aspirin and thrombolysis in STEMI
- PURSUIT, PRISM, EPIC, CAPTURE = GP-IIb/IIIa inhibitors in NSTEMI
- HORIZONS AMI trial: Bivalirudin (direct thrombin inhibitor) superiority compared with combined heparin and GP-IIb/IIIa inhibitors in STEMI.

Ischaemic heart disease (continued)

- *Primary PCI*[4] with goal <90 min if available *or thrombolysis* (see below) with goal of 30 min.
- *Thrombolysis*: Using fibrinolytics such as streptokinase or rtPA (alteplase, reteplase, tenecteplase) if within 12 h of chest pain with ECG changes (ST elevation, new-onset LBBB or posterior infarction) and not contraindicated.[5] *Rescue PCI*: If continued pain or ST elevation after thrombolysis (<50% ↓ of the initial ST-segment elevation on a follow-up ECG 60–90 min after fibrinolytic therapy).

Secondary Prevention: Antiplatelet agents (aspirin and clopidogrel), ACE inhibitors, β-blockers and statins. Control other risk factors (smoking, diabetes, hypertension).

Advice: Not to drive for 1 month following MI. Education by cardiac rehabilitation team: lifestyle changes (e.g. exercise, stop smoking, changing diet).

CABG for patients with left main stem or three-vessel disease.

COMPLICATIONS At risk of MI and other vascular diseases (e.g. stroke, peripheral vascular disease). Cardiac injury can lead secondarily to heart failure and arrhythmias.

Early complications of MI (24–72 h): Death, cardiogenic shock, heart failure, ventricular arrhythmias, heart block, pericarditis, myocardial rupture, thromboembolism.

Late complications of MI: Ventricular wall (or septum) rupture, valvular regurgitation, ventricular aneurysms, tamponade, Dressler's syndrome (pericarditis), thromboembolism.

PROGNOSIS

ACS: TIMI score (range 0–7) can be used for risk stratification (high scores are associated with high risk of cardiac events within 30 days), consists of:

(1) >65 years;
(2) known coronary artery disease;
(3) aspirin in last 7 days;
(4) severe angina (>2 episodes in 24 h);
(5) ST deviation >1 mm;
(6) elevated troponin levels;
(7) >3 coronary artery disease risk factors (hypertension, hyperlipidaemia, family history, diabetes, smoking).

Killip classification of acute MI:

Class I: no evidence of heart failure.
Class II: mild to moderate heart failure (S_3, crepitations <one-half way up the posterior lung fields, or jugular venous distension).
Class III: overt pulmonary oedema.
Class IV: cardiogenic shock.

The higher the Killip class on presentation, the greater the subsequent mortality.

---

[4]Other indications of primary PCI: typical and persistent symptoms and new or presumably new left bundle branch block; patients presenting 12–24 h after symptom onset, with persistent ischaemic symptoms, severe heart failure, haemodynamic or electrical instability.

[5]*Absolute contraindications to thrombolysis*: History of intracranial haemorrhage/vascular lesion/neoplasm, ischaemic stroke within 3 months, suspected aortic dissection, active bleeding or bleeding diathesis, significant closed-head or facial trauma within 3 months. *Relative contraindications*: Systolic BP > 180 mmHg, ischaemic stroke >3 months previously, dementia, traumatic or cardiopulmonary resuscitation >10 min, major surgery (within <3 weeks), recent internal bleeding (within 2–4 weeks), non-compressible vascular puncture, pregnancy, active peptic ulcer, current use of anticoagulants, for streptokinase: prior exposure or allergic reaction.

Mitral regurgitation

DEFINITION   Retrograde flow of blood from LV to left atrium during systole.

AETIOLOGY   Mitral valve damage or dysfunction:
* rheumatic heart disease (most common);
* infective endocarditis;
* mitral valve prolapse (prolapse of mitral valve leaflets into the left atrium during systole);
* papillary muscle rupture or dysfunction (secondary to ischaemic heart disease or cardiomyopathy);
* chordal rupture and floppy mitral valve associated with connective tissue diseases (e.g. pseudoxanthoma elasticum[1], osteogenesis imperfecta,[2] Ehlers–Danlos syndrome,[3] Marfan syndromes, SLE).

Functional mitral regurgitation may be secondary to left ventricular dilation.

EPIDEMIOLOGY   Affects ~5% of adults. Mitral valve prolapse is more common in young females.

HISTORY
Acute MR: May present with symptoms of left ventricular failure.
Chronic MR: May be asymptomatic or present with exertional dyspnoea, palpitations if in AF and fatigue.
Mitral valve prolapse: Asymptomatic or atypical chest pain or palpitations.

EXAMINATION   Pulse may be normal or irregularly irregular (AF).
Apex beat may be laterally displaced and thrusting (left ventricular dilation).
Pansystolic murmur, loudest at apex, radiating to axilla (palpable as a thrill). S_1 is soft; S_3 may be heard (rapid ventricular filling in early diastole).
Signs of left ventricular failure in acute mitral regurgitation.
Mitral valve prolapse: Mid-systolic click and late systolic murmur. The click moves towards the first heart sound on standing and moves away on lying down.

INVESTIGATIONS
ECG: Normal or may show AF or broad bifid p wave (p mitrale) indicating delayed activation of left atrium due to left atrial enlargement.
CXR: Acute mitral regurgitation may produce signs of left ventricular failure. Chronic mitral regurgitation shows left atrial enlargement, cardiomegaly (caused by left ventricular dilation) or mitral valve calcification in rheumatic cases.
Echocardiography: Every 6–12 months for moderate–severe MR to assess the LV ejection fraction and end-systolic dimension.

MANAGEMENT
Surgical: Indicated in patients with chronic MR with symptoms or LV enlargement or dysfunction, pulmonary hypertension, or new-onset AF.

---

[1]**Pseudoxanthoma elasticum**: Collagen/elastic tissue disorder characterized by yellow papules on the skin in the flexures, ischaemic heart disease, GI bleeding and angioid streaks on fundoscopy (caused by degeneration of Bruch's membrane).

[2]**Osteogenesis imperfecta**: Group of autosomally dominant inherited disorders caused by mutations in type I collagen gene causing brittle, deformed bones, blue sclerae, hypermobile joints and heart valve disorders.

[3]**Ehlers–Danlos syndrome**: A group of genetic disorders due to defects in type III collagen resulting in joint hypermobility and skin hyperelasticity and fragility. Spontaneous rupture of arteries is the most serious cardiovascular complication.

Mitral regurgitation (continued)

Mitral valve repair: May occasionally be feasible.

Mitral valve replacement: Mechanical valve with lifelong anticoagulation in patients <65 years with long-standing AF. Bioprosthetic valve in patients with a contraindication to warfarin or ≥65 years of age (since limited durability of bioprosthetic valve is less of an issue). The choice of valve in patients <65 years who are in sinus rhythm relies on patient preference. Discuss the risks of warfarin compared to the likelihood of repeat valve replacement in the future.

Medical:

Functional MR due to LV dysfunction: ACE inhibitors and/or angiotensin II receptor blockers. Optimal medical therapy of heart failure. In appropriate patients, CRT.

Mitral valve prolapse and symptomatic patients with primary MR (e.g. rheumatic or myxomatous): ↓ systolic pressure (β-blockers, diuretic).

Treatment of atrial fibrillation (See Atrial Fibrillation).

Anticoagulation with warfarin (target INR: 2–3): In patients with AF, history of systemic embolism or rheumatic mitral valve disease with left atrial thrombus. Antibiotic prophylaxis is no longer recommended in the absence of prosthetic repair or replacement for those undergoing dental or other invasive procedures.

Advice: Patients with severe MR, LV enlargement, pulmonary hypertension or ↓ left ventricular systolic function at rest should not participate in any competitive sports. Patients treated with long-term anticoagulation therapy should not engage in contact sports.

COMPLICATIONS Left atrial enlargement and AF (and resultant systemic embolism), pulmonary oedema, pulmonary hypertension, right heart failure, infective endocarditis.

PROGNOSIS Prognosis depends on aetiology, severity and state of left ventricular function. Acute mitral regurgitation resulting from rupture of a cusp or papillary muscle has a poor prognosis. Rheumatic mitral regurgitation may slowly deteriorate over 10–20 years.

Mitral stenosis

DEFINITION   Mitral valve narrowing causing obstruction to blood flow from the left atrium to the ventricle.

AETIOLOGY   Most common cause is rheumatic heart disease (90%).
Rarer causes are congenital mitral stenosis, SLE, rheumatoid arthritis, endocarditis and atrial myxoma (rare cardiac tumour).

EPIDEMIOLOGY   Incidence is declining in industrialized countries because of declining incidence of rheumatic fever.

HISTORY   May be asymptomatic.
Presents with fatigue, shortness of breath on exertion or lying down (orthopnoea). Palpitations (related to AF).
Rare symptoms: Cough, haemoptysis, hoarseness caused by compression of the left laryngeal nerve by an enlarged left atrium.

EXAMINATION   May have peripheral or facial cyanosis (malar flush).
Pulse: May be 'thready' or irregularly irregular (AF).
Palpation: Apex beat is undisplaced and tapping. Parasternal heave (right ventricular hypertrophy and pulmonary hypertension)
Auscultation: Loud first heart sound with opening snap.
Mid-diastolic murmur (presystolic accentuation if in sinus rhythm).
Evidence of pulmonary oedema on lung auscultation (if decompensated).

INVESTIGATIONS
ECG: May be normal, broad bifid p wave (p mitrale) caused by left atrial hypertrophy, AF or evidence of right ventricular hypertrophy in cases of severe pulmonary hypertension.
CXR: Left atrial enlargement, cardiac enlargement, pulmonary congestion; mitral valve may be calcified in rheumatic cases.
Echocardiography: To assess functional and structural impairments. Transoesophageal gives better valve visualization.
Cardiac catheterization: Measures severity of heart failure.

MANAGEMENT
Medical: Anticoagulation for AF. Treat dyspnoea and heart failure with diuretics. Antibiotic cover for dental/invasive procedures. Cardioversion of AF may be considered.
Surgical: Mitral valvuloplasty, valvotomy or replacement if severe.

COMPLICATIONS   AF and systemic embolism, pulmonary oedema, pulmonary hypertension and right heart failure, infective endocarditis.

PROGNOSIS   Significantly worse if pulmonary hypertension or right heart failure develops.

Myocarditis

DEFINITION   Acute inflammation and necrosis of cardiac muscle (myocardium).

AETIOLOGY   Usually unknown (idiopathic).
Infection:
Viruses: e.g. Coxsackie B, echovirus, EBV, CMV, adenovirus, influenza.
Bacterial: e.g. post-streptococcal, tuberculosis, diphtheria, Lyme disease.
Fungal: e.g. candidiasis.
Protozoal: e.g. trypanosomiasis (Chagas disease).
Helminths: e.g. trichinosis.

Non-infective: Systemic disorders (e.g. SLE, sarcoidosis, polymyositis), hypersensitivity myocarditis (e.g. sulphonamides).
Drugs: Chemotherapy agents (e.g. doxorubicin, streptomycin)
Others: Cocaine abuse, heavy metals, radiation.

EPIDEMIOLOGY   True incidence is unknown, as many cases are not detected at the time of acute illness. Coxsackie B virus is a common cause in Europe and the USA. Chagas disease is a common cause in South America.

HISTORY   Prodromal 'flu-like' illness, fever, malaise, fatigue, lethargy.
Breathlessness (pericardial effusion/myocardial dysfunction).
Palpitations.
Sharp chest pain (suggesting associated pericarditis).

EXAMINATION   Signs of concurrent pericarditis or complications: heart failure, arrhythmia.

INVESTIGATIONS
Blood: FBC ($\uparrow$ WCC in infective causes), U&E, $\uparrow$ ESR or CRP, cardiac enzymes (may be $\uparrow$). To identify the cause (viral or bacterial serology, antistreptolysin O titre, ANA, serum ACE, TFT).
ECG: Non-specific T wave and ST changes, widespread saddle-shaped ST elevation in pericarditis.
CXR: May be normal or show cardiomegaly with or without pulmonary oedema.
Pericardial fluid drainage: Measure glucose, protein, cytology, culture and sensitivity.
Echocardiography: Assesses systolic/diastolic function, wall motion abnormalities, pericardial effusion.
Myocardial biopsy: Rarely required (result does not influence management).

MANAGEMENT
Supportive: Bed rest, treatment of complications (heart failure, arrhythmias), pericardial drainage for compromising pericardial effusion.
Steroids and immunosuppressants have been used in severe cases but are of unproven benefit.
Surgical: Cardiac transplantation for severe cases.

COMPLICATIONS   Severe cases can lead to chronic inflammation, cardiac failure. Resolution of inflammation with different degrees of residual dilated cardiomyopathy, arrhythmias and death.

PROGNOSIS   Usually mild and self-limiting. Recovery is variable in patients with severe acute myocarditis.

Pericarditis

DEFINITION   Inflammation of the pericardium, may be acute, subacute or chronic.

AETIOLOGY
- Idiopathic;
- infective (commonly, coxsackie B, echovirus, mumps virus, streptococci, fungi, staphylococci, TB);
- connective tissue disease (e.g. sarcoid, SLE, scleroderma);
- post-myocardial infarction (24–72 h) in up to 20% of patients;
- Dressler's syndrome (weeks to months after acute MI);
- malignancy (lung, breast, lymphoma, leukaemia, melanoma);
- metabolic (myxoedema, uraemia);
- radiotherapy;
- thoracic surgery;
- drugs (e.g. hydralazine, isoniazid).

EPIDEMIOLOGY   Uncommon. The clinical incidence is <1 in 100 hospital admissions. More common in males.

HISTORY
Chest pain: Sharp and central, which may radiate to neck or shoulders. Aggravated by coughing, deep inspiration and lying flat. Relieved by sitting forward.
Dyspnoea, nausea.

EXAMINATION   Fever, pericardial friction rub (best heard lower left sternal edge, with patient leaning forward in expiration), heart sounds may be faint in the presence of an effusion.
Cardiac tamponade: ↑ JVP, ↓ BP and muffled heart sounds (Beck's triad). Tachycardia, pulsus paradoxus (reduced systolic BP by >10 mmHg on inspiration).
Constrictive pericarditis (chronic): ↑ JVP with inspiration (Kussmaul's sign), pulsus paradoxus, hepatomegaly, ascites, oedema, pericardial knock (rapid ventricular filling), AF.

INVESTIGATIONS
ECG: Widespread ST elevation that is saddle-shaped.
Echocardiogram: For assessment of pericardial effusion and cardiac function.
Blood: FBC, U&E, ESR, CRP, cardiac enzymes (usually normal). Where appropriate: blood cultures, ASO titres, ANA, rheumatoid factor, TFT, Mantoux test, viral serology.
CXR: Usually normal (globular heart shadow if >250 mL effusion). Pericardial calcification can be seen in constrictive pericarditis (best seen on lateral CXR or CT).

MANAGEMENT
Acute: Cardiac tamponade treated by emergency pericardiocentesis.
Medical: Treat the underlying cause, NSAIDs for relief of pain and fever.
Recurrent: Low-dose steroids, immunosuppressants or colchicine.
Surgical: Surgical excision of the pericardium (pericardiectomy) in constrictive pericarditis.

COMPLICATIONS   Pericardial effusion, cardiac tamponade, cardiac arrythmias.

PROGNOSIS   Depends on underlying cause. Good prognosis in viral cases (recovery within ~2 weeks), poor in malignant pericarditis. Pericarditis may be recurrent (particularly in those caused by thoracic surgery).

Pulmonary hypertension

DEFINITION   A consistently increased pulmonary arterial pressure (>20 mmHg) under resting conditions.

AETIOLOGY
Primary: Idiopathic.
Secondary: Left heart disease (mitral valve disease, left ventricular failure, left atrial myxoma/thrombosis), chronic lung disease (COPD), recurrent pulmonary emboli, ↑ pulmonary blood flow (ASD, VSD, patent ductus arteriosus), connective tissue disease (e.g. SLE, systemic sclerosis), drugs (e.g. amiodarone).

EPIDEMIOLOGY   Primary pulmonary hypertension is usually seen in young females.

HISTORY   Dyspnoea (on exertion), chest pain, syncope, tiredness.
Symptoms of the underlying cause (e.g. chronic cough).

EXAMINATION   ↑ JVP (Prominent a wave in the JVP waveform).
Palpation: Left parasternal heave (right ventricular hypertrophy).
Auscultation: Loud pulmonary component of S_2 (S_3/S_4 may be heard), an early diastolic murmur (Graham–Steell murmur) caused by pulmonary regurgitation may be present, if tricuspid regurgitation develops (large cv wave and pansystolic murmur).
Signs of the underlying condition, or right heart failure in severe cases.

INVESTIGATIONS
CXR: Cardiomegaly (right ventricular enlargement, right atrial dilation), prominent main pulmonary arteries (which taper rapidly), signs of the cause (e.g. COPD, calcified mitral valves).
ECG: Right ventricular hypertrophy (right-axis deviation, prominent R wave in V_1, T inversion in V_1, V_2), right atrial enlargement (peaked P wave in II, called 'P pulmonale'); limb leads exhibit low voltage (R < 5 mm) in COPD.
Echocardiography: To visualize right ventricular hypertrophy or dilation and possible underlying cause.
Lung function tests: To assess for chronic lung disease.
VQ scan: To assess for pulmonary embolism.
Cardiac catheterization: To assess severity, right heart pressures and response to vasodilators.
High resolution CT-thorax: Images pulmonary arteries and to diagnose lung disease.
Lung biopsy: Assesses structural lung changes.

MANAGEMENT
Medical: Treat secondary cause. For primary pulmonary hypertension, consider:
• anticoagulation (warfarin);
• calcium channel antagonists (e.g. verapamil, nifedipine);
• prostacycline analogues (e.g. iloprost);
• endothelial receptor antagonist (bosentan) blocks vasoconstriction, but teratogenic, so only indicated in NYHA III or IV patients;
• phosphodiesterase inhibitor (e.g. sildenafil) promotes pulmonary smooth muscle relaxation reducing pulmonary hypertension.

Surgical: Heart and lung transplantation may be an option for younger patients.

COMPLICATIONS   Right heart failure, arrhythmias (AF, VT, VF), sudden death.

PROGNOSIS   Chronic and incurable with unpredictable survival rate. Length of survival has improved to up to 15–20 years.

Rheumatic fever

DEFINITION An inflammatory multisystem disorder, occurring following group A β-haemolytic streptococci (GAS) infection.

AETIOLOGY The pathogenic mechanisms remain incompletely understood. Streptococcal pharyngeal infection is required, and genetic susceptibility may be present. Molecular mimicry is thought to play an important role in the initiation of the tissue injury (antibodies directed against GAS antigens cross-react with host antigens).

EPIDEMIOLOGY Peak incidence: between 5 and 15 years. More common in the Far East, Middle East, eastern Europe and South America. The mean incidence is 19/100 000. Despite ↓ incidence over time in the West, the incidence rates remain relatively high in non-Western countries.

HISTORY 2–5 weeks after GAS infection.
General: Fever, malaise, anorexia. *Joints*: Painful, swollen, ↓ movement/function. *Cardiac*: Breathlessness, chest pain, palpitations.

EXAMINATION
Duckett Jones criteria: Positive diagnosis if at least two major criteria, or one major plus two minor criteria are present.
Major criteria:
• Arthritis: Migratory or fleeting polyarthritis with swelling, redness and tenderness of large joints.
• Carditis: New murmur, e.g. Carey Coombs murmur (mid-diastolic murmur due to mitral valvulitis). Pericarditis, pericardial effusion or rub, cardiomegaly, cardiac failure, ECG changes (*see* Investigations).
• Chorea (Sydenham's): Rapid, involuntary, irregular movements with flowing or dancing quality. May be accompanied by slurred speech. More common in females.
• Nodules: Small firm painless subcutaneous nodules seen on extensor surfaces, joints and tendons.
• *Erythema marginatum* (20% cases): Transient erythematous rash with raised edges, seen on trunk and proximal limbs. They may form crescent- or ring-shaped patches.

Minor criteria:
• Pyrexia;
• previous rheumatic fever;
• arthralgia (only if arthritis is not present as major criteria);
• recent streptococcal infection (supported by positive throat cultures or ↑ antistreptolysin O titre);
• ↑ inflammatory markers (ESR, CRP or WCC);
• ↑ PR and QT intervals on ECG (only if carditis not present as major criteria).

INVESTIGATIONS
Blood: FBC (↑ WCC), ESR/CRP (↑), ↑ or rising antistreptolysin O titre.
Throat swab: Culture for GAS, rapid streptococcal antigen test.
ECG: Saddle-shaped ST elevation and PR segment depression (features of pericarditis), arrhythmias.
Echocardiogram: Pericardial effusion, myocardial thickening or dysfunction, valvular dysfunction.

MANAGEMENT
Strict bed rest: (∼ 4 weeks) Gradual mobilization with clinical improvement.

Rheumatic fever (continued)

Anti-inflammatory drugs: High-dose aspirin or, for more severe carditis, consider corticosteroids.

Antibiotics: Eradicate residual streptococcal infection using oral penicillin V for 10 days. Long-term antibiotics to prevent recurrence is necessary (e.g. long-acting benzathine penicillin G intramuscularly every 4 weeks, switch to oral prophylaxis in young adulthood). Prophylaxis in the setting of carditis should continue usually for 10 years. The risk for GAS exposure and severity of valvular disease should then be reviewed.

Carditis: Treat heart failure if present.

Chorea: May be controlled with diazepam or haloperidol.

Valve surgery: If valvular disease cannot be managed with medical therapy alone.

COMPLICATIONS   Recurrence, may be precipitated by streptococcal infection, more common in patients with residual cardiac damage. Chronic rheumatic valvular disease: scarring, deformation and dysfunction (usually mitral or aortic) after 10–20 years; more common in those with carditis as part of acute rheumatic fever.

PROGNOSIS   Acute rheumatic fever may last up to 3 months if untreated. ♀ more likely to develop mitral stenosis.

Note: Post-streptococcal reactive arthritis is a reactive arthritis that occurs ~1–2 weeks after GAS pharyngitis. Patients have marked arthritis with poor response to aspirin/NSAIDs, tenosynovitis, renal abnormalities and lower ESR and CRP than acute rheumatic fever. Secondary prophylaxis is given for up to 1 year and discontinued, unless there is evidence of valvular disease.

Tricuspid regurgitation

DEFINITION   Tricuspid regurgitation is backflow of blood from the right ventricle to the right atrium during systole.

AETIOLOGY

Congenital: Ebstein anomaly (malpositioned tricuspid valve), cleft valve in ostium primum defect.

Functional: Consequence of right ventricular dilation (e.g. in pulmonary hypertension), valve prolapse.

Rheumatic heart disease: Associated with other valvular disease.

Infective endocarditis: Common in IV drug users. Usually staphylococcal.

Other: Carcinoid syndrome, trauma, cirrhosis (long-standing), iatrogenic (e.g. radiotherapy to the thorax).

EPIDEMIOLOGY   The epidemiology differs with various causes. Infective endocarditis probably most common cause.

HISTORY   Fatigue, breathlessness, palpitations, headaches, nausea, anorexia, epigastric pain made worse by exercise, jaundice, lower limb swelling.

EXAMINATION

Pulse: May be irregularly irregular due to AF (may occur with right atrial enlargement).

Inspection: ↑ JVP with giant v waves which may oscillate the earlobe. This is caused by transmission of right ventricular pressure to the great veins. There may be giant a wave, if the patient is in sinus rhythm.

Palpation: Parasternal heave.

Auscultation: Pansystolic murmur heard best at the lower left sternal edge, louder on inspiration (Carvallo sign). Loud P2 component of second heart sound.

Chest: Pleural effusion. Causes of pulmonary hypertension (e.g. emphysema).

Abdomen: Palpable liver (tender, smooth, pulsatile), ascites.

Legs: Pitting oedema.

INVESTIGATIONS

Blood: FBC, LFT, cardiac enzymes, blood cultures.

ECG: Tall P wave (right atrial hypertrophy) if in sinus rhythm. Changes indicative of other cardiac disease.

CXR: Right-sided enlargement of cardiac shadow.

Echocardiography: Extent of regurgitation estimated by colour flow Doppler. May be able to detect tricuspid valve abnormality (e.g. prolapse), right ventricular dilation.

Right heart catheterization: Rarely necessary but may be considered to assess pulmonary artery pressure.

MANAGEMENT

Medical: Treat the underlying condition, e.g. infective endocarditis or functional regurgitation caused by pulmonary hypertension. Diuretics may be given for fluid retention.

Surgery: Annuloplasty, plication or, rarely, replacement. Repair of the valve only in very severe tricuspid regurgitation, when the required doses of diuretics are large enough to cause metabolic consequences. Surgical removal of the valve may be required to eradicate the source of infection in IV drug users with infective endocarditis.

COMPLICATIONS   Heart failure, hepatic fibrosis.

PROGNOSIS   Prognosis varies depending on the underlying cause.

Acute respiratory distress syndrome (ARDS)

DEFINITION   Syndrome of acute and persistent lung inflammation with increased vascular permeability. Characterized by:
- acute onset;
- bilateral infiltrates consistent with pulmonary oedema;
- hypoxaemia: $PaO_2/FiO_2 \leq 200$ mmHg regardless of the level of positive end-expiratory pressure (PEEP);
- no clinical evidence for $\uparrow$ left atrial pressure (pulmonary capillary wedge pressure (PCWP) ≤ 18 mmHg).
- ARDS is the severe end of the spectrum of 'acute lung injury' (ALI).

AETIOLOGY   Severe insult to the lungs or other organs induces the release of inflammatory mediators, increased capillary permeability, pulmonary oedema, impaired gas exchange and $\downarrow$ lung compliance. Common causes include: sepsis, aspiration, pneumonia, pancreatitis, trauma/burns, transfusion (massive, transfusion-related lung injury), transplantation (bone marrow, lung) and drug overdose/reaction.
Patients progress through three pathologic stages: exudative, proliferative and fibrotic stage.

EPIDEMIOLOGY   Annual UK incidence ~ 1 in 6000.

HISTORY   Rapid deterioration of respiratory function, dyspnoea, respiratory distress, cough, symptoms of aetiology.

EXAMINATION   Cyanosis, tachypnoea, tachycardia, widespread inspiratory crepitations. Hypoxia refractory to oxygen treatment.
Signs are usually bilateral but may be asymmetrical in early stages.

INVESTIGATIONS
CXR: Bilateral alveolar and interstitial shadowing.
Blood: FBC, U&E, LFT, ESR/CRP, amylase, clotting, ABG, blood culture, sputum culture.
Plasma BNP < 100 pg/mL may distinguish ARDS/ALI from heart failure, but higher levels can neither confirm heart failure nor exclude ARDS/ALI in critically ill patients.
Echocardiography: Severe aortic or mitral valve dysfunction or $\downarrow$ LVEF favours haemodynamic oedema over ARDS.
Pulmonary artery catheterization: PCWP ≤ 18 mmHg (however $\uparrow$ PCWP does not exclude ARDS as patients with ARDS may have concomitant left ventricular dysfunction).
Bronchoscopy: If the cause cannot be determined from the history, and to exclude differentials, e.g. diffuse alveolar haemorrhage (frothy blood in all airways, haemosiderin-laden macrophage from lavage fluid), lavage fluid for microbiology (mycobacteria, *Legionella pneumophila*, Pneumocystis, respiratory viruses) and cytology (eosinophils, viral inclusion bodies and cancer cells).

MANAGEMENT
Respiratory support: Supplemental oxygen (FiO_2: 50–60%). Almost all patients require intubation and mechanical ventilation.
Fully supported volume limited and pressure limited modes are both acceptable. The tidal volume, respiratory rate, PEEP and FiO_2 are managed according to the strategy of low tidal volume ventilation (LTVV). The rationale for LTVV is that smaller tidal volumes are less likely to generate alveolar overdistension and ventilator-associated lung injury. LTVV frequently requires '*permissive hypercapnic ventilation*', a ventilatory strategy that accepts alveolar hypoventilation in order to maintain a low alveolar pressure and minimize the complications of alveolar overdistension. The lowest plateau airway pressure possible should be targeted.
Sedation and analgesia: To improve tolerance of mechanical ventilation and to $\downarrow$ oxygen consumption. Neuromuscular blockade should be used only when sedation alone is inadequate.

Acute respiratory distress syndrome (ARDS) (continued)

Fluid management: Conservative strategy, as long as hypotension and organ hypoperfusion can be avoided (target a central venous pressure of <4 mmHg), blood transfusion if Hb < 7 g/dL, no evidence for inotropes cardiac function is normal.

Nutritional support: Enteral feedings are preferred, control of blood glucose.

Treat the cause: e.g. antibiotics for sepsis.

Prophylaxis/treat complications: e.g. nosocomial pneumonia, deep vein thrombosis (DVT) and gastrointestinal bleeding.

COMPLICATIONS   Respiratory failure, death. Complications related to mechanical ventilation, e.g. barotraumas (pneumothorax, subcutaneous emphysema) or intensive care (nosocomial pneumonia).

PROGNOSIS   Highly variable depending on cause but generally poor. Mortality ∼ 60% (mostly from sepsis). ↑ Mortality with ↑ age, sepsis and steroid treatment prior to the onset of ARDS. ARDS associated with trauma has a lower mortality.

Aspergillus lung disease

DEFINITION   Lung disease associated with Aspergillus fungal infection.

AETIOLOGY   Inhalation of the ubiquitous Aspergillus (usually *Aspergillus fumigates*) spores can produce three different clinical pictures:
1. **Aspergilloma**: Growth of an *A. fumigatus* mycetoma ball in a preexisting lung cavity (e.g. post-TB, old infarct or abscess).
2. **Allergic bronchopulmonary aspergillosis (ABPA)**: Aspergillus colonization of the airways (usually in asthmatics) leads to IgE- and IgG-mediated immune responses. Proteolytic enzymes and mycotoxins released by fungi, CD4/Th2 cells producing IL-4 and IL-5 and mediating eosinophilic inflammation, and IL-8 mediated neutrophilic inflammation result in airway damage and central bronchiectasis.

Invasive aspergillosis: Invasion of Aspergillus into lung tissue and fungal dissemination. Secondary to immunosuppression (e.g. neutropaenia, steroids, haematopoietic stem cell/solid organ transplantation, AIDS).

EPIDEMIOLOGY   Uncommon. Most common in elderly and immunocompromised.

HISTORY
Aspergilloma: Asymptomatic, haemoptysis, which may be massive.
ABPA: Difficult to control asthma, recurrent episodes of pneumonia with wheeze, cough, fever and malaise.
Invasive aspergillosis: Dyspnoea, rapid deterioration, septic picture.

EXAMINATION   Tracheal deviation in large aspergillomas.
Dullness in affected lung, ↓ breath sounds, wheeze (in ABPA).
Cyanosis may develop in invasive aspergillosis.

INVESTIGATIONS
Aspergilloma: *CXR*: Round opacity may be seen with a crescent of air around it (usually in the upper lobes).
CT or MR imaging if CXR does not clearly delineate a cavity.
Cultures of the sputum may be negative if there is no communication between the cavity and the bronchial tree. Also Aspergillus is a common colonizer of an abnormal respiratory tract.
ABPA:
Immediate skin test reactivity to Aspergillus antigens.
Eosinophilia.
↑ *Serum total IgE.*
↑ *Serum specific IgE and IgG to A. fumigatus* or precipitating serum antibodies to *A. fumigates*.
CXR: Transient patchy shadows, collapse, distended mucus-filled bronchi producing tubular shadows ('gloved fingers' appearance). Signs of complications: Fibrosis in upper lobes (similar to tuberculosis), parallel-line shadows and rings (bronchiectasis).
CT: Lung infiltrates, central bronchiectasis.
Lung function tests: Reversible airflow limitation, ↓ lung volumes/gas transfer in progressive cases.
Invasive aspergillosis: Detection of Aspergillus in cultures or by histologic examination (septated hyphae with acute angle branching). Diagnosis may be made in patients with risk factors, suggestive clinical findings and microscopic evidence of septate hyphae on examination of either *bronchoalveolar lavage fluid* or *sputum* or a positive *serum galactomannan* or *beta-D-glucan assay* (constituents of Aspergillus cell walls).
Chest CT scan may show nodules surrounded by a ground-glass appearance (halo sign) in invasive pulmonary aspergillosis (haemorrhage into the tissue surrounding the area of fungal invasion).

Aspergillus lung disease (continued)

MANAGEMENT

Aspergilloma: Surgical resection for large aspergillomas if uncontrolled or symptomatic (recurrent haemoptysis). Adjunctive itraconazole or voriconazole, if there is concern for residual disease following surgery, or tissue invasion beyond the confines of the cavity.

ABPA: Combination of steroids and itraconazole. Monitor LFTs. The usual duration of therapy is 3–6 months. Inhaled steroids and broncholdilators may help control symptoms of asthma. The response is monitored with serial measurement of the serum total IgE level.

Invasive aspergillosis: ↓ Immunosuppression if possible. Voriconazole (initially IV, when stabilized orally). Monitor serum voriconazole trough concentrations. If intolerant of voriconazole, use liposomal amphotericin B. Add caspofungin in patients who do not respond. Continue antifungal therapy until all signs, symptoms and radiographic evidence of the infection have resolved for at least 2 weeks. Debridement is essential in the treatment of Aspergillus sinusitis.

COMPLICATIONS

Aspergilloma: Secondary bacterial infection, massive haemoptysis or haemorrhage.

ABPA: Worsening of asthma, bronchiectasis, lobar collapse, lung fibrosis or respiratory failure.

Invasive aspergillosis: Septic shock, respiratory failure.

PROGNOSIS Grave prognosis for invasive aspergillosis. Good prognosis for ABPA and aspergillomas but bronchospasm and haemoptysis can still lead to death.

Asthma

DEFINITION   Chronic inflammatory airway disease characterized by variable reversible airway obstruction, airway hyper-responsiveness and bronchial inflammation.

AETIOLOGY

Genetic factors: Positive family history, twin studies. Almost all asthmatic patients show some atopy (tendency of T lymphocyte (Th$_2$) cells to drive production of IgE on exposure to allergens). Linkages to multiple chromosomal locations point to 'genetic heterogeneity'.

Environmental factors: House dust mite, pollen, pets (e.g. urinary proteins, furs), cigarette smoke, viral respiratory tract infection, *Aspergillus fumigatus* spores, occupational allergens (isocyanates, epoxy resins).

PATHOLOGY/PATHOGENESIS

Early phase (up to 1 h): Exposure to inhaled allergens in a presensitized individual results in cross-linking of IgE antibodies on the mast cell surface and release of histamine, prostaglandin D2, leukotrienes and TNF-α. These mediators induce smooth muscle contraction (bronchoconstriction), mucous hypersecretion, oedema and airway obstruction.

Late phase (after 6–12 h): Recruitment of eosinophils, basophils, neutrophil and Th2 lymphocytes and their products results in perpetuation of the inflammation and bronchial hyper-responsiveness.

Structural cells (bronchial epithelial cells, fibroblasts, smooth muscle and vascular endothelial cells), may also release cytokines, profibrogenic and proliferative growth factors, and contribute to the inflammation and altered function and proliferation of smooth muscle cells and fibroblasts ('airway remodeling').

EPIDEMIOLOGY   Affects 10% of children and 5% of adults. The prevalence of asthma appears to be increasing. $\female = \male$. Acute asthma is a very common medical emergency and still responsible for 1000–2000 deaths/year in the UK.

HISTORY   Episodes of wheeze, breathlessness, cough; worse in the morning and at night. Ask about interference with exercise, sleeping, days off school and work.

In an acute attack it is important to ask whether the patient has been admitted to hospital because of his/her asthma, or to ITU, as a gauge of potential severity.

Precipitating factors: Cold, viral infection, drugs (β-blockers, NSAIDs), exercise, emotions.

May have a history of allergic rhinitis, urticaria, eczema, nasal polyps, acid reflux and family history.

EXAMINATION   Tachypnoea, use of accessory muscles, prolonged expiratory phase, polyphonic wheeze, hyperinflated chest.

Severe attack: PEFR < 50% predicted, pulse > 110/min, respiratory rate > 25/min, inability to complete sentences.

Life-threatening attack: PEFR < 33%, silent chest, cyanosis, bradycardia, hypotension, confusion, coma.

INVESTIGATIONS

Acute: Peak flow, pulse oximetry, ABG, CXR (to exclude other diagnoses, e.g. pneumothorax, pneumonia), FBC ($\uparrow$ WCC if infective exacerbation), CRP, U&Es, blood and sputum cultures.

Chronic: *PEFR monitoring*: There is often a diurnal variation with a morning 'dip'.

Pulmonary function test: Obstructive defect, with improvement after a trial of a β_2-agonist.

Blood: Eosinophilia, IgE level, *Aspergillus* antibody titres (*see* allergic Aspergillus lung disease).

Skin prick tests: May help in the identification of allergens.

Asthma (continued)

MANAGEMENT

Acute:

- Resuscitate, monitor O_2 sats, ABG and PEFR.
- High-flow oxygen.
- Nebulized β_2-agonist bronchodilator salbutamol (5 mg, initially continuously, then 2–4 hourly), ipratropium (0.5 mg qds).
- Steroid therapy (100–200 mg IV hydrocortisone, followed by 40 mg oral prednisolone for 5–7 days).
- If no improvement: IV magnesium sulphate. Consider IV aminophylline infusion or IV salbutamol.
- Summon anaesthetic help if patient is getting exhausted (PCO_2 increasing).
  Treat any underlying cause (e.g. infection, pneumothorax). Give antibiotics if there is evidence of chest infection (purulent sputum, abnormal CXR, ↑ WCC, fever). Monitor electrolytes closely (bronchodilators and aminophyline ↓ K^+).
- May need ventilation in severe attacks. If not improving or patient tiring, involve ITU early.

Discharge: When PEF > 75% predicted or patient's best, diurnal variation < 25%, inhaler technique checked, stable on discharge medication for 24 h, patient owns a PEF meter and has steroid and bronchodilator therapy. Arrange follow-up.

Chronic 'stepwise' therapy: Start on the step appropriate to initial severity and step up or down to control symptoms. Treatment should be reviewed every 3–6 months.

Step 1: Inhaled short-acting β_2-agonist as needed. If used >1/day, move to Step 2.

Step 2: As Step 1 plus regular inhaled low-dose steroids (400 mcg/day).

Step 3: As Step 2 plus inhaled long-acting β_2-agonist (LABA). If inadequate control with LABA, ↑ steroid dose (800 mcg/day). If no response to LABA, stop and ↑ steroid dose (800 mcg/day).

Step 4: ↑ Inhaled steroid dose (2000 mcg/day), add a fourth drug, e.g. leukotriene receptor antagonist, SR theophylline or β_2-agonist tablet.

Step 5: Addition of regular oral steroids. Maintain high-dose inhaled steroid. Consider other treatments to minimize the use of oral steroids. Refer for specialist care.

Advice: Educate on proper inhaler technique and routine monitoring of peak flow. Develop an individualized management plan, with emphasis on avoidance of provoking factors.

COMPLICATIONS   Growth retardation, chest wall deformity (e.g. pigeon chest), recurrent infections, pneumothorax, respiratory failure, death.

PROGNOSIS   Many children improve as they grow older. Adult-onset asthma is usually chronic.

Bronchiectasis

DEFINITION   Lung airway disease characterized by chronic bronchial dilation, impaired mucuociliary clearance and frequent bacterial infections.

AETIOLOGY   Severe inflammation in the lung causes fibrosis and dilation of the bronchi. This is followed by pooling of mucus, predisposing to further cycles of infection, damage and fibrosis to bronchial walls.
- Causes of bronchiectasis.
- Idiopathic in ~50% of cases.
- Post-infectious: After severe pneumonia, whooping cough, tuberculosis.
Host defence defects: e.g. Kartagener's syndrome,[1] cystic fibrosis, immunoglobulin deficiency, yellow-nail syndrome.[2]
- Obstruction of bronchi: Foreign body, enlarged lymph nodes.
- Gastric reflux disease.
- Inflammatory disorders: e.g. rheumatoid arthritis.

EPIDEMIOLOGY   Most often arises initially in childhood, incidence has ↓ with use of antibiotics, approximately 1 in 1000 per year.

HISTORY   Productive cough with purulent sputum or haemoptysis.
Breathlessness, chest pain, malaise, fever, weight loss.
Symptoms usually begin after an acute respiratory illness.

EXAMINATION   Finger clubbing; Coarse creptitations (usually at the bases) which shift with coughing; Wheeze.

INVESTIGATIONS
Sputum: Culture and sensitivity, common organisms in acute exacerbations: *Pseudomonas aeruginosa, Haemophilus influenzae, Staphylococcus aureus, Streptococcus pneumoniae, Klebsiella, Moraxella catarrhalis*, Mycobacteria.
CXR: Dilated bronchi may be seen as parallel lines radiating from hilum to the diaphragm ('tramline shadows'). It may also show fibrosis, atelectasis, pneumonic consolidations, or it may be normal.
High-resolution CT: Dilated bronchi with thickened walls. Best diagnostic method.
Bronchography (rarely used): To determine extent of disease before surgery (radio-opaque contrast injected through the cricoid ligament or via a bronchoscope).
Other: Sweat electrolytes (*see* Cystic fibrosis), serum immunoglobulins (~10% of adults have some immune deficiency), sinus X-ray (30% have concomitant rhinosinusitis), mucociliary clearance study.

MANAGEMENT   *Treat acute exacerbations* with two IV antibiotics with efficacy for *Pseudomonas*. Prophylactic courses of antibiotics (oral or aerosolized) for those with frequent (≥3/year) exacerbations.
Inhaled corticosteroids (e.g. fluticasone) have been shown to reduce inflammation and volume of sputum, although it does not affect the frequency of exacerbations or lung function.
Bronchodilators may be considered in patients with responsive disease.
Maintain hydration with adequate oral fluid intake.

---

[1] Kartagener's syndrome is caused by immotile cilia and is characterized by a combination of chronic sinusitis, infertility and situs inversus.

[2] Yellow-nail syndrome is characterized by pleural effusions, lymphoedema and yellow dystrophic nails. Approximately 40% will also have bronchiectasis.

Bronchiectasis (continued)

Consider flu vaccination.

Physiotherapy: Cornerstone of management is sputum and mucus clearance techniques (e.g. postural drainage). Patients are taught to position themselves so the lobe to be drained is uppermost, ~20 min twice daily. Some studies show that these techniques reduce frequency of acute exacerbations and aids recovery.

Bronchial artery embolization: For life-threatening haemoptysis due to bronchiectasis.

Surgical: Various surgical options include localized resection, lung or heart–lung transplantation.

COMPLICATIONS Life-threatening haemoptysis, persistent infections, empyema, respiratory failure, cor pulmonale, multi-organ abscesses.

PROGNOSIS Most patients continue to have the symptoms after 10 years.

Chronic obstructive pulmonary disease (COPD)

DEFINITION   Chronic, progressive lung disorder characterized by airflow obstruction, with the following.

Chronic bronchitis: Chronic cough and sputum production on most days for at least 3 months per year over 2 consecutive years; and/or

Emphysema: Pathological diagnosis of permanent destructive enlargement of air spaces distal to the terminal bronchioles.

AETIOLOGY   Bronchial and alveolar damage as a result of environmental toxins (e.g. cigarette smoke). A rare cause is α1-antitrypsin deficiency (<1%) but should be considered in young patients or in those who have never smoked. Overlaps and may co-present with asthma.

Chronic bronchitis: Narrowing of the airways resulting from bronchiole inflammation (bronchiolitis) and bronchi with mucosal oedema, mucous hypersecretion and squamous metaplasia.

Emphysema: Destruction and enlargement of the alveoli. This results in loss of the elastic traction that keeps small airways open in expiration. Progressively larger spaces develop, termed bullae (diameter is >1 cm).

EPIDEMIOLOGY   Very common (prevalence up to 8%). Presents in middle age or later. More common in males, but likely to change with ↑ female smokers.

HISTORY   Chronic cough and sputum production (*see* Definition).
Breathlessness, wheeze, ↓ exercise tolerance.

EXAMINATION

Inspection: May have respiratory distress, use of accessory muscles, barrel-shaped overinflated chest, ↓ cricosternal distance, cyanosis.

Percussion: Hyper-resonant chest, loss of liver and cardiac dullness.

Auscultation: Quiet breath sounds, prolonged expiration, wheeze, rhonchi and crepitations sometimes present.

Signs of CO_2 retention: Bounding pulse, warm peripheries, flapping tremor of the hands (asterixis). In late stages, signs of right heart failure (e.g. right ventricular heave, raised JVP, ankle oedema).

INVESTIGATIONS

Spirometry and pulmonary function tests: Obstructive picture as reflected by ↓ PEFR, ↓ FEV_1: FVC ratio (mild, 60–80%; moderate, 40–60%; severe, <40%), ↑ lung volumes and carbon monoxide gas transfer coefficient ↓ when significant alveolar destruction.

CXR: May appear normal or show hyperinflation (>6 ribs visible anteriorly, flat hemidiaphragms), ↓ peripheral lung markings, elongated cardiac silhouette.

Blood: FBC (↑ Hb and PCV as a result of secondary polycythemia).

ABG: May show hypoxia (↓ PaO_2), normal or ↑ $PaCO_2$.

ECG and echocardiogram: For cor pulmonale (*see* Cardiac failure).

Sputum and blood cultures: In acute exacerbations for treatment.

Consider α1-antitrypsin levels in young patients or minimal smoking history.

MANAGEMENT[1]   *Stop smoking.*

Bronchodilators: Short-acting β_2-agonists (e.g. salbutamol) and anticholinergics (e.g. ipratropium), delivered by inhalers or nebulizers. Long-acting bronchodilators should be used if >2 exacerbations per year.

Steroids: Inhaled beclometasone should be considered for all with FEV_1 <50% predicted or those with >2 exacerbations per year. Regular oral steroids should be avoided but may be necessary for maintenance.

---

[1]Refer to http://www.nice.org.uk/nicemedia/pdf/CG012_niceguideline.pdf (NICE 2004 guidelines) for complete information.

Chronic obstructive pulmonary disease (COPD) (continued)

Pulmonary rehabilitation.

Oxygen therapy (only for those who stop smoking): Long-term home oxygen therapy has been shown to improve mortality. Indications are:

- $PaO_2 < 7.3$ kPa on air during a period of clinical stability.
- PaO_2 7.3–8.0 kPa and signs of secondary polycythaemia, nocturnal hypoxaemia, peripheral oedema or pulmonary hypertension.

Oxygen concentrators are more economical if being used for >8 h/day.

Treatment of acute infective exacerbations:

Provide 24% O_2 via non-variable flow Venturi mask.

Increase slowly if no hypercapnia and still hypoxic (measured by ABG).

Corticosteroids (oral or inhaled) are of proven benefit.

Start empirical antibiotic therapy (follow local policy) if evidence of infection.

Respiratory physiotherapy is essential to clear sputum.

Consider non-invasive ventilation in severe cases.

Prevention of infective exacerbations: Pneumococcal and influenza vaccination.

COMPLICATIONS Acute respiratory failure, infections (particularly *Streptococcus pneumoniae, Haemophilus influenzae*), pulmonary hypertension and right heart failure, pneumothorax (resulting from bullae rupture), secondary polycythaemia.

PROGNOSIS High level of morbidity. Three-year survival rate of 90% if age <60 years and FEV_1 >50% predicted; 75% if >60 years and FEV_1 40–49% predicted.

Cystic fibrosis

DEFINITION   Autosomal recessive inherited multi-system disease characterized by recurrent respiratory tract infections, pancreatic insufficiency, malabsorption and male infertility.

AETIOLOGY   Caused by a defective CFTR gene on chromosome 7q, which encodes a cAMP-dependent Cl^- channel. This channel regulates Na^+ and Cl^- concentrations in exocrine secretions, especially in the lung and pancreas. Any loss of function mutations results in thick viscous secretions. Greater than 800 mutations reported, most common is ΔF508 phenylalanine deletion (75% cases in UK).
At birth, the lung is normal histologically but as the lung matures there is mucous gland hyperplasia, recurrent infection leads to fibrosis, consolidation and bronchiectasis.

EPIDEMIOLOGY   Most common life-threatening autosomal inherited condition in Caucasians. Incidence is 1 in 2500 live births. In UK, 1 in 25 are carriers.

HISTORY
Lung: Recurrent chest infections, chronic cough, wheeze, sputum, haemoptysis.
Gut: Meconium ileus (in neonates), steatorrhoea (caused by ↑ fat in the stool).
Other: Chronic sinusitis, nasal polyps, male infertility, arthritis.

EXAMINATION
Chest: Chest wall deformities, coarse crepitations and wheeze.
Signs of malnutrition: Anaemia, weight loss, signs of vitamin deficiencies, slow growth, failure to thrive in children, delayed puberty in adolescents.
Other: Clubbing, nasal polyps, signs of diabetes, hepatomegaly.

INVESTIGATIONS
Sweat test: Pilocarpine iontophoresis (low electrical current) stimulates sweat secretion which is collected and analyzed for Na^+ and Cl^- (Cl^- levels >60 mmol is diagnostic of cystic fibrosis).
Neonatal screening: Standard day 6 Guthrie heal prick, blood is tested for immunoreactive trypsin (raised by 2–5× in babies with cystic fibrosis).
CXR: May be normal in mild disease or show increased bronchial markings, ring shadows, fibrosis (often upper zone). Consolidation or bronchiectasis in more advanced cases.
Pancreatic assessment: Faecal elastase, faecal fat content, GTT, HbA1c.
Genetic analysis: For CFTR mutations. Rarely necessary.
Lung function tests: To assess lung function and for long-term prognosis.

MANAGEMENT
Multidisciplinary specialist care is necessary.
Respiratory:
- Chest physiotherapy (postural drainage, regular exercise), positive expiratory pressure masks;
- bronchodilator therapy (if responsive);
- nebulized recombinant human deoxyribonuclease (rhDNase) and hypertonic saline can be used to assist in mucociliary clearance and may reduce pulmonary exarcebations;
- antibiotic prophylaxis and aggressive treatment of infections (especially *Pseudomonas*);
- influenza vaccination.

GI: Adequate nutritional intake is vital, using high-calorie oral supplements and oral pancreatic enzyme replacement, vitamin (especially fat-soluble) supplements.
Endocrine: Insulin replacement therapy if diabetes develops.
Surgical: Single lung or heart–lung transplants is an option in end-stage disease (5-year survival is 55%).

COMPLICATIONS   Recurrent chest infections, bronchiectasis (particularly *Haemophilus*, *Staphylococcus* and *Pseudomonas*).

Cystic fibrosis (continued)

Malabsorption, meconium ileus, intussusception, rectal prolapse.
Diabetes mellitus Type I (30% by late teens).
Male infertility (females are fertile but conception may be difficult).
Gallstones.

PROGNOSIS   Life expectancy is in the third decade, but steadily improving. Those with pancreatic insufficiency and those colonized by *Pseudomonas* have poorer prognosis. Gene replacement therapy may be possible in the future.

Extrinsic allergic alveolitis

DEFINITION   Interstitial inflammatory disease of the distal gas-exchanging parts of the lung caused by inhalation of organic dusts. Also known as hypersensitivity pneumonitis.

AETIOLOGY   Inhalation of antigenic organic dusts containing microbes (bacteria, fungi or amoebae) or animal proteins induce a hypersensitivity response (a combination of type III antigen–antibody complex hypersensitivity reaction and a type IV granulomatous lymphocytic inflammation) in susceptible individuals. Examples:

Farmer's lung: Mouldy hay containing thermophilic actinomycetes.

Pigeon/budgerigar fancier's lung: Bloom on bird feathers and excreta.

Mushroom worker's lung: Compost containing thermophilic actinomycetes.

Humidifier lung: Water-containing bacteria and *Naegleria* (amoeba).

Maltworker's lung: Barley or maltings containing *Aspergillus clavatus*.

EPIDEMIOLOGY   Uncommon, 2% of occupational lung diseases, 50% of reported cases affect farm workers (incidence is about 4–10 in 100 000/year), marked geographical variation reflecting dependence on occupational causes.

HISTORY

Acute: Presents 4–12 h post-exposure. Reversible episodes of dry cough, dyspnoea, malaise, fever, myalgia. Wheeze and productive cough may develop on repeat high-level exposures.

Chronic: Poorly reversible manifestation in some, slowly ↑ breathlessness and ↓ exercise tolerance, weight loss. Exposure is usually chronic, low level and there may be no history of previous acute episodes.

Full occupational history and enquiry into hobbies and pets important.

EXAMINATION

Acute: Rapid shallow breathing, pyrexia, inspiratory crepitations.

Chronic: Fine inspiratory crepitations (*see* Cryptogenic fibrosing alveolitis). Finger clubbing is rare.

INVESTIGATIONS

Blood: FBC (neutrophilia, lymphopenia), ABG (↓ PO_2, ↓ PCO_2).

Serology: Precipitating IgG to fungal or avian antigens in serum; however, these are not diagnostic as are often found in asymptomatic individuals.

CXR: Often normal in acute episodes, may show 'ground glass' appearance with alveolar shadowing or nodular opacities in the middle and lower zones. In chronic cases, fibrosis is prominent in the upper zones.

High-resolution CT-thorax: Detects early changes before CXR. Patchy 'ground glass' shadowing and nodules.

Pulmonary function tests: Restrictive ventilatory defect (↓ FEV1, ↓ FVC with preserved or increased ratio), ↓ TLCO.

Bronchoalveolar lavage: Increased cellularity with ↑ CD8 + suppressor T cells. Lung biopsy (transbronchial or thorascopic).

MANAGEMENT

Advice: Complete avoidance of exposure to the antigen (e.g. change of work practice or hobby), if this is problematic, then minimize exposure and encourage use of respiratory protection masks.

Medical:

Acute flare: Spontaneous recovery usually within 1–2 days, high-dose corticosteroids for 2–4 weeks may accelerate recovery but do not appear to affect long-term outcome.

Chronic disease: Trial of high-dose oral prednisolone for 1 month may be carried out, this is gradually reduced, or stopped if no objective response demonstrated.

Extrinsic allergic alveolitis (continued)

General: Regular follow-up to monitor lung function. Environmental assessment is necessary for risk posed to others. In UK, farmer's lung patients are entitled to compensation, depending on the degree of disability.

COMPLICATIONS Progressive lung fibrosis, pulmonary hypertension, right heart failure.

PROGNOSIS The acute form generally resolves if further exposure is prevented, with chronic disease some patients will improve while a minority progress to lung fibrosis.

Idiopathic fibrosing alveolitis

DEFINITION Inflammatory condition of the lung resulting in fibrosis of alveoli and interstitium. Previously known as 'cryptogenic fibrosing alveolitis'.

AETIOLOGY In a genetically predisposed host (e.g. with telomerase/surfactant protein mutations), recurrent injury to alveolar epithelial cells may result in secretion of cytokines and growth factors (e.g. TNF-α, IL-1 and MCP-1) which cause fibroblast activation, recruitment, proliferation, differentiation into myofibroblasts and ↑ collagen synthesis and deposition. Profibrogenic molecules, e.g. PDGF and TGF-β, are secreted by inflammatory, epithelial and endothelial cells.

Certain drugs can produce a similar illness (e.g. bleomycin, methotrexate and amiodarone).

Histological patterns: Usual interstitial pneumonia (UIP: patchy interstitial fibrosis, later: 'honeycomb' lung). Desquamative interstitial pneumonia (DIP: diffuse intra-alveolar accumulation of macrophages, mild thickening of alveolar septa, lymphoid aggregates) and non-specific interstitial pneumonia (NSIP).

Risk factors: Smoking (in 75%), occupational exposure to metal (steel, brass, lead) or wood (pine) in ~20% cases; chronic microaspiration, animal and vegetable dusts.

EPIDEMIOLOGY Rare. Prevalence in UK is ~6 in 100 000. ♂:♀ is 2 : 1. Mean age 67 years.

HISTORY Gradual onset of progressive dyspnoea on exertion.
Dry irritating cough. No wheeze.
Symptoms may be preceded by a viral-type illness.
Fatigue and weight loss are common.
Full occupational and drug history is important.

EXAMINATION Finger clubbing (~50%).
Bibasal fine late inspiratory crepitations.
Signs of right heart failure in advanced stages (e.g. right ventricular heave, raised JVP, peripheral oedema).

INVESTIGATIONS

Blood: ABG (normal in early disease, but ↓ PO_2 on exercise; normal Pco_2 which rises in late disease). One-third have rheumatoid factor or antinuclear antibodies.

CXR: Usually normal at presentation. Early disease may feature small lung fields and 'ground glass' shadowing. Later, there is reticulonodular shadowing (especially at bases), signs of cor pulmonale and eventually, in advanced disease, honeycombing.

High-resolution CT: More sensitive in early disease than CXR. Affecting mainly lower zones and subpleural areas, with reticular densities, honeycombing and traction bronchiectasis.

Pulmonary function tests: Restrictive ventilatory defect (↓ FEV_1, ↓ FVC with preserved or increased ratio), ↓ lung volumes, ↓ lung compliance and ↓ TLCO.

Bronchoalveolar lavage: To exclude infections and malignancy.

Lung biopsy: Gold standard for diagnosis but may not be appropriate.

Echocardiography: To look for pulmonary hypertension.

MANAGEMENT No curative treatment available.

Combination of azathioprine, oral glucocorticoids and high-dose acetylcysteine, reassess the response (symptoms, lung function tests) every 3 months. After 3–6 months of treatment, if there is no evidence of a response, treatment is discontinued. Immunosuppressant therapy may not be offered to patients with severe loss of lung function or extensive fibrosis on high-resolution chest CT.

Supportive care: Home oxygen may be necessary. Pulmonary rehabilitation. Opiates in terminal stages for relieving distressing breathlessness. Psychosocial support is necessary because of poor long-term prognosis.

Acute exacerbation: Broad-spectrum antibiotics and high-dose glucocorticoids.

Idiopathic fibrosing alveolitis (continued)

Surgical: Single lung transplantation. Lung transplantation may be an option for patients with progressive disease and minimal comorbidities.

COMPLICATIONS Right heart failure. Lung cancer (12%). Pulmonary embolus. Death from respiratory failure.

PROGNOSIS Poor; mean survival is only about 3 years. Good prognostic factors:
Clinical: Young age, female, response to steroids.
Radiological: Predominantly 'ground glass' shadowing.
Histology: DIP and NSIP better response to treatment than UIP.

Lung cancer, non-small cell

DEFINITION Primary malignant neoplasm of the lung. WHO classification of broncho-carcinoma: Small cell (20%; *see* separate topic) and non-small cell (80%).

Histological types of non-small cell lung cancer include: Squamous cell carcinoma, adeno-carcinoma, large cell carcinoma and adenosquamous carcinoma.

AETIOLOGY Factors such as smoking (active or passive) are thought to ultimately cause genetic alterations that result in neoplastic transformation. Other risk factors include occupational exposures (polycyclic hydrocarbons, asbestos, nickel, chromium, cadmium, radon) and atmospheric pollution.

Tumours generally arise in main or lobar bronchi. Adenocarcinomas tend to occur more peripherally.

EPIDEMIOLOGY Most common fatal malignancy in the West (18% of cancer mortality worldwide), 35 000 deaths per year (UK), $3\times$ more common in men (but increasing in women).

HISTORY May be asymptomatic with radiographic abnormality found (5%).

Due to primary: Cough, haemoptysis, chest pain, recurrent pneumonia.

Due to local invasion: e.g. brachial plexus (Pancoast tumour, in the apex of the lung) causing pain in the shoulder or arm, left recurrent laryngeal nerve (hoarseness and bovine cough), oesophagus (dysphagia), heart (palpitations/arrhythmias).

Due to metastatic disease or paraneoplastic phenomena: Weight loss, fatigue, fits, bone pain or fractures, neuromyopathies.

EXAMINATION There may be no signs. Fixed monophonic wheeze. Signs of collapse, consolidation or pleural effusion.

Due to local invasion: Superior vena cava compression (facial congestion, distension of neck veins, upper limb oedema). Brachial plexus (wasting of the small muscles of the hand). Sympathetic chain (Horner's syndrome: pupillary miosis, ptosis and facial anhydrosis).

Due to paraneoplastic phenomena: Hypertrophic osteoarthropathy: clubbing, painful swollen wrists/ankles (periosteal new bone formation). Dermatological signs (*see* Complications).

Due to metastases: Supraclavicular lymphadenopathy, hepatomegaly.

INVESTIGATION

Diagnosis: CXR (coin lesions, lobar collapse, pleural effusion, features of lymphangitis carcinomatosis[1]). Sputum cytology, bronchoscopy with brushings or biopsy, CT- or ultrasound-guided percutaneous biopsy, lymph node biopsy.

TNM staging: Based on tumour size, nodal involvement and metastatic spread, using CT chest, CT or MRI head and abdomen (or ultrasound), bone scan, PET scan. Invasive methods like mediastinoscopy or video-assisted thoracoscopy may be used.

Bloods: FBC, U&Es, Ca^{2+} (hypercalcaemia is common), AlkPhos ($\uparrow$ bone metastases), LFT.

Pre-op: ABG, pulmonary function tests ($FEV_1 > 80\%$ predicted to tolerate a pneumonecto-my, lung resection is contraindicated if $FEV_1 < 30\%$ predicted), V/Q scan, ECG, echo-cardiogram and general anaesthetic assessment.

MANAGEMENT Multidisciplinary discussion on tumour staging and optimal treatment modality. Important considerations are resectibility of the tumour (stages I and II disease, selectively IIIa) and operability (whether a patient is fit enough to undergo surgery). Frank discussion with the patient about the risks/benefits and the prognosis is vital. Only $\sim$14% cases are considered for surgery.

---

[1] Lymphangitis carcinomatosis is the diffuse infiltration and obstruction of pulmonary parenchymal lymphatic channels by tumour. Eighty percent are caused by adenocarcinomas. CXR shows a reticulo-nodular opacification, but best seen with high-resolution CT. Very poor prognosis.

Lung cancer, non-small cell (continued)

Surgery: Aimed at curative resection but often not appropriate.

Non-operable: Combined modality therapy with radiotherapy and chemotherapy improves survival. Docetaxel is a commonly used chemotherapy. Biological therapy in the form of erlotinib (epidermal growth factor receptor, EGFR, tyrosine kinase inhibitor) is a second-line chemotherapy agent.

Palliation and terminal care: Includes laser therapy to bronchial tumours, endobronchial stents, management of complications and pain control.

COMPLICATION   Local invasion. Metastases (commonly liver, bones, brain, adrenals). Pneumonia, pleural effusion, lung collapse. Paraneoplastic syndromes (squamous cell carcinomas are associated with hypercalcaemia of malignancy). Skin: Acanthosis nigricans (pigmented thickened skin in axilla or neck), herpes zoster, dermatomyositis, thrombophlebitis migrans.

PROGNOSIS   Depends on stage, but generally poor. Overall 5-year survival <5%. After resection for early stage disease ~25% 5-year survival. Mortality of lobectomy is <2%, and mortality for pneumonectomy is 8%.

Lung cancer, small cell

DEFINITION   Malignant neoplasm of neuroendocrine Kulchitsky cells of the lung with early dissemination. Also known as oat cell carcinoma.

AETIOLOGY   Smoking. Occupational and environmental exposures (see Lung cancer, non-small cell).

EPIDEMIOLOGY   Accounts for 20% of lung cancers.

HISTORY   May be asymptomatic with radiographical abnormality found.
Due to primary tumour: Cough, haemoptysis, dyspnoea, chest pain.
Due to metastatic disease: Weight loss, fatigue, bone pain.
Due to paraneoplastic syndromes: Weakness, lethargy, seizures, muscle fatiguability.

EXAMINATION   May be no signs or a fixed wheeze on auscultation of the chest.
Signs of lobar collapse or pleural effusion.
Signs of metastases, e.g. supraclavicular lymphadenopathy or hepatomegaly.
Signs of paraneoplastic syndrome.

INVESTIGATIONS
Diagnosis: Sputum cytology, bronchoscopy with brushings and biopsy or percutaneous biopsy, thoracoscopy.
Staging: CT of chest, abdomen, head. Isotope bone scan.
Other: Lung function tests, FBC, U&E, Ca^{2+}, AlkPhos, LFT.

MANAGEMENT
Limited disease: Combination chemotherapy and radiotherapy. Cisplatin and etoposide is a common regimen and chest irradiation results in a 5% improvement in 3-year survival. Prophylactic cranial irradiation also improves survival in those who achieve a complete remission or have limited stage disease.
Extensive disease: Chemotherapy, e.g. cisplatin and etoposide.
Palliation: Radiotherapy to metastasis.

COMPLICATIONS   Pneumonia, superior vena caval compression.
Metastases: Most commonly to brain, liver, adrenals, skin.
Endocrine: Ectopic ACTH (1%): Cushing's syndrome; ectopic ADH production (7–10%): SIADH; hypercalcaemia (bony metastases or PTH-related peptide secretion).
Skin: *See also* Lung cancer, non-small cell.
Eaton–Lambert myasthenic syndrome (<1%).

PROGNOSIS   Poor. Even with limited disease, 5-year survival rate is only 15–20%. Small cell carcinoma is often disseminated by the time of presentation.

Obstructive sleep apnoea

DEFINITION   Characterized by recurrent collapse of the pharangeal airway and apnoea (defined as cessation of airflow for >10 s) during sleep, followed by arousal from sleep. Also known as Pickwickian syndrome.

AETIOLOGY   Obstructive apnoeas occur when the upper airway narrows because of collapse of the soft tissues of the pharynx when tone in pharangeal dilators decreases during sleep. Associated with:
• excessive weight gain, smoking, alcohol or sedative use;
• enlarged tonsils or adenoids in children; and
• macroglossia, Marfan's syndrome, craniofacial abnormalities.

EPIDEMIOLOGY   Common. Affects 5–20% of men, 2–5% of women >35 years. Prevalence increases with age.

HISTORY   Excessive daytime sleepiness (at work, driving).
Unrefreshing or restless sleep.
Morning headaches or dry mouth, difficulty concentrating, irritability or mood changes.
Partner reporting snoring, nocturnal apnoeic episodes or nocturnal choking.

EXAMINATION   Large tongue, enlarged tonsils, long or thick uvula, retrognathia (pulled back jaws).
Neck circumference (>42 cm males, >40 cm females) is strongly correlated with presence of disease.
Obesity and hypertension is common.

INVESTIGATIONS   Video recording of episodes.
Sleep study: Managed by sleep study centre for polysomnography or diagnostic sleep studies with monitoring of airflow, respiratory effort, pulse oximetry and heart rate.
Blood: Thyroid function tests, ABG.

MANAGEMENT
Mild: Advice on sleep positions (sleep on side rather than on back), weight loss, smoking cessation, avoidance of alcohol, sedatives and late night meals.
Moderate: Mandibular advancement splints.
Severe: Nasal or face-mask CPAP uses positive pressure to maintain patency of upper airways and prevents their closure.
Surgery: Used in severe cases with variable success (e.g. removal of nasal polyps, correction of deviated nasal septum uvulopalatopharyngoplasty).
Public health: Patient is advised to inform DVLA.

COMPLICATIONS   Risk of accidents when driving or working. Worsening of congestive heart failure. Linked to ↑ risk of coronary artery disease and stroke.

PROGNOSIS   Short-term prognosis good with symptom improvement with CPAP. Compliance with advice or CPAP may be poor in long term.

Pneumoconiosis

DEFINITION   Fibrosing interstitial lung disease caused by chronic inhalation of mineral dusts.
Simple: Coalworker's pneumoconiosis or silicosis (symptom-free).
Complicated: Pneumoconiosis (progressive massive fibrosis) results in loss of lung function.
Asbestosis: A pneumoconiosis in which diffuse parenchymal lung fibrosis occurs as a result of prolonged exposure to asbestos.

AETIOLOGY   Caused by inhalation of particles of coal dust, silica or asbestos (two main types of fibre: white asbestos and blue asbestos or crocidolite, the latter is more toxic).

ASSOCIATIONS/RISK FACTORS   Occupational exposure: in coal mining, quarrying, iron and steel foundries, stone cutting, sandblasting, insulation industry, plumbers, ship builders. Risk depends on extent of exposure, size and shape of particles and individual susceptibility, as well as co-factors such as smoking and TB.

EPIDEMIOLOGY   Incidence ↑ in developing countries, disability and mortality from asbestosis will ↑ for the next 20–30 years.

HISTORY   Occupational history is important, there may be a long latency between disease exposure and expression.
Asymptomatic: Picked up on routine CXR (simple coal or silica pneumoconiosis).
Symptomatic: There is usually insidious onset of shortness of breath and a dry cough. Occasionally, black sputum (melanoptysis) is produced in coalworker's pneumoconiosis. Workers exposed to asbestos may develop pleuritic chest pain many years after first exposure as a result of acute asbestos pleurisy.

EXAMINATION   Examination may be normal.
Decreased breath sounds in coalworker's pneumoconiosis or silicosis.
End-inspiratory crepitations and clubbing in asbestosis.
Signs of a pleural effusion or right heart failure (cor pulmonale).

PATHOLOGY/PATHOGENESIS   *Complicated disease*: There are large nodules in the lung, consisting of dust particles (coal or silica) surrounded by layers of collagen and dying macrophages. Mechanisms of damage include:
1. direct cytotoxicity by particles;
2. particle ingestion by macrophages results in activation and excessive free radical production causing lipid peroxidation and cell injury; and
3. proinflammatory cytokines and growth factors from macrophages and epithelial cells stimulate fibroblast proliferation and eventual scarring.

Asbestosis: Asbestos bodies consisting of fibres coated with an iron-containing protein are seen in fibrotic areas, especially in the lung bases.

INVESTIGATIONS
CXR:
Simple: Micronodular mottling is present.
Complicated: Nodular opacities in the upper lobes, micronodular shadowing, eggshell calcification of hilar lymph nodes is characteristic of silicosis. In asbestosis, there is often bilateral lower zone reticulonodular shadowing and pleural plaques, visible as white lines when calcified, often most obvious on the diaphragmatic pleura or as 'holly leaf' patterns.

CT scan: Fibrotic changes can be visualized early.
Bronchoscopy: Visualizes changes. Allows for bronchoalveolar lavage.
Lung function tests: Restrictive ventilatory defect, impaired gas diffusion.

Pneumoconiosis (continued)

MANAGEMENT

General: Prevention of exposure. Avoidance of further exposure.

Medical: No specific treatment other than supportive care, e.g. oxygen or trial of inhaled steroids, and the treatment of complications.

Advice: Patients are entitled to compensation for occupational lung diseases.

COMPLICATIONS Progressive massive fibrosis, emphysema, cor pulmonale, Caplan's syndrome, end-stage respiratory failure, benign and malignant pleural effusions, lung carcinoma and mesothelioma (malignancy of pleura, seen especially with blue asbestos, crocidolite, exposure).

PROGNOSIS Not curable. Lifespan shortened with complicated disease. Prognosis is poor if malignancy develops.

Pneumonia

DEFINITION   Infection of distal lung parenchyma. Several ways of categorization:
- community-acquired, hospital-acquired or nosocomial;
- aspiration pneumonia, pneumonia in the immunocompromised;
- typical and atypical (*Mycoplasma, Chlamydia, Legionella*).

AETIOLOGY
Community-acquired: *Streptococcus pneumoniae* (70%), *Haemophilus influenzae* and
  Moraxella catarrhalis (COPD), *Chlamydia pneumonia* and *Chlamydia psittaci* (contact
  with birds/parrots), *Mycoplasma pneumonia* (periodic epidemics), *Legionella* (anywhere
  with air conditioning), *Staphylococcus aureus* (recent influenza infection, IV drug users),
  Coxiella burnetii (Q fever, rare), TB (may present as pneumonia; *see* Tuberculosis).
Hospital-acquired: Gram-negative enterobacteria (*Pseudomonas, Klebsiella*), anaerobes
  (aspiration pneumonia).
Risk factors: Age, smoking, alcohol, pre-existing lung disease, immunodeficiency, contact
  with pneumonia.

EPIDEMIOLOGY   Incidence ~5–11 in 1000 (25–44 in 1000 in elderly). Community-
acquired causes >60 000 deaths/year in the UK.

HISTORY   Fever, rigors, sweating, malaise, cough, sputum (yellow, green or rusty in *S.
  pneumoniae*), breathlessness and pleuritic chest pain, confusion (severe cases, elderly,
  Legionella).
Atypical pneumonia: Headache, myalgia, diarrhoea/abdominal pain.

EXAMINATION   Pyrexia, respiratory distress, tachypnoea, tachycardia, hypotension,
  cyanosis.
↓ Chest expansion, dullness to percussion, ↑ tactile vocal fremitus, bronchial breathing
  (inspiration phase lasts as long as expiration phase), coarse crepitations on affected side.
Chronic suppurative lung disease (empyema, abscess): Clubbing.

INVESTIGATIONS
Blood: FBC (abnormal WCC), U&E (↓ Na$^+$, especially with *Legionella*), LFT, blood cultures
  (sensitivity 10–20%), ABG (assess pulmonary function), blood film (RBC agglutination by
  Mycoplasma caused by cold agglutinins; *see* Anaemia, haemolytic).
CXR: Lobar or patchy shadowing, may lag behind clinical signs, pleural effusion, *Klebsiella*
  often affects upper lobes, repeat 6–8 weeks (if abnormal suspect underlying pathology,
  e.g. lung cancer). May detect complications: Abscess (cavitation and air-fluid level).
Sputum/pleural fluid: Microscopy, culture and sensitivity, acid-fast bacilli.
Urine: *Pneumococcus* and *Legionella* antigens.
Atypical viral serology: ↑ Antibody titres between acute and convalescent samples
  (>2 weeks post-onset).
Bronchoscopy (and bronchoalveolar lavage): If *Pneumocystis carinii* pneumonia is
  suspected, or when pneumonia fails to resolve or when there is clinical progression.

MANAGEMENT   Refer to British Thoracic Society Guidelines 2001 and the 2004 update).
Assess severity (*see* Prognosis; if ≥1 feature present, manage in hospital).
Start empirical antibiotics:
- Oral amoxicillin (0 markers);
- oral or IV amoxicillin and erythromycin (1 marker);
- IV cefuroxime/cefotaxime/co-amoxiclav and erythromycin (>1 marker);
- add metronidazole, if aspiration, lung abscess or empyema suspected;
- switch to appropriate antibiotic as per sensitivity.

Levofloxacin and moxifloxacin can provide useful alternatives in selected hospitalized patients
with community-acquired pneumonia.

Pneumonia (continued)

Supportive treatment:

- Oxygen (maintain $PO_2 > 8\,kPa$, start with 28% O_2 in COPD to avoid hypercapnia);
- parenteral fluids for dehydration or shock, analgesia, chest physiotherapy;
- CPAP, BiPAP or ITU care for respiratory failure;
- surgical drainage may be needed for empyema/abscesses.

Discharge planning:

Presence of two or more features of clinical instability (↑ temperature, heart rate, respiratory rate and ↓ BP, oxygen saturation, mental status and oral intake) predict a significant chance of re-admission or mortality. Thus this assessment should be considered when planning for discharge.

Non-resolving pneumonia: Consider other causes (see Table 1).

Prevention: Pneumococcal, *H. influenzae* type B vaccination in vulnerable groups (e.g. elderly, splenectomized).

COMPLICATIONS   Pleural effusion, empyema (pus in the pleural cavity), localized suppuration → lung abscess[1] (especially staphylococcal, *Klebsiella* pneumonia, presenting with swinging fever, persistent pneumonia, copious/foul-smelling sputum), septic shock, ARDS, acute renal failure.

M. pneumonia: Erythema multiforme, myocarditis, haemolytic anaemia, meningoencephalitis, transverse myelitis, Guillain–Barré syndrome.

Table 1

Causes of 'non-resolving pneumonia'

Unusual pathogens, e.g. *Chlamydia psittaci*, *C. burnetii*, *Mycobacterium tuberculosis*, Nocardia, *Actinomyces israelii*, fungi (Aspergillus, histoplasmosis, coccidioidomycosis, blastomycosis)

Pulmonary embolism

Malignancy: Bronchogenic carcinoma, bronchoalveolar cell carcinoma, lymphoma

Inflammatory: Vasculitis, Wegener's granulomatosis, sarcoidosis, systemic lupus erythematosus

Congestive heart failure

Drug toxicity

Diffuse alveolar haemorrhage

Bronchiolitis obliterans-organizing pneumonia

Eosinophilic pneumonia

Acute interstitial pneumonia

Pulmonary alveolar proteinosis

---

[1] May also be secondary to obstruction (e.g. malignancies), infarction or septic emboli (staphylococcal).

PROGNOSIS Most resolve with treatment (1–3 weeks). High mortality of severe pneumonia (community-acquired 5–10%; hospital-acquired 30%, 50% in those in ITU). Markers of severe pneumonia (CURB-65 score):

- **C**onfusion
- **U**rea > 7 mmol/L
- **R**espiratory rate ≥ 30/min
- **B**P: Systolic <90 mm Hg or diastolic ≤60 mm Hg
- Age ≥ **65** years

Other markers are hypoxia < 8 kPa, WCC < 4 or > 20 × 10^9/mm^3, age > 50 years.

Pneumothorax

DEFINITION   Air in the pleural space (the potential space between visceral and parietal pleura). Other variants depend on the substance in the pleural space (e.g. blood: haemothorax; lymph: chylothorax).

Tension pneumothorax: Emergency when a functional valve lets air enter the pleural space during inspiration, but not leave during expiration.

AETIOLOGY

Spontaneous: In individuals with previously normal lungs, typically tall thin males. Probably caused by rupture of a subpleural bleb.

Secondary: Pre-existing lung disease (COPD, asthma, TB, pneumonia, lung carcinoma, cystic fibrosis, diffuse lung disease).

Traumatic: Penetrating injury to chest, often iatrogenic causes, e.g. during subclavian or jugular venous cannulation, thoracocentesis, pleural or lung biopsy, or positive pressure-assisted ventilation.

Risk factors: Collagen disorders (e.g. Marfan's disease and Ehlers–Danlos syndrome).

EPIDEMIOLOGY   Annual incidence of spontaneous pneumothorax is 9 in 100 000. Mainly affects 20–40 year olds. Four times more common in males.

HISTORY   May be asymptomatic if pneumothorax is small.
Sudden onset breathlessness or chest pain, especially on inspiration.
Distress with rapid shallow breathing if tension pneumothorax.

EXAMINATION   Signs may be absent if small.
Signs of respiratory distress with reduced expansion, hyper-resonance to percussion, ↓ breath sounds.

Tension: Severe respiratory distress, tachycardia, hypotension, cyanosis, distended neck veins, tracheal deviation away from side of pneumothorax.

INVESTIGATIONS

CXR: A pneumothorax is seen as a dark area of film where lung markings do not extend to. Fluid level may be seen if there is blood present. In small pneumothoraces, expiratory films may make it more prominent.

ABG: May be necessary to determine if there is any hypoxaemia, particularly in secondary disease.

MANAGEMENT

Tension pneumothorax (emergency): Maximum O_2, insert large-bore needle into second intercostal space, midclavicular line, on side of pneumothorax to relieve pressure, insert chest drain soon after.

Small pneumothorax (<2 cm lung-pleural margin): If there is no underlying lung disease, pleural fluid or clinical compromise, reassure, analgesia if required and **moderate pneumothorax (>2 cm lung-pleural margin):**

- *Aspiration using large-bore cannula or catheter with three-way tap*: Inserted into the second intercostal space in the midclavicular line. Up to 2.5 L of air can be aspirated (stop if patient repeatedly coughs or resistance is felt). Follow-up CXR should be performed just after, 2 h and 2 weeks later. Advised to avoid diving.
- *Chest drain with water seal*: If aspiration fails or if there is fluid in the pleural cavity or after decompression of a tension pneumothorax. It is inserted into the fourth to sixth intercostal space in midaxillary line.

Recurrent pneumothoraces: Chemical pleurodesis (visceral and parietal pleura fusion with tetracycline or talc). Surgical pleurectomy.

Advice: Avoiding air travel until follow-up CXR confirms resolution of pneumothorax. Avoid diving unless bilateral surgical pleurectomy.

COMPLICATIONS   Recurrent pneumothoraces, bronchopleural fistula.

PROGNOSIS   After one spontaneous pneumothorax, at least 20% will have another, with the frequency increasing with repeated pneumothoraces.

Pulmonary embolism

DEFINITION Occlusion of pulmonary vessels, most commonly by a thrombus that has travelled to the vascular system from another site.

AETIOLOGY Thrombus (>95% originating from DVT of the lower limbs and rarely from right atrium in patients with AF). Other agents that can embolize to pulmonary vessels include amniotic fluid embolus, air embolus, fat emboli, tumour emboli and mycotic emboli from right-sided endocarditis. Groups at risk include surgical patients, immobility, obesity, OCP, heart failure, malignancy.

EPIDEMIOLOGY Relatively common, especially in hospitalized patients, they occur in 10–20% of those with a confirmed proximal DVT.

HISTORY Depends on the size and site of the pulmonary embolus:
Small: May be asymptomatic.
Moderate: Sudden onset dyspnoea, cough, haemoptysis and pleuritic chest pain.
Large (or proximal): All of the above plus severe central pleuritic chest pain, shock, collapse, acute right heart failure or sudden death.
Multiple small recurrent: Symptoms of pulmonary hypertension.

EXAMINATION
Clinical probability assessment: Various scales can predict probability to guide further investigation and management. Use local guidelines (Table 2).
Severity of pulmonary embolism (PE) can be assessed based on associated signs:
Small: Often no clinical signs. Earliest sign is tachycardia or tachypnoea.
Moderate: Tachypnoea, tachycardia, pleural rub, low saturation O_2 (despite oxygen supplementation).
Massive PE: Shock, cyanosis, signs of right heart strain (↑ JVP, left parasternal heave, accentuated S2 heart sound).
Multiple recurrent PE: Signs of pulmonary hypertension and right heart failure.

INVESTIGATIONS
Low probability: Use D-dimer blood test (cross-linked fibrin degradation products, highly sensitive but poor specificity).

Table 2

Well's Score (>4 high probability, ≤3 probability)		Revised Geneva Score (≥11 high probability, 4–10 intermediate probability, ≤3 low probability)	
Clinically suspected DVT	3.0	>65 years	1
PE is most likely diagnosis	3.0	Recent surgery or fracture (1 month)	2
Recent surgery (4 weeks)	1.5	Previous DVT/PE	3
Immobilization	1.5	Active malignancy	2
Tachycardia	1.5	Unilateral leg pain	3
History of DVT or PE	1.5	Haemoptysis	2
Haemoptysis	1.0	Heart rate > 75–94/min	3
Malignancy	1.0	Heart rate > 95/min	5
		Unilateral leg oedema and tenderness	4

DVT, deep vein thrombosis; PE, pulmonary embolism.

High probability: Requires imaging.
Additional initial investigations:
Bloods: ABG, consider thrombophilia screen.
ECG: May be normal or more commonly show a tachycardia, right axis deviation or RBBB. Classical SI, QIII, TIII pattern is relatively uncommon.
CXR: Often normal but to exclude other differential diagnoses.

Spiral CT pulmonary angiogram: First-line investigation of choice. Poor sensitivity for small emboli, but very sensitive for medium to large emboli.
Ventilation-perfusion (VQ) scan: Administration of IV 99mTc macro-aggregated albumin and inhalation of 81 krypton gas. This identifies any areas of ventilation and perfusion mismatch that would indicate infarcted lung. Not suitable if there is an abnormal CXR or coexisting lung disease due to difficulty in interpretation.
Pulmonary angiography: Gold standard, but invasive. Rarely necessary.
Doppler USS of the lower limb: To examine for venous thrombosis.
Echocardiogram: May show right heart strain.

MANAGEMENT
Primary prevention: Graduated pressure stockings (TEDs) and heparin prophylaxis in those at risk (e.g. undergoing surgery). Early mobilization and adequate hydration post-surgery.
If haemodynamically stable: O_2, anticoagulation with heparin or LMW heparin, changing to oral warfarin therapy (INR 2–3) for a minimum of 3 months. Analgesics for pain.
If haemodynamically unstable (massive PE): Resuscitate, give oxygen, IV fluid resuscitation, thrombolysis with tPA can be considered on clinical grounds alone if cardiac arrest is imminent (50 mg bolus of tPA).
Surgical or radiological: Embolectomy (when thrombolysis is contraindicated). IVC filters (Greenfield filter) may be inserted for recurrent pulmonary emboli despite adequate anticoagulation or when anticoagulation is contraindicated.

COMPLICATIONS   Death, pulmonary infarction, pulmonary hypertension, right heart failure.

PROGNOSIS   Thirty percent untreated mortality, 8% with treatment (due to recurrent emboli or underlying disease). Patients have ↑ risk of future thromboembolic disease.

Achalasia

DEFINITION   An oesophageal motility disorder, characterized by loss of peristalsis and failure of relaxation of the lower oesophageal sphincter (LOS).

AETIOLOGY   Degeneration of ganglion cells of the myenteric plexus in the oesophagus due to an unknown cause. Oesophageal infection with *Trypanosoma cruzi* seen in Central and South America produces a similar disorder (Chagas' disease).

EPIDEMIOLOGY   Annual incidence is about 1 in 100 000. Usual presentation age: 25–60 years.

HISTORY   Insidious onset and gradual progression of:
- intermittent dysphagia involving solids and liquids;
- difficulty belching;
- regurgitation (particularly at night);
- heartburn;
- chest pain (atypical/cramping, retrosternal);
- weight loss.

EXAMINATION   May reveal signs of complications (*see* the following text).

INVESTIGATIONS
CXR may show a widened mediastinum and double right heart border (dilated oesophagus), an air-fluid level in the upper chest and absence of the normal gastric air bubble.
Barium swallow: Dilated oesophagus which smoothly tapers down to the sphincter (beak-shaped).
Endoscopy: To exclude malignancy which can mimic achalasia.
Manometry:
- Elevated resting LOS pressure (>45 mmHg);
- incomplete LOS relaxation;
- absence of peristalsis in the distal (smooth muscle portion) of the oesophagus.

Serology for antibodies against *T. cruzi* if Chagas' disease is suggested by epidemiology and symptoms. Blood film might detect parasites.

MANAGEMENT
Pneumatic balloon dilation of the LOS: Up to 80% short-term success rate, 2–6% risk of oesophageal perforation.
Surgical myotomy via an abdominal or thoracic approach: The LOS is weakened by cutting its muscle fibres using a modified Heller approach. Surgery can be complicated by reflux oesophagitis and some surgeons combine it with a fundoplication procedure to prevent reflux. More recently, laparoscopic and thoracoscopic techniques have been used to perform the myotomy.
Botulinum toxin injected into the LOS inhibits acetylcholine release from the excitatory neurons that increase smooth muscle tone. The long-term safety and efficacy remain uncertain.
Medical treatment: Nitrates and calcium channel blockers (e.g. nifedipine) may be used to relax the smooth muscle of the LOS. Medical treatment is often ineffective, and may be associated with side effects (e.g. headache, hypotension) and tachyphylaxis.

COMPLICATIONS   If untreated, aspiration pneumonia, malnutrition and weight loss may result. Increased risk of oesophageal malignancy: 15 times that of the general population (on average 15 years after diagnosis).

PROGNOSIS   Good if treated. If untreated, oesophageal dilation may worsen causing pressure on mediastinal structures.

Coeliac disease

DEFINITION Inflammatory disease caused by intolerance to gluten, causing chronic intestinal malabsorption.

AETIOLOGY Sensitivity to the gliadin component of the cereal protein, gluten, triggers an immunological reaction in the small intestine leading to mucosal damage and loss of villi. Ten percent risk of first-degree relatives being affected and there is a clear genetic susceptibility associated with HLA-B8, DR3 and DQW2 haplotypes.

EPIDEMIOLOGY UK prevalence is 1 in 2000. One in 300 in the west of Ireland; rare in East Asia.

HISTORY
May be asymptomatic.
Abdominal discomfort, pain and distention.
Steatorrhoea (pale bulky stool, with offensive smell and difficult to flush away), diarrhoea.
Tiredness, malaise, weight loss (despite normal diet).
Failure to 'thrive' in children, amenorrhoea in young adults.

EXAMINATION
Signs of anaemia: Pallor.
Signs of malnutrition: Short stature, abdominal distension and wasted buttocks in children.
    Triceps skinfold thickness gives an indication of fat stores.
Signs of vitamin or mineral deficiencies (e.g. osteomalacia, easy bruising).
Intense, itchy blisters on elbows, knees or buttocks (dermatitis herpetiformis).

INVESTIGATIONS
Blood: FBC ($\downarrow$ Hb), iron and folate, U&E, albumin, Ca^{2+} and phosphate.
Serology: Testing for IgG anti-gliadin (AGA), IgA and IgG anti-endomysial transglutaminase antibodies can be diagnostic. As IgA deficiency is common (1 in 50 with coeliac disease), immunoglobulin levels should also be measured to avoid false negatives.
Stool: Culture to exclude infection, faecal fat tests for steatorrhoea.
D-xylose test: Reduced urinary excretion after an oral xylose load indicates small bowel malabsorption.
Endoscopy: Direct visualization shows villous atrophy in the small intestine (particularly the jejunum and ileum) giving the mucosa a flat smooth appearance. Biopsy shows villous atrophy with crypt hyperplasia of the duodenum. The epithelium adopts a cuboidal appearance, and there is an inflammatory infiltrate of lymphocytes and plasma cells in the lamina propria.

MANAGEMENT
Advice: Withdrawal of gluten from the diet, with avoidance of all wheat, rye and barley products. Education and expert dietary advice is essential. The Coeliac Society offers patient support and advice.
Medical: Vitamin and mineral supplements. Oral corticosteroids may be used if the disease does not subside with gluten withdrawal.

COMPLICATIONS Iron, folate and Vitamin B12 deficiency, osteomalacia, ulcerative jejunoileitis, gastrointestinal lymphoma (particularly T cell), bacterial overgrowth. Rarely, can cause cerebellar ataxia.

PROGNOSIS With strict adherence to gluten-free diet, most patients make a full recovery. Symptoms usually resolve within weeks. Histological changes may take longer to resolve. A gluten-free diet needs to be followed for life.

Colonic polyps

DEFINITION   A protuberance into the lumen from the normally flat colonic mucosa.

AETIOLOGY   Classified into neoplastic and non-neoplastic:
Neoplastic polyps include adenomas (~two-thirds of all colonic polyps) and adenocarcinomas.
Non-neoplastic polyps include hyperplastic polyps, inflammatory pseudopolyps (islands of residual intact colonic mucosa resulting from mucosal ulceration and regeneration that occurs in inflammatory bowel disease), and hamartomatous polyps, e.g. in Peutz-Jeghers syndrome (autosomal dominant disorder associated with mucocutaneous pigmentation of lips and gums) and Cronkhite-Canada syndrome (associated with alopecia, nail atrophy, cutaneous hyperpigmentation and watery diarrhoea).
Multiple colonic polyps occur in familial adenomatous polyposis (FAP) and its variants such as Turcot's syndrome (FAP associated with glioblastomas or medulloblastomas) and Gardner's syndrome (FAP associated with osteomas, soft-tissue tumours, sebaceous cysts). These are autosomal dominant diseases caused by mutations in the adenomatous polyposis coli (*APC*) gene.

EPIDEMIOLOGY   Common. Prevalence is >50% of those over 60 years old. FAP occurs in approximately 1/10 000 to 1/30 000 live births.

HISTORY   Usually asymptomatic.
May cause a change in bowel habit, tenesmus if in the rectum.
Mucoid diarrhoea.
PR bleeding (in case of polyp ulceration).
Symptoms of anaemia.

EXAMINATION   Usually no findings on examination.
May be palpable on PR examination if low in rectum.
Associated features of the syndromes mentioned above.

INVESTIGATIONS
Blood: FBC (look for microcytic anaemia).
Stool: Occult or frank blood in stool.
Endoscopy: Colonoscopy is the gold standard investigation. For multiple polyposis syndromes, an upper GI endoscopy is necessary to look for upper GI polyps. Polyps removed need to be histologically examined to determine their malignant potential.

MANAGEMENT   Colonoscopic polypectomy for small isolated polyps. Large polyps may have to be surgically resected. In multiple polyposis syndromes (particularly FAP), early colectomy is recommended to reduce risk of malignancy.
Follow-up: The timing of the next follow-up colonoscopy depends on the number, size and histology of polyps, family history, preferences of the patient and judgment of the physician. Guidelines suggest:
for 1–2 small (< 1 cm) tubular adenomas with low-grade dysplasia: 5 years;
for 3–10 adenomas, or any adenoma ≥1 cm, with villous features, or high-grade dysplasia: 3 years;
for >10 adenomas: < 3 years;
for a large (>2 cm) sessile polyp: 2–6 months to ensure complete removal.

Genetic screening of relatives may be necessary in multiple polyposis syndromes.

COMPLICATIONS   Malignant change, with highest risk in villous adenomas and multiple polyposis syndromes. Risk of bowel obstruction with very large polyps.

PROGNOSIS   Good if detected and treated before any malignant change.

Colorectal carcinoma

DEFINITION   Malignant adenocarcinoma of the large bowel.

AETIOLOGY   Environmental and genetic factors have been implicated. A sequence from epithelial dysplasia leading to adenoma and then carcinoma is thought to occur, involving accumulation of genetic changes in oncogenes (e.g. APC, K-ras) and tumour suppressor genes (e.g. p53, DCC). Sixty percent occur in the rectum and sigmoid colon; 15–20% in the ascending colon; and the remainder in the transverse and descending colon.
Some inherited conditions are associated with high rates of colorectal carcinoma[1].
Chronic bowel inflammation (e.g. inflammatory bowel disease) also increases the risk of colorectal carcinoma.

EPIDEMIOLOGY   Second most common cause of cancer death in the West. Twenty thousand deaths per year in the UK. Average age at diagnosis 60–65 years.

HISTORY   Symptoms will depend on the location of the tumour.
Left-sided colon and rectum: Change in bowel habit, rectal bleeding or blood/mucous mixed in with stools. Rectal masses may also present as tenesmus (sensation of incomplete emptying after defecation).
Right-sided colon: Later presentation, with symptoms of anaemia, weight loss and non-specific malaise or, more rarely, lower abdominal pain.
Up to 20% of tumours will present as an emergency with pain and distension caused by large bowel obstruction, haemorrhage or peritonitis as a result of perforation.

EXAMINATION   Anaemia may be only sign, particularly in right-sided lesions.
Abdominal mass, low-lying rectal tumours may be palpable on rectal examination.
Metastatic disease: Hepatomegaly, 'shifting dullness' of ascites.

INVESTIGATIONS
Blood: FBC (for anaemia), LFT, tumour markers (CEA to monitor treatment response or disease recurrence).
Stool: Occult or frank blood in stool (can be used as a screening test).
Endoscopy: Sigmoidoscopy, colonoscopy. Allows visualization and biopsy. Polypectomy can also be performed if isolated small carcinoma in situ.
Barium contrast studies: 'Apple core' stricture on barium enema.
Abdominal ultrasound scan for hepatic metastases.
Other staging investigations include CXR, CT or MRI, endorectal ultrasound.

MANAGEMENT
Surgery: Surgery is the only curative treatment. Operation depends on circumstances.
Caecum, ascending colon, proximal transverse colon: Right hemicolectomy.
Distal transverse colon, descending colon: Left hemicolectomy.
Sigmoid colon: Sigmoid colectomy.
High rectum: Anterior resection.
Low rectum: Abdo-perineal resection and end colostomy formation.
Emergency: Hartmann's procedure (proximal colostomy, resection of tumour and oversew of distal stump).
Survival in rectal tumours is improved if total mesorectal excision (removal of surrounding fascia). Isolated hepatic metastases may be successfully resected.
Radiotherapy: May be given in a neoadjuvent setting to downstage rectal tumours prior to resection or as adjuvant therapy to reduce risk of recurrence.
Chemotherapy: Used as adjuvant therapy in Dukes' C, or sometimes B. 5-Fluorouracil, oxaliplatin and irinotecan are common drugs in first-line chemotherapy protocols; newer agents like cetuximab (monoclonal against EGFR-receptor) and bevacizumab (monoclonal against VEGF) may be considered in metastatic disease or in the context of clinical trials.

COMPLICATIONS   Bowel obstruction or perforation, fistula formation. Recurrence. Metastatic disease.

PROGNOSIS   Prognosis varies depending on Dukes' staging (Table 3).

Table 3

Dukes' stage	Extent of spread	5-year survival (%)
A	Confined to bowel wall	80–90
B	Breached serosa, negative lymph nodes	60
C	Breached serosa, positive lymph nodes	30
D	Distant metastases	< 5

[1] Inherited (autosomal dominant) disorders: Hereditary non-polyposis colorectal cancer (HNPCC) caused by mutations in mismatch repair genes (1–5% of colorectal cancers), FAP caused by mutation in the APC gene.

Crohn's disease

DEFINITION   Chronic granulomatous inflammatory disease that can affect any part of the gastrointestinal tract. Grouped with ulcerative colitis and together they are known as inflammatory bowel disease.

AETIOLOGY   Cause has not yet been elucidated, but thought to involve an interplay between genetic and environmental factors.
Inflammation can occur anywhere along GI tract (40% involving the terminal ileum) and 'skip' lesions with inflamed segments of bowel interspersed with normal segments is not unusual.

EPIDEMIOLOGY   Annual UK incidence is 5–8 in 100 000. Prevalence is 50–80 in 100 000. Affects any age but peak incidence is in the teens or twenties.

HISTORY   Crampy abdominal pain (caused by inflammation, fibrosis or bowel obstruction). Diarrhoea (may be bloody or steatorrhoea).
Fever, malaise, weight loss.
Symptoms of complications.

EXAMINATION   Weight loss, clubbing, signs of anaemia.
Aphthous ulceration of the mouth.
Perianal skin tags, fistulae and abscesses.
Signs of complications (eye disease, joint disease, skin disease).

INVESTIGATIONS
Blood: FBC ($\downarrow$ Hb, $\uparrow$ platelets, $\uparrow$ WCC), U&E, LFTs ($\downarrow$ albumin), $\uparrow$ ESR, CRP ($\uparrow$ or may be normal), haematinics to look for deficiency states: ferritin, Vitamin B12 and red cell folate.
Stool microscopy and culture: To exclude infective colitis.
AXR: For evidence toxic megacolon.
Erect CXR: If risk of perforation.
Small bowel barium follow-through: May reveal fibrosis/strictures (string sign of Kantor), deep ulceration (rose thorn), cobblestone mucosa.
Endoscopy (OGD, colonoscopy) and biopsy: May help to differentiate between ulcerative colitis and Crohn's disease, useful monitoring for malignancy and disease progression. Mucosal oedema and ulceration with 'rose-thorn' fissures (cobblestone mucosa), fistulae, abscesses. Transmural chronic inflammation with infiltration of macrophages, lymphocytes and plasma cells. Granulomas with epithelioid giant cells may be seen in blood vessels or lymphatics.
Radionuclide-labelled neutrophil scan: Localization of inflammation (when other tests are contraindicated).

MANAGEMENT
Acute exacerbation: Fluid resuscitation, IV or oral corticosteroids, 5-ASA analogues (e.g. mesalazine, sulfasalazine) may induce a remission in colonic Crohn's disease. Analgesia. Elemental diet may induce remission (more often used in children). Parenteral nutrition may be necessary. Monitor markers of activity (fluid balance, ESR, CRP, platelets, stool frequency, Hb and albumin). Assess for complications.
Long term:
- Steroids: For treating acute exacerbations.
- 5-ASA analogues (e.g. sulfasalazine, mesalazine): $\downarrow$ relapses. Useful for mild-to-moderate disease.
- Immunosuppression: Using steroid-sparing agents (e.g. azathioprine, 6-mercaptopurine, methotrexate) to $\downarrow$ relapses.
- Anti-TNF agents (e.g. infliximab, adalimumab): Very effective agents in achieving and maintaining remission. Usually reserved for refractory cases.

Advice: Stop smoking, dietician referral. Education and advice (e.g. from inflammatory bowel disease nurse specialists).

Surgery: Indicated for failure of medical treatment, failure to thrive in children or the presence of complications. This involves resection of affected bowel and stoma formation, although there is a risk of disease recurrence.

COMPLICATIONS

GI: Haemorrhage, bowel strictures, perforation, fistulae (between bowel, bladder, vagina), perianal fistulae and abscess, GI carcinoma (5% risk in 10 years), malabsorption.

Extraintestinal features: Uveitis, episcleritis, gallstones, kidney stones, arthropathy, sacroiliitis, ankylosing spondylitis, erythema nodosum and pyoderma gangrenosum, amyloidosis.

PROGNOSIS   Chronic relapsing condition. Two-thirds will require surgery at some stage and two-thirds of these >1 surgical procedure.

Diverticular disease

DEFINITION

Diverticulosis: The presence of diverticulae outpouchings of the colonic mucosa and submucosa through the muscular wall of the large bowel.

Diverticular disease: Diverticulosis associated with complications, e.g. haemorrhage, infection, fistulae.

Diverticulitis: Acute inflammation and infection of colonic diverticulae.

Hinchey classification of acute diverticulitis: Ia: phlegmon, Ib and II: localized abscesses, III: perforation with purulent peritonitis or IV: faecal peritonitis.

AETIOLOGY A low-fibre diet leads to loss of stool bulk. Consequently, high colonic intraluminal pressures must be generated to propel the stool, leading to herniation of the mucosa and submucosa through the muscularis.

Pathogenesis: Diverticulae are most common in the sigmoid and descending colon but can be right sided. Absent from the rectum. Diverticulae consist of herniated mucosa and submucosa through the muscularis, particularly at sites of nutrient artery penetration. Proposed diverticular obstruction by inspissated faeces can lead to bacterial overgrowth, toxin production and mucosal injury and diverticulitis, perforation, pericolic phlegmon, abscess, ulceration and fistulation or stricture formation.

EPIDEMIOLOGY Common, 60% of people living in industrialized countries will develop colonic diverticula, rare < 40years. Right-sided diverticula are more common in Asia.

HISTORY Often asymptomatic (80–90%). Complications include: pr bleeding, diverticulitis: typically, left iliac fossa or lower abdominal pain, fever. Diverticular fistulation into bladder: pneumaturia, faecaluria and recurrent UTI.

EXAMINATION Diverticulitis: Tender abdomen; signs of local or generalized peritonitis if perforation has occurred.

INVESTIGATIONS

Bloods: FBC, ↑ WCC and ↑ CRP in diverticulitis, check clotting and cross-match if bleeding.

Barium enema (+ / − air contrast): Demonstrates the presence of diverticulae with a sawtooth appearance of lumen, reflecting pseudohypertrophy of circular muscle (should not be performed in acute setting as there is a danger of perforation).

Flexible sigmoidoscopy and colonoscopy: Diverticulae can be seen and other pathology (e.g. polyps or tumour) can be excluded.

In an acute setting: CT scan for evidence of diverticular disease and complications.

MANAGEMENT

Asymptomatic: Soluble high-fibre diet (20–30 g/day). Probiotics and anti-inflammatories (mesalazine) are under investigation for preventing recurrent flares of diverticulitis.

GI bleed: PR bleeding is often managed conservatively with IV rehydration, antibiotics, blood transfusion if necessary. Angiography and embolization or surgery if severe.

Diverticulitis: Treated by IV antibiotics and IV fluid rehydration and bowel rest. Localized collections or abscesses may be treated by radiologically sited drains.

Surgery: May be necessary with recurrent attacks or when complications develop, e.g. perforation and peritonitis. Surgical treatment can be by open or laparoscopic approaches. Open: Hartmann's procedure (resection and stoma) or one-stage resection and anastomosis (risk of leak) ± defunctioning stoma. More recently, laparoscopic drainage, peritoneal lavage and drain placement can be effective.

COMPLICATIONS Diverticulitis, pericolic abscess, perforation, faecal peritonitis, colonic obstruction, fistula formation (bladder, small intestine, vagina), haemorrhage.

PROGNOSIS Ten to 25% of patients will have one or more episodes of diverticulitis. Of these, 30% will have a second episode.

Gallstones

DEFINITION   Stone formation in the gallbladder.

AETIOLOGY
Mixed stones: Contain cholesterol, calcium bilirubinate, phosphate and protein (80%). Associated with older age, female, obesity, parenteral nutrition, drugs (OCP, octreotide), family history, ethnicity (e.g. Pima Indians), interruption of the enterohepatic recirculation of bile salts (e.g. Crohn's disease), terminal ileal resection.
Pure cholesterol stones (10%): Similar associations as mixed stones.
Pigment stones (10%): Black stones made of calcium bilirubinate (↑ bilirubin secondary to haemolytic disorders, cirrhosis), brown stones due to bile duct infestation by liver fluke *Clonorchis sinensis*. Associated with haemolytic disorders (e.g. sickle cell, thalassemia, hereditary spherocytosis).

EPIDEMIOLOGY   Very common (UK prevalence ∼ 10%), more common with age, 3× more females in younger population but equal sex ratio after 65 years.

HISTORY   Asymptomatic (90%): Found incidentally.
Biliary colic: Sudden onset, severe right upper quadrant or epigastric pain, constant in nature. May radiate to right scapula, often precipitated by a fatty meal. Can last hours, may be associated nausea and vomiting.
Acute cholecystitis: Patient systemically unwell, fever, prolonged upper abdominal pain that may be referred to the right shoulder (due to diaphragmatic irritation).
Ascending cholangitis: Classical association between right upper quadrant pain, jaundice and rigors (Charcot's triad). If combined with hypotension and confusion, it is known as Reynold's pentad.

EXAMINATION
Biliary colic: Right upper quadrant or epigastric tenderness.
Acute cholecystitis: Tachycardia, pyrexia, right upper quadrant or epigastric tenderness. There may be guarding +/− rebound. Murphy's sign is elicited by placing a hand at the costal margin in the RUQ and asking the patient to breathe deeply. Patient stops breathing as the inflamed gallbladder descends and contacts the palpating fingers.
Ascending cholangitis: Pyrexia, right upper quadrant pain, jaundice.

INVESTIGATIONS
Bloods: FBC (↑ WBC in cholecystitis or cholangitis), LFT (↑ AlkPhos, ↑ bilirubin in ascending cholangitis; there may be ↑ transaminases), blood cultures, amylase (risk of pancreatitis).
USS: Demonstrates gallstones (acoustic shadow within the gallbladder), ↑ thickness of gallbladder wall and can examine for presence of dilatation of biliary tree indicative of obstruction.
AXR: Gallstones are infrequently radio-opaque (10%).
Other imaging: Erect CXR (to exclude perforation as a differential diagnosis), CT scanning, magnetic resonance cholangiopancreatography (MRCP) or endoscopic retrograde cholangiopancreatography (ERCP).

MANAGEMENT
Mild symptoms: Conservative, avoidance of fat in diet.
Sever biliary colic: Admission, IV fluids, analgesia, antiemetics and antibiotics if there are signs of infection (cholecystitis or cholangitis).
If symptoms fail to improve or worsen, a localized abscess or empyema should be suspected. This can be drained percutaneously by cholecystostomy and pigtail catheter.
If there is evidence of obstruction, urgent biliary drainage by ERCP or percutaneous transhepatic cholangiogram.
Surgical: Laparoscopic cholecystectomy ± on table cholangiogram. In acute setting, performed within 72 h of symptom onset, or after several weeks for inflammation to settle.

Gallstones (continued)

COMPLICATIONS

Stones within gallbladder: Biliary colic, cholecystitis, mucocoele or gallbladder empyema, porcelain gallbladder, predisposition to gallbladder cancer (rare).

Stones outside gallbladder: Obstructive jaundice, pancreatitis, ascending cholangitis, perforation and pericholecystic abscess or bile peritonitis, cholecystenteric fistula, gallstone ileus, Mirizzi syndrome (common hepatic duct obstruction by an extrinsic compression from an impacted stone in the cystic duct), Bouveret's syndrome (gallstones causing gastric outlet obstruction).

Of cholecystectomy: Bleeding, infection, bile leak, bile duct injury (0.3% laparoscopic, 0.2% open), post-cholecystectomy syndrome (persistant dyspeptic symptoms), port-site hernias.

PROGNOSIS   In most cases gallstones are benign and do not cause significant problems (2% with gallstones develop symptoms annually). If they become symptomatic, surgery is an effective treatment.

Gastric carcinoma

DEFINITION   Gastric malignancy, most commonly adenocarcinoma, more rarely lymphoma, leiomyosarcoma.

AETIOLOGY   Most cases are probably caused by environmental insults in genetically predisposed individuals that lead to mutation and subsequent unregulated cell growth. Risk factors include:
- *Helicobacter pylori* infection;
- atrophic gastritis;
- diet high in smoked, processed foods and nitrosamines;
- smoking;
- alcohol.

EPIDEMIOLOGY   Common cause of cancer death worldwide, with highest incidence in Asia, especially Japan. Sixth most common cancer in UK (annual incidence is 15 in 100 000). ♂ : ♀ ~ 2 : 1. Age > 50 years.
Cancer of the antrum/body is becoming less common, while that of the cardia and gastro-oesophageal junction is increasing.

HISTORY   In the early phases, it is often asymptomatic.
Early satiety or epigastric discomfort.
Weight loss, anorexia, nausea and vomiting.
Haematemesis, melaena, symptoms of anaemia.
Dysphagia (tumours of the cardia).
Symptoms of metastases, particularly abdominal swelling (ascites) or jaundice (liver involvement).

EXAMINATION   Physical examination may be normal.
Epigastric mass. Abdominal tenderness. Ascites.
Signs of anaemia.
Many eponymous signs:
Virchow's node/Troisier's sign: Lymphadenopathy in left supraclavicular fossa.
Sister Mary Joseph node: Metastatic nodule on umbilicus.
Krukenberg's tumour: Ovarian metastases.

INVESTIGATIONS
Upper GI endoscopy: With multiquadrant biopsy of all gastric ulcers.
Blood: FBC (for anaemia), LFT.
CT/MRI: Staging of tumour and planning of surgery.
Ultrasound of liver: Staging of tumour.
Bone scan: Staging of tumour.
Endoscopic ultrasound: Assesses depth of invasion and lymph node spread.
Laparoscopy: May be needed to determine if tumour is resectable.

MANAGEMENT
Surgery: Various surgical techniques, depending on size and tumour site.
Bilroth I partial gastrectomy: Excision of tumour and distal stomach. Duodenal stump is anastomosed with remainder of stomach.
Bilroth II partial gastrectomy: Excision of tumour and distal stomach. Duodenal stump is oversewn and remainder of the stomach is anastomosed to jejunum (gastrojejunostomy). Suitable for antral tumours.
Total gastrectomy: Removal of stomach and spleen. Oesophagojejunostomy. Suitable for large tumours.
Ivor–Lewis gastrectomy: Proximal gastrectomy and distal oesophagectomy, with oesophagoantrostomy and pyloroplasty. Suitable for cardial or fundal tumours.

Gastric carcinoma (continued)

Roux-en-Y reconstruction: Duodenal stump oversewn. Distal duodenum anastomosed to jejunum.

Medical: Adjunctive combined chemoradiotherapy reduces relapse and improves survival. Commonly used agents include 5-fluorouracil, epirubicin, platinum agents and capecitabine.

Palliative: Debulking surgery. Gastrojejunostomy and stenting to bypass obstruction and maintain enteral nutrition. Coeliac plexus nerve block to reduce pain.

COMPLICATIONS Dysphagia, gastric outlet obstruction, upper GI haemorrhage, iron-deficiency anaemia. Early and late complications of gastrectomy (e.g. dumping syndrome, diarrhoea, deficiencies of vitamin B12).

PROGNOSIS Generally poor with < 10% overall 5-year survival. About 50% in those with early disease undergoing resection.

Gastroenteritis

DEFINITION   Acute inflammation of the lining of the GI tract, manifested by nausea, vomiting, diarrhoea and abdominal discomfort.

AETIOLOGY   Can be caused by viruses, bacteria, protozoa or toxins contained in contaminated food or water.

Viral: Rotavirus, adenovirus, astrovirus, calcivirus, Norwalk virus, small round structured viruses.

Bacterial: *Campylobacter jejuni*, *Escherichia coli* (particularly 0157), *Salmonella*, *Shigella*, *Vibrio cholerae*, *Listeria*, *Yersinia enterocolitica*.

Protozoal: *Entamoeba histolytica*, *Cryptosporidium parvum*, *Giardia lamblia*.

Toxins: From *Staphylococcus aureus*, *Clostridium botulinum*, *Clostridium perfringens*, *Bacillus cereus*, mushrooms, heavy metals, seafood.

Commonly contaminated foods: Improperly cooked meat (*S. aureus*, *C. perfringens*), old rice (*B. cereus*, *S. aureus*), eggs and poultry (*Salmonella*), milk and cheeses (*Listeria*, *Campylobacter*), canned food (botulism).

Depending on the organism or toxin, there are different pathogenic mechanisms.

Non-inflammatory mechanisms: e.g. *V. cholerae*, enterotoxigenic *E. coli* produce enterotoxins that cause enterocytes to secrete water and electrolytes.

Inflammatory mechanisms: e.g. *Shigella*, enteroinvasive *E. coli* release cytotoxins and invade and damage the epithelium, with greater invasion and bacteraemia in the case of *Salmonella typhi*.

EPIDEMIOLOGY   Common, and often under-reported, a serious cause of morbidity and mortality in the developing world.

HISTORY   Sudden onset nausea, vomiting, anorexia.

Diarrhoea (bloody or watery), abdominal pain or discomfort, fever and malaise.

Enquire about recent travel, antibiotic use and recent food intake (how cooked, source and whether anyone else ill).

Time of onset: Toxins (early; 1–24 h), bacterial/viral/protozoal (12 h or later).

Effect of toxin: Botulinum causes paralysis; mushrooms can cause fits, renal or liver failure.

EXAMINATION   Diffuse abdominal tenderness, abdominal distension and bowel sounds are often increased.

If severe, pyrexia, dehydration, hypotension, peripheral shutdown.

INVESTIGATIONS

Blood: FBC, blood culture (helps identification if bacteraemia present), U&Es (dehydration).

Stool: Faecal microscopy for polymorphs, parasites, oocysts, culture, electron microscopy (used to diagnose viral infections). Analysis for toxins, particularly for pseudomembranous colitis (*Clostridium difficile* toxin).

AXR or ultrasound: To exclude other causes of abdominal pain.

Sigmoidoscopy: Often unnecessary unless inflammatory bowel disease needs to be excluded.

MANAGEMENT   Bed rest, fluid and electrolyte replacement with oral rehydration solution (containing glucose and salt). IV rehydration may be necessary in those with severe vomiting. Most infections are self-limiting. Antibiotic treatment is only warranted if severe or the infective agent has been identified (e.g. ciprofloxacin against *Salmonella*, *Shigella*, *Campylobacter*).

Typhoid fever: *See* 'Shorter topics'.

Botulism: Botulinum antitoxin IM and manage in ITU.

Public health: Often a notifiable disease. Educate on basic hygiene and cooking.

Gastroenteritis (continued)

COMPLICATIONS   Dehydration, electrolyte imbalance, prerenal failure. Secondary lactose intolerance (particularly in infants). Sepsis and shock (particularly *Salmonella* and *Shigella*). Haemolytic uraemic syndrome is associated with toxins from *E. coli* 0157. Guillian–Barré syndrome may occur weeks after recovery from *Campylobacter* gastroenteritis.

Botulism: Respiratory muscle weakness or paralysis.

PROGNOSIS   Generally good, as the majority of cases are self-limiting.

Gastro-oesophageal reflux disease (GORD)

DEFINITION   Inflammation of the oesophagus caused by reflux of gastric acid and/or bile.

AETIOLOGY   Disruption of mechanisms that prevent reflux (physiological LOS, mucosal rosette, acute angle of junction, intra-abdominal portion of oesophagus). Prolonged oesophageal clearance contributes to 50% of cases.

EPIDEMIOLOGY   Common, prevalence 5–10% adults.

HISTORY   Substernal burning discomfort or 'heartburn' aggravated by lying supine, bending or large meals and drinking alcohol. Pain relieved by antacids.
Waterbrash. Regurgitation of gastric contents.
Aspiration may result in voice hoarseness, laryngitis, nocturnal cough and wheeze ± pneumonia (rare).
Dysphagia (caused by formation of peptic stricture after long-standing reflux).

EXAMINATION   Usually normal. Occasionally, epigastric tenderness, wheeze on chest auscultation, dysphonia.

INVESTIGATIONS
Upper GI endoscopy, biopsy and cytological brushings: To confirm the presence of oesophagitis, exclude the possibility of malignancy (all patients >45 years).
Barium swallow: To detect hiatus hernia, peptic stricture, extrinsic compression of the oesophagus can be visualized.
CXR: Not specifically for GORD. Incidental finding of hiatus hernia (gastric bubble behind cardiac shadow).
Twenty-four hour oesophageal pH monitoring: pH probe placed in lower oesophagus determines the temporal relationship between symptoms and oesophageal pH.

MANAGEMENT
Advice: Lifestyle changes, weight loss, elevating head of bed, avoid provoking factors, stopping smoking, lower fat meals, avoiding large meals late in the evening.
Medical: Antacids and alginates, H2 antagonists (e.g. ranitidine) or proton pump inhibitors (e.g. lansoprazole) are sufficient for most patients.
Endoscopy: Annual endoscopic surveillance for Barrett's oesophagus; may be necessary for stricture dilation or stenting.
Surgery: Antireflux surgery for those with symptoms despite optimal medical management or in those intolerant of medication.
Nissen fundoplication (fundus of the stomach is wrapped around the lower oesophagus and held with seromuscular sutures) helps reduce any hiatus hernia and reduce reflux.

COMPLICATIONS   Oesophageal ulceration, peptic stricture, anaemia, Barrett's oesophagus[1] and oesophageal adenocarcinoma. Associated with asthma and chronic laryngitis.

PROGNOSIS   Fifty percent respond to lifestyle measures alone. In patients who require drug therapy withdrawal is often associated with relapse. Twenty percent of patients undergoing endoscopy for GORD have Barrett's oesophagus.

---

[1] Barrett's oesophagus is characterized by metaplasia of oesophageal squamous epithelium and replacement with columnar epithelium. This is a premalignant condition with an increased risk of dysplasia and adenocarcinoma.

Irritable bowel syndrome (IBS)

DEFINITION   A functional bowel disorder defined as recurrent episodes (in the absence of detectable organic pathology) of abdominal pain/discomfort for ≥6 months of the previous year, associated with two of the following:[1]
- altered stool passage;
- abdominal bloating;
- symptoms made worse by eating;
- passage of mucous.

AETIOLOGY   Unknown. Visceral sensory abnormalities, gut motility abnormalities, psychosocial factors (particularly stress), food intolerance (e.g. lactose) are all implicated.

EPIDEMIOLOGY   Common, prevalence 10–20% of adults. More common in ♀ (2 : 1 ratio to ♂).

HISTORY   ≥6 month history abdominal pain (often colicky, in the lower abdomen and relieved by defecation or flatus).
Altered bowel frequency with ≥3 bowel motions daily or ≤3 motions weekly.
Abdominal bloating.
Change in stool consistency.
Passage with urgency or straining. Tenesmus.
Screen for 'red flag' alarm symptoms:
- weight loss;
- anaemia;
- PR bleeding;
- late onset (≥60 years).

Presence of any of the above requires referral to exclude colonic malignancy.

EXAMINATION   Normally nothing on examination. In some cases the abdomen may appear distended and be mildly tender to palpation in one or both iliac fossa.

INVESTIGATIONS   Diagnosis mainly from history but it may be vital to exclude organic pathology.
Blood: FBC (for anaemia), LFT, ESR, CRP, TFT. Anti-endomysial or anti-transglutaminase antibodies (to exclude coeliac disease).
Stool examination: Microscopy and culture for parasites, cysts and infection.
Ultrasound: To exclude gallstone disease.
Hydrogen breath test: To exclude dyspepsia associated with *Helicobacter pylori*.
Endoscopy: Upper GI endoscopy, sigmoidoscopy or colonoscopy if other pathologies suspected.

MANAGEMENT
Advice: Explanation and support with establishment of a positive doctor–patient relationship. Dietary modification (e.g. reducing dietary insoluble fibre) may help with constipation, other approaches include exclusion diets and use of probiotics.
Medical: According to the predominant symptoms:
- antispasmodics (e.g. mebeverin, buscopan);
- prokinetic agents (e.g. domperidone, metoclopramide);
- antidiarrhoeals (e.g. loperamide);
- laxatives (e.g. lactulose);
- low-dose tricyclic antidepressants (may ↓ visceral awareness).

Psychological therapies: Often beneficial (e.g. cognitive–behavioural therapy, relaxation and psychotherapy).

---

[1] For guidelines on diagnosis and management, *see* NICE 2008 guidelines on www.nice.org.uk.

COMPLICATIONS Physical and psychological morbidity. ↑ Incidence of colonic diverticulosis.

PROGNOSIS A chronic relapsing and remitting course, often exacerbated by psychosocial stresses.

Ischaemic colitis

DEFINITION   Inflammation of the colon caused by decreased colonic blood supply.

AETIOLOGY   Occlusion of large vessels by thrombosis/embolism (↑ risk with atherosclerosis, AF). Iatrogenic ligation (particularly in abdominal aortic aneurysm surgery). Hypovolaemia. In younger patients may be caused by small vessel vasculitis, vasospasm (e.g. cocaine) or hypercoagulable states.
No specific cause may be identified.
Ischaemia leads to mucosal inflammation, oedema, necrosis and ulceration. The splenic flexure, the watershed between superior and inferior mesenteric artery territories, is the most common area affected.

EPIDEMIOLOGY   Most commonly in the elderly (60–80 years) with equal gender distribution.

HISTORY   Symptoms may be acute or chronic in onset.
Crampy abdominal pain, may be post-prandial ('gut claudication') giving 'food fear'. Fever, nausea, bloody diarrhoea.

EXAMINATION   There may be a paucity of signs.
Abdominal distension and tenderness, local peritonism (worse on left).
Fever and tachycardia, depending on severity of insult.
Proctoscopy typically shows normal rectal mucosa with blood from a higher source.

INVESTIGATIONS
Blood: FBC (↑ WCC), ↑ CRP, U&Es, LFTs, ↑ LDH, ↑ CK, ↑ lactate, ABG (metabolic acidosis), clotting screen. Evaluation for hypercoagulability in younger patients and those with recurrent colonic ischemia.
Stool: Cultures for *Salmonella*, *Shigella*, *Campylobacter*, *Yersinia*, *E. coli* O157:H7, assay *Clostridium difficile* toxins (to exclude infective colitis).
AXR: Large bowel wall thickening or diffuse dilation, air in bowel wall, thumbprinting (submucosal oedema).
CXR (erect): Air under diaphragm in cases of perforation.
CT: Thickening of colonic wall, irregular lumen, intramural air, portal or mesenteric venous air, occlusion in larger blood vessels.
Colonoscopy: Usually without bowel preparation (to avoid reducing blood flow due to dehydration). May show: pale mucosa, petechial bleeding, bluish haemorrhagic nodules, cyanotic mucosa, mucosal friability and haemorrhagic ulcerations. Segmental distribution, abrupt transition between injured and non-injured mucosa and rectal sparing, favour ischemia rather than inflammatory bowel disease.
Angiography: May be normal or show attenuated flow or site of occlusion.

MANAGEMENT
Conservative management: IV fluids, nil orally, broad-spectrum antibiotics that cover enteric bacteria (e.g. cephalosporin and metronidazole). Specific treatment of the cause of the vascular insufficiency. Nasogastric tube if an ileus is present. Cardiac function and oxygenation should be optimized.
Surgical: Colonic resection may be required in cases of gangrenous or perforated bowel.
Long term: Follow-up colonoscopy is used to assess recovery or stricture formation.

COMPLICATIONS   Acute ischaemia can lead to gangrene (15%), perforation, sepsis and, occasionally, toxic megacolon or pyocolon. Segmental ulcerating colitis, stricture formation with intestinal obstruction.

PROGNOSIS   Outcome depends on severity, extent and timing of ischaemic insult and comorbidities. The majority of cases settle with conservative measures.

Oesophageal carcinoma

DEFINITION   Malignant tumour arising in the oesophageal mucosa. Two major histological types: squamous cell carcinoma and adenocarcinoma.

AETIOLOGY

Squamous: Alcohol, tobacco, certain nutritional deficiencies (vitamins, trace elements), HPV infection, achalasia, Paterson–Kelly (Plummer–Vinson) syndrome, tylosis (Howel–Evans syndrome), scleroderma, coeliac disease, lye stricture, history of previous thoracic radiotherapy or upper aerodigestive squamous cancer, dietary nitrosamines.

Adenocarcinoma: GORD, Barrett's oesophagus (intestinal metaplasia of the distal oesophageal mucosa with ~0.5–0.7% incidence of adenocarcinoma per year).

Pathology: Squamous cell carcinomas are more common in the mid-upper oesophagus. Adenocarcinoma usually develops in the lower oesophagus or, increasingly, the gastro-oesophageal junction. Barretts intestinal metaplasia can progress to low-grade dysplasia, high-grade dysplasia and invasive carcinoma. Spread is typically initially direct (oesophagus has no serosa) and longitudinal via an extensive network of submucosal lymphatics to tracheobronchial, mediastinal, coeliac, gastric or cervical nodes. Rare oesophageal tumours include lymphoma, melanoma and leiomyosarcoma.

EPIDEMIOLOGY   Eighth most common malignancy (UK 7000–8000 per year). 3–4 : 1 male : female. Worldwide squamous carcinoma is more common (95%), with considerable geographical variation (high incidence in northern China, Iran, southern Russia). Adenocarcinoma is more common in westernized countries (65% cases in the UK) and increasing by 5–10% per year. Peak incidence 60–70 years.

HISTORY   Early: symptomatic/symptoms of reflux. Later: dysphagia, initially worse for solids, regurgitation, cough or choking after food, pain (odynophagia), weight loss, fatigue, voice hoarseness (may indicate recurrent laryngeal nerve palsy).

EXAMINATION   No physical signs may be evident, signs of weight loss. With metastatic disease there may be supraclavicular lymphadenopathy, hepatomegaly. Respiratory signs may be due to aspiration or direct tracheobronchial involvement.

INVESTIGATIONS

Endoscopy: Tumour location and biopsy. Early high-grade dysplasia and cancer detection is improved by endoscopic techniques such as narrow band imaging or magnification, staging.

Imaging: Barium swallow, CT (chest, abdomen, pelvis), PET can detect previously occult distant metastases.

Other: Bronchoscopy (if risk of trancheobronchial invasion), bone scan is symptoms of bony involvement. Laparoscopy and peritoneal washings, thoracoscopy. Careful cardiac and respiratory assessment if surgery planned.

MANAGEMENT

Best managed at specialist centres with multidisciplinary expertise. For early (mucosal) localized disease endoscopic therapies are increasing, e.g. endoscopic mucosal resection, endoscopic submucosal dissection. Surgical: only ~30% are suitable for surgical resection. Neoadjuvant chemoradiotherapy (e.g. cisplatin, 5-fluorouracil) can be beneficial in downstaging tumours prior to surgery.

Surgery: Operative approach depends on tumour location and extent of proposed lymphadenectomy. Minimally invasive approaches are increasingly used, i.e. laparoscopic and thorascopic dissection.

Radiotherapy/chemotherapy: Squamous cell carcinomas are more radiosensitive than adenocarcinomas. Radical radio or chemoradiotherapy can be performed in localized disease in patients are unfit for surgery. Neoadjuvent and adjuvant chemotherapy using a cisplatin-based regimen is used where tolerated.

Oesophageal carcinoma (continued)

Palliation: Is tailored to individual patient's tumour and symptoms. Luminal recannulization can be achieved by expandable stents or laser ablation or photodynamic therapy techniques. Radiotherapy and/or chemotherapy is associated with variable response rates, e.g. epirubicin, cisplatin and 5-fluorouracil.

COMPLICATIONS

Of tumour: Malnutrition, aspiration pneumonia, haematemesis, oesophageobronchial fistula, of metastatic disease: ascites, pleural effusions.

Of oesophagectomy: Mortality $< 5\%$ in specialized centres, morbidity up to 40%: pulmonary complications are the most common, e.g. atelectasis, pneumonia, serious complications include anastomotic leakage (5–15%) or conduit failure, others: chylothorax, recurrent laryngeal nerve damage.

PROGNOSIS Depends on stage, overall 5-year survival is 20–25%, for advanced disease 5-year survival $< 5\%$.

Pancreatic cancer

DEFINITION   Malignancy arising from the exocrine or endocrine tissues of the pancreas.

AETIOLOGY   Unknown cause. Five to 10% have a familial component, hereditary syndromes include BRCA2 mutation, familial atypical multiple mole melanoma (CDKN2A), Peutz-Jeghers (STK11/LKB1), hereditary pancreatitis (PRSS1), MEN, HNPCC, FAP, Gardner, von Hippel–Lindau syndromes. Precursor lesions include pancreatic intraductal neoplasia, intraductal pancreatic mucinous neoplasm and mucinous cystic neoplasm.

EPIDEMIOLOGY   Increasing in incidence (8–12/100 000), worldwide eighth cause of cancer deaths. 2× more males, peak age 60–80 years.

HISTORY   Clinical diagnosis of pancreatic cancer is often difficult as the initial symptoms are often quite non-specific. These include anorexia, malaise, weight loss, nausea. Later, jaundice, epigastric pain.

EXAMINATION   Signs of weight loss, epigastric tenderness or mass.
Jaundice and a palpable gallbladder (Courvoisier's law).[1]
In patients with metastatic spread, there may be hepatomegaly.
Trousseau's sign is an associated superficial thrombophlebitis.

PATHOLOGY/PATHOGENESIS   Seventy-five percent occur within the head or neck of the pancreas (where it can present as a periampullary tumour), 15–20% occur in the body and 5–10% occur in the tail. Spread is local and to the liver. Eighty percent are adenocarcinomas, other types include adenosquamous, mucinous cystadenocarcinomas. Endocrine tumours include insulinomas, glucagonomas and gastrinomas.

INVESTIGATIONS
Bloods: Tumour markers CA19-9 and CEA can be elevated (former more specific, but neither are diagnostic). If causing obstructive jaundice, ↑ bilirubin, ↑ ALP, clotting may be deranged.
Imaging: Ultrasound, endoscopic ultrasound and FNA, CT, MRI, PET and laparoscopy are all useful in staging the disease. ERCP may allow biopsy/bile cytology ± stenting.
Other: Staging laparoscopy or intraoperative ultrasound.

MANAGEMENT
Medical: Most patients with disease who are not amenable to curative resection undergo palliative management. This may involve chemotherapy, e.g. gemcitabine, cisplatin or the epidermal growth factor receptor antagonist, erlotinib. Pain relief by medical analgesia, radiotherapy or coeliac plexus block. For obstructive jaundice, endoscopic stent insertion or a surgical choledochojejunostomy. For duodenal obstruction, endoscopic stenting or a gastrojejunostomy.
Surgery: Less than 20% of patients are suitable, tumours on the body and tail are often unresectable at presentation.
Pancreaticoduodenectomy (Whipple's procedure): For tumours of the head (no vascular involvement or metastases). Involves en bloc resection of the pancreatic head, 1st–3rd parts of the duodenum; the distal antrum; and the distal common bile duct. The GI tract is reconstructed with a gastrojejunostomy. The common bile duct and residual pancreas are anastomosed into a segment of small bowel.
Pylorus-preserving pancreaticoduodenectomy: Sparing the pylorus allows for more physiological emptying of the stomach.

COMPLICATIONS   Unresectable disease, pain, obstructive jaundice, pruritus, cholangitis, diabetes, splenic vein thrombosis, malignant ascites.

---

[1] *Courvoisier's law*: Palpable gallbladder with painless jaundice is unlikely to be caused by gallstones.

Pancreatic cancer (continued)

From surgery: Anastomotic leaks, bleeding, collections, pancreatic fistulas, brittle diabetes.

PROGNOSIS   Fewer than 5% of all patients are alive at 5 years. The median survival of all patients after initial diagnosis is 4–6 months. In patients able to undergo a successful curative resection the median survival ranges from 12 to 19 months, and the 5-year survival rate is 15–20%. Patients with periampullary and endocrine tumours have a better prognosis.

Pancreatitis, acute

DEFINITION   An acute inflammatory process of the pancreas with variable involvement of other regional tissues or remote organ systems.
Mild: Associated with minimal organ dysfunction and uneventful recovery.
Severe: Associated with organ failure and/or local complications such as necrosis, abscess or pseudocyst (1992 Atlanta classification).

AETIOLOGY   Insult results in activation of pancreatic proenzymes within the duct/acini resulting in tissue damage and inflammation.
Most common: Gallstones, alcohol (80% cases).
Others: Drugs (e.g. steroids, azathioprine, thiazides, valproate), trauma, ERCP or abdominal surgery, infective (e.g. mumps, EBV, CMV, coxsackie B, mycoplasma), hyperlipidaemia, hyperparathyroidism, anatomical (e.g. pancreas divisum, annular pancreas), idiopathic.

EPIDEMIOLOGY   Common. Annual UK incidence ~10/10 000. Peak age is 60 years; in males, alcohol-induced is more common while in females, principal cause is gallstones.

HISTORY   Severe epigastric or abdominal pain (radiating to back, relieved by sitting forward, aggravated by movement).
Associated with anorexia, nausea and vomiting.
There may be a history of gallstones or alcohol intake.

EXAMINATION   Epigastric tenderness, fever. Shock, tachycardia, tachypnoea.
↓ Bowel sounds (due to ileus).
If severe and haemorrhagic, Turner's sign (flank bruising) or Cullen's sign (periumbilical bruising).

INVESTIGATIONS
Bloods: ↑ Amylase (usually >3× normal but does not correlate with severity), FBC (↑ WCC), U&Es, ↑ glucose, ↑ CRP, ↓ Ca^{2+}, LFTs (maybe deranged if gallstone pancreatitis or alcohol), ABG (for hypoxia or metabolic acidosis).
USS: For gallstones or biliary dilatation.
Erect CXR: There may be pleural effusion. Mainly for excluding other causes.
AXR: To exclude other causes of acute abdomen. Psoas shadow may be lost.
CT scan: If diagnostic uncertainty or if persisting organ failure, signs of sepsis or deterioration for severe cases. Scoring system (Balthazar score): combination of grade of pancreatitis and degree of necrosis.

MANAGEMENT
Assessment of severity: The two most validated scales are:
(1) Modified Glasgow[1] combined with CRP (>210 mg/L).
(2) APACHE-II score (*see Gut* 1998;42(Suppl. 2):S1–13).

Alternatively, there is the older Ranson's criteria.[2]

---

[1] Modified Glasgow criteria (≥3 indicates severe disease):
(**P**) pO2 < 8 kPa	(u**R**) Urea > 16 mmol/L
(**A**) Age > 55	(**En**z) LDH > 600
(**N**) WCC > 15 × 109/L	(**A**) Albumin > 32 g/L
(**C**) Ca^{2+} < 2 mmol/L	(**S**ugar) Glucose > 10 mmol/L

[2] **Ranson's criteria (only for alcoholic pancreatitis):**
On admission: WCC < 16 × 109/L, age > 55, AST > 250, LDH > 350, glucose > 11 mmol/L.
During first 48 h: pO2 < 8 kPa, Ca^{2+} < 2 mmol/L, urea > 16 mmol/L, base deficit > 4, haematocrit fall > 10%, fluid sequestration > 600 mL.

Pancreatitis, acute (continued)

Medical: Fluid and electrolyte resuscitation, urinary catheter and NG tube if vomiting. Analgesia and blood sugar control. Early HDU or intensive care support. Meta-analysis has shown reduced infective complications and mortality in severe pancreatitis with enteral, as opposed to parenteral, feeding. Prophylactic antibiotics have not been shown to reduce mortality, unless infective pancreatic necrosis develops.

ERCP and sphincterotomy: For gallstone pancreatitis, cholangitis, jaundice or dilated common bile duct, ideally within 72 h. All patients should undergo definitive management of gallstones during same admission or within 2 weeks.

Early detection and treatment of complications: e.g. if persistent symptoms and >30% pancreatic necrosis or signs of sepsis should undergo image guided fine needle aspiration for culture (BSG guidelines).

Surgical: Patient with necrotizing pancreatitis should be managed in a specialist unit. Minimal access or open necresectomy (drainage and debridement of all necrotic tissue).

COMPLICATIONS

Local: Pancreatic necrosis, pseudocyst (peripancreatic fluid collection persisting >4 weeks), abscess, ascites, pseudoaneurysm or venous thrombosis.

Systemic: Multiorgan dysfunction, sepsis, renal failure, ARDS, DIC, hypocalcemia, diabetes.

Long term: Chronic pancreatitis (with diabetes and malabsorption).

PROGNOSIS Twenty percent follow severe fulminating course with high mortality (infected pancreatic necrosis associated with 70% mortality), 80% run milder course (but still 5% mortality).

Pancreatitis, chronic

DEFINITION   Chronic inflammatory disease of the pancreas characterized by irreversible parenchymal atrophy and fibrosis leading to impaired endocrine and exocrine function and recurrent abdominal pain.

AETIOLOGY   Alcohol (70%). Idiopathic in 20%.
Rare: Recurrent acute pancreatitis, ductal obstruction, pancreas divisum, hereditary pancreatitis, tropical pancreatitis, autoimmune pancreatitis, hyperparathryroidism, hypertriglyceridemia.

EPIDEMIOLOGY   Annual UK incidence ~1/100 000; prevalence ~3/100 000. Mean age 40–50 years in alcohol-associated disease.

HISTORY   Recurrent severe epigastric pain, radiating to back, relieved by sitting forward, can be exacerbated by eating or drinking alcohol. Over many years, weight loss, bloating and pale offensive stools (steatorrhoea).

EXAMINATION   Epigastric tenderness. Signs of complications, e.g. weight loss, malnutrition.

PATHOLOGY/PATHOGENESIS   Disruption of normal pancreatic glandular architecture due to chronic inflammation and fibrosis, calcification, parenchymal atropy, ductal dilatation, cyst and stone formation. Pancreatic stellate cells are thought to play a role, converting from quiescent fat storing cells to myofibroblast-like cells forming extracellular matrix, cytokines and growth factors in response to injury. Pain is associated with raised intraductal pressures and inflammation.

INVESTIGATIONS
Bloods: Glucose ($\uparrow$ may indicate endocrine dysfunction), glucose tolerance test. Amylase and lipase (usually normal), $\uparrow$ immunoglobulins, especially IgG4 in autoimmune pancreatitis.
USS: Percutaneous or endoscopic: can show hyperechoic foci with post-acoustic shadowing.
ERCP or MRCP: Early changes include main duct dilatation and stumping of branches. Late manifestations are duct strictures with alternating dilatation ('chain of lakes' appearance).
AXR: Pancreatic calcification may be visible.
CT scan: Pancreatic cysts, calcification.
Tests of pancreatic exocrine function: Faecal elastase.

MANAGEMENT
General: Treatment is mainly symptomatic and supportive, e.g. dietary advice, abstinence from alcohol and smoking, treatment of diabetes, oral pancreatic enzyme replacements, e.g. Creon, analgesia for exacerbations of pain. Chronic pain management may need specialist input. The sensory nerves to the pancreas transverse the coeliac ganglia and splanchnic nerves, coeliac plexus block (CT or EUS-guided neurolysis) and transthoracic splanchnicectomy offer variable degrees of pain relief.
Endoscopic therapy: Sphincterotomy, stone extraction, dilatation or stenting of strictures. Extracorporeal shock-wave lithotripsy is sometimes used for fragmentation of larger pancreatic stones prior to endoscopic removal.
Surgical: May be indicated if medical management has failed. Options include lateral pancreaticojejunal drainage (modified Puestow procedure), resection (pancreaticoduodenectomy or Whipple's) or limited resection of the pancreatic head (Beger procedure) or combined opening of the pancreatic duct and excavation of the pancreatic head (Frey procedure).

COMPLICATIONS
Local: Pseudocysts, biliary duct stricture, duodenal obstruction, pancreatic ascites, pancreatic carcinoma.

Pancreatitis, chronic (continued)

Systemic: Diabetes, steatorrhoea, reduced quality of life, chronic pain syndromes and dependence on strong analgesics.

PROGNOSIS   Difficult to predict as pain may improve, stabilize or worsen. Surgery improves symptoms in 60–70% but results are often not sustained. Life expectancy can be reduced by 10–20 years.

Peptic ulcer disease

DEFINITION Ulceration of areas of the GI tract caused by exposure to gastric acid and pepsin. Most commonly gastric and duodenal (can also occur in oesophagus and Meckel's diverticulum).

AETIOLOGY Cause is an imbalance between damaging action of acid and pepsin and mucosal protective mechanisms. There is a strong correlation with *Helicobacter pylori* infection, but it is unclear how the organism causes formation of ulcers.

Common: Very strong association with *H. pylori* (present in 95% of duodenal and 70–80% of gastric ulcers), NSAID use.

Rare: Zollinger–Ellison syndrome.

EPIDEMIOLOGY Common. Annual incidence is about 1–4/1000. More common in males. Duodenal ulcers have a mean age in the thirties, while gastric ulcers have a mean age in the fifties. *H. pylori* is usually acquired in childhood and the prevalence is roughly equivalent to age in years.

HISTORY Epigastric abdominal pain: relieved by antacids.
Symptoms have a variable relationship to food:
- if worse soon after eating, more likely to be gastric ulcers;
- if worse several hours later, more likely to be duodenal.

May present with complications (e.g. haematemesis, melaena).

EXAMINATION May be no physical findings.
Epigastric tenderness.
Signs of complications (e.g. anaemia, succession splash in pyloric stenosis).

INVESTIGATIONS
Bloods: FBC (for anaemia), amylase (to exclude pancreatitis), U&Es, clotting screen (if GI bleeding), LFT, cross-match if actively bleeding. Secretin test; if Zollinger–Ellison syndrome is suspected: IV secretin causes a rise in serum gastrin in ZE patients but not controls.
Endoscopy: Four quadrant gastric ulcer biopsies to rule out malignancy; duodenal ulcers need not be biopsied.
Rockall scoring (*see* Gastrointestinal haemorrhage, upper): For severity after a GI bleed. Less than 3 carries good prognosis, >8 have a high risk of mortality.
Testing for *H. pylori*:

- ^{13}C-Urea breath test: Radio-labelled urea given by mouth and detection of ^{13}C in the expired air.
- Serology: IgG antibody against *H. pylori*, confirms exposure but not eradication.
- Stool antigen test. Campylobacter-like organism test: Gastric biopsy is placed with a substrate of urea and a pH indicator. If *H. pylori* is present, ammonia is produced from the urea and there is a colour change (yellow to red).

Histology of biopsies: Difficult to visualize *H. pylori* so of limited value.

MANAGEMENT
Acute: Resuscitation if perforated or bleeding (IV colloids/crystalloids), close monitoring of vital signs, and proceeding endoscopic or surgical treatment.
Patients with upper GI bleeding should be treated with IV PPI (e.g. omeprazole or pantoprazole) at presentation until the cause of bleeding is confirmed. Patients with actively bleeding peptic ulcers or ulcers with high-risk stigmata (e.g. visible vessel or adherent clot) should continue IV PPI. Switch to oral PPI If there is no rebleeding within 24 hours.
Endoscopy: Haemostasis by injection sclerotherapy, laser or electrocoagulation.
Surgery: If perforated or ulcer-related bleeding cannot be controlled.

Peptic ulcer disease (continued)

H. pylori eradication with 'triple therapy' for 1–2 weeks: Various combinations are recommended made up of one proton pump inhibitors and two antibiotics (e.g. clarithromycin + amoxicillin, metronidazole + tetracycline).

If not associated with H. pylori: Treat with PPIs or H2-antagonists. Stop NSAID use (especially diclofenac), use misoprostol (prostaglandin E1 analogue), if NSAID use is necessary.

COMPLICATIONS   Rate of major complication is 1% per year including haemorrhage (haematemesis, melaena, iron-deficiency anaemia), perforation, obstruction/pyloric stenosis (due to scarring, penetration, pancreatitis).

PROGNOSIS   Overall lifetime risk ~10%. Generally good as peptic ulcers associated with H. pylori can be cured by eradication.

Pseudomembranous colitis

DEFINITION Large bowel inflammation with mucosal destruction and inflammatory exudates forming pseudomembranes on the bowel wall associated with toxin-releasing *Clostridium difficile* bacilli.

AETIOLOGY The organism responsible is *C. difficile*, a Gram-positive anaerobic bacillus. Colonic overgrowth of these toxin-forming bacteria is associated with disturbance of gut microflora, nearly always brought about by antibiotic use. In rare cases, it may occur without antibiotic use.

C. difficile releases two potent toxins: toxin A (enterotoxin) and toxin B (cytotoxin). Toxin A inactivates Rho-GTPase (epithelial cytoplasmic protein), causing intestinal hypersecretion, disaggregation of epithelial actin microfilaments and cell death. Both toxins also disrupt intercellular tight junctions.

Associations/Risk factors: Antibiotics, especially clindamycin, ampicillin and broad-spectrum cephalosporins.

EPIDEMIOLOGY *C. difficile* is commonly carried asymptomatically (2% of the population). Pseudomembranous colitis is common in hospitals, where there is both increased carriage of *C. difficile* and antibiotic use.

HISTORY
History of antibiotic use.
Onset of watery diarrhoea, which may become bloody, associated with crampy abdominal pain.

EXAMINATION
Pyrexia, abdominal tenderness.
In severe cases, toxic megacolon or perforation may occur.

INVESTIGATIONS
Blood: FBC (↑ WCC), ↑ CRP, U&Es (electrolyte status), lactate, blood culture (excludes other organisms).
Stools: Demonstration of *C. difficile* toxin by ELISA. (Note: Stool culture is only useful in excluding other enteric infections.)
Sigmoidoscopy/colonoscopy: Visualizes colitis and pseudomembranes (mucus and fibrin).

MANAGEMENT If the clinical suspicion is high, empiric therapy is appropriate before diagnosis is confirmed, Treatment of *C. difficile* is not indicated in asymptomatic patients who have a positive toxin assay.

Medical: Oral metronidazole or vancomycin for 10–14 days, or longer if diarrhoea persists. Discontinue other antibiotics. Supportive treatment to replenish fluid and electrolyte loss.

First relapse: Consider other causes for the patient's symptoms. Repeat treatment as above. Second relapse: tapering vancomycin (over 6 weeks) plus probiotics (e.g. *Saccharomyces boulardii*) started during the final week of vancomycin and continued for two additional weeks.

In critically ill patients: oral vancomycin plus IV metronidazole.

Infection control practices: Isolate and barrier nurse; hand hygiene must include soap and water, as alcohol-based agents do not kill *C. difficile* spores.

Surgery: Subtotal colectomy with ileostomy. Urgent for patients ≥65 years of age, with $WCC \geq 20 \times 10^9$/L, or plasma lactate between 2.2 and 5 mEq/L. Surgery is also advisable in the setting of peritoneal signs, severe ileus or toxic megacolon.

COMPLICATIONS Toxic megacolon, perforation. Intestinal perforation. Septic shock.

PROGNOSIS Recovery is prompt with treatment; 25% relapse on stopping treatment.

Ulcerative colitis

DEFINITION Chronic relapsing and remitting inflammatory disease affecting the large bowel.

AETIOLOGY/ASSOCIATIONS Unknown. Suggested hypotheses include genetic susceptibility (chromosomes 12, 16), immune response to bacterial or self-antigens, environmental factors, altered neutrophil function, abnormality in epithelial cell integrity. Positive family history of IBD (~15%). Associated with ↑ serum pANCA, primary sclerosing cholangitis.

EPIDEMIOLOGY Prevalence: 1/1500 (in developed world). Higher prevalence in Ashkenazi Jews, Caucasians. Uncommon before the age of 10 years, peak onset age 20–40 years. Equal sex ratio up to age 40, then higher in males.

HISTORY Bloody or mucous diarrhoea (stool frequency related to severity of disease). Tenesmus and urgency. Crampy abdominal pain before passing stool, weight loss, fever. Symptoms of extra GI manifestations.

EXAMINATION Signs of iron-deficiency anaemia, dehydration. Clubbing. Abdominal tenderness, tachycardia. Blood, mucus and tenderness on PR examination. Signs of extra GI manifestations.

INVESTIGATIONS
Bloods: FBC (↓ Hb, ↑ WCC), ↑ ESR or CRP, ↓ albumin, cross-match if severe blood loss, LFT.
Stool: Culture as infectious colitis is a differential diagnosis. Faecal calprotectin – marker for disease severity.
AXR: To rule out toxic megacolon (*see* Toxic megacolon).
Flexible sigmoidoscopy or colonoscopy (and biopsy): Determines severity, histological confirmation, detection of dysplasia.
Barium enema: Mucosal ulceration with granular appearance and filling defects (pseudo-polyps), featureless narrowed colon, loss of haustral pattern (leadpipe or hosepipe appearance). Colonoscopy and barium enema may be dangerous in acute exacerbations (risk of perforation).

MANAGEMENT
Markers of activity: ↓ Hb, ↓ alb, ↑ ESR or CRP and diarrhoea frequency (< 4 per day is mild, 4–6 per day is moderate, >6 per day is severe), bleeding, fever.
Acute exacerbation: IV rehydration, IV corticosteroids, antibiotics, bowel rest, parenteral feeding may be necessary, and DVT prophylaxis. Monitor fluid balance and vital signs closely. If toxic megacolon develops, low threshold for proctocolectomy and ileostomy as perforation has a mortality of 30%.
- *Mild disease*: Oral or rectal 5-aminosalicylic acid derivatives, e.g. sulphasalazine and/or rectal steroids.
- *Moderate to severe disease*: Oral steroids and oral 5-ASA. Immunosuppression with azathioprine, cyclosporine, 6-mercaptopurine, infliximab (anti-TNF monoclonal antibody).

Advice: Patient education and support. Treatment of complications. Regular colonoscopic surveillance.
Surgical: Indicated for failure of medical treatment, presence of complications or prevention of colonic carcinoma. Proctocolectomy with ileostomy or an ileo-anal pouch formation.

COMPLICATIONS

Gastrointestinal: Haemorrhage, toxic megacolon, perforation, colonic carcinoma (in those with extensive disease for >10 years), gallstones and PSC.

Extra-gastrointestinal manifestations (10–20%): Uveitis, renal calculi, arthropathy, sacroiliitis, ankylosing spondylitis, erythema nodosum, pyoderma gangrenosum, osteoporosis (from steroid treatment), amyloidosis.

PROGNOSIS A relapsing and remitting condition, with normal life expectancy.

Poor prognostic factors (ABCDEF): Albumin (< 30 g/L), blood PR, CRP raised, dilated loops of bowel, eight or more bowel movements per day, fever (>38 °C in first 24 h).

Hepatitis, alcoholic

DEFINITION   Inflammatory liver injury caused by chronic heavy intake of alcohol.

AETIOLOGY   One of the three forms of liver disease caused by excessive intake of alcohol, a spectrum that ranges from alcoholic fatty liver (steatosis) to alcoholic hepatitis and chronic cirrhosis. In alcoholic hepatitis, the liver histopathology shows centrilobular ballooning degeneration and necrosis of hepatocytes, steatosis, neutrophilic inflammation, cholestasis, Mallory hyaline inclusions (eosinophilic intracytoplasmic aggregates of cytokeratin intermediate filaments) and giant mitochondria.

EPIDEMIOLOGY   Ten to 35% of heavy drinkers develop this form of liver disease.

HISTORY   May remain asymptomatic and undetected unless they present for other reasons. May be mild illness with nausea, malaise, epigastric or right hypochondrial pain and a low-grade fever.
May be more severe with jaundice, abdominal discomfort or swelling, swollen ankles or GI bleeding. Women tend to present with more florid illness than men. There is a history of heavy alcohol intake (~15–20 years of excessive intake necessary for development of alcoholic hepatitis). There may be trigger events (e.g. aspiration pneumonia or injury).

EXAMINATION
Signs of alcohol excess: Malnourished, palmar erythema, Dupuytren's contracture, facial telangiectasia, parotid enlargement, spider naevi, gynaecomastia, testicular atrophy, hepatomegaly, easy bruising.
Signs of severe alcoholic hepatitis: Febrile (50% of patients), tachycardia, jaundice (>50% of patients), bruising, encephalopathy (e.g. hepatic foetor, liver flap, drowsiness, unable to copy a five-pointed star, disoriented), ascites (30–60% of patients), hepatomegaly (liver is usually mild–moderately enlarged and may be tender on palpation), splenomegaly.

INVESTIGATIONS
Blood: *FBC:* ↓ Hb, ↑ MCV, ↑ WCC, ↓ platelets. LFT (↑ transaminases, ↑ bilirubin, ↓ albumin, ↑ AlkPhos, ↑ GGT). *U&E:* Urea and K^+ levels tend to be low, unless significant renal impairment. *Clotting:* Prolonged PT is a sensitive marker of significant liver damage.
Ultrasound scan: For other causes of liver impairment (e.g. malignancies).
Upper GI endoscopy: To investigate for varices.
Liver biopsy: Percutaneous or transjugular (in the presence of coagulopathy) may be helpful to distinguish from other causes of hepatitis.
Electroencephalogram: For slow-wave activity indicative of encephalopathy.

MANAGEMENT
Acute: Thiamine, Vitamin C and other multivitamins (initially parenterally). Monitor and correct K^+, Mg^{2+} and glucose abnormalities. Ensure adequate urine output. Treat encephalopathy with oral lactulose and phosphate enemas. Ascites is managed by diuretics (spironolactone with or without frusemide (furosemide)) or therapeutic paracentesis. Glypressin and *N*-acetylcysteine for hepatorenal syndrome.
Nutrition: Nutritional support with oral or nasogastric feeding is important with increased caloric intake. Protein restriction should be avoided unless the patient is encephalopathic. Total enteral nutrition may also be considered as this improves mortality rate. Nutritional supplementation and vitamins (B group, thiamine, folic acid) should be started parenterally initially and then continued orally after.
Steroid therapy: Meta-analyses show that steroids reduce short-term mortality for severe alcoholic hepatitis.
Long-term: *See* Alcohol dependence.

COMPLICATIONS   Acute liver decompensation, hepatorenal syndrome (renal failure secondary to advanced liver disease), cirrhosis (*see* Liver failure).

Hepatitis, alcoholic (continued)

PROGNOSIS Mortality in first month is about 10%; 40% in first year. If alcohol intake continues, most progress to cirrhosis within 1–3 years. Various validated prognostic scores can be used:

Maddrey's discriminant function (MDF):

$$MDF = (bilirubin/17) + (prolongation of PT \times 4.6)$$

If MDF > 32, this indicates >50% 30-day mortality.

Glasgow alcoholic hepatitis score (GAHS):

	1	2	3
Age (years)	<50	≥50	–
WCC (10^9/L)	<15	≥15	–
Urea (mmol/L)	<5	≥5	–
PT ratio	<1.5	1.5–2.0	>2.0
Bilirubin (μmol/L)	<125	125–250	>250

If GAHS ≥ 9 from Day 1 to 9, this indicates >50% 30-day mortality.

Cirrhosis

DEFINITION End-stage of chronic liver damage with replacement of normal liver architecture with diffuse fibrosis and nodules of regenerating hepatocytes. *Decompensated* when there are complications such as ascites, jaundice, encephalopathy or GI bleeding (*see* Liver failure).

AETIOLOGY
Chronic alcohol misuse: Most common UK cause.
Chronic viral hepatitis: Hepatitis B/C are the most common causes worldwide.
Autoimmune hepatitis.
Drugs: e.g. methotrexate, hepatotoxic drugs.
Inherited: α_1-Antitrypsin deficiency, haemochromatosis, Wilson's disease, galactosaemia, cystic fibrosis.
Vascular: Budd–Chiari syndrome or hepatic venous congestion.
Chronic biliary diseases: Primary biliary cirrhosis (PBC), primary sclerosing cholangitis (PSC), biliary atresia.
Cryptogenic: In 5–10%.
Non-alcoholic steatohepatitis (NASH) ↑ risk of developing cirrhosis. NASH is associated with obesity, diabetes, total parenteral nutrition, short bowel syndromes, hyperlipidaemia and drugs, e.g. amiodarone, tamoxifen.
Decompensation can be precipitated by infection, GI bleeding, constipation, high-protein meal, electrolyte imbalances, alcohol and drugs, tumour development or portal vein thrombosis.

EPIDEMIOLOGY Among the top 10 leading cause of deaths worldwide.

HISTORY Early non-specific symptoms: Anorexia, nausea, fatigue, weakness, weight loss.
Symptoms caused by ↓ liver synthetic function: Easy bruising, abdominal swelling, ankle oedema.
Reduced detoxification function: Jaundice, personality change, altered sleep pattern, amenorrhoea.
Portal hypertension: Abdominal swelling, haematemesis, PR bleeding or melaena.

EXAMINATION Stigmata of chronic liver disease: **A**sterixis ('liver flap'). **B**ruises. **C**lubbing. **D**upuytren's contracture. **E**rythema (palmar). Jaundice, gynaecomastia, leukonychia, parotid enlargement, spider naevi, scratch marks, ascites ('shifting dullness' and fluid thrill), enlarged liver (shrunken and small in later stage), testicular atrophy, caput medusae (dilated superficial abdominal veins), splenomegaly (indicating portal hypertension).

INVESTIGATIONS
Blood: *FBC:* ↓ Hb, ↓ platelets as a result of hypersplenism. *LFTs:* May be normal or often ↑ transaminases, AlkPhos, GGT, bilirubin, ↓ albumin. *Clotting:* Prolonged PT (↓ synthesis of clotting factors). *Serum AFP:* ↑ In chronic liver disease, but high levels may suggest hepatocellular carcinoma.
Other investigations: To determine the cause, e.g. viral serology (HBsAg, HBsAb, HCV ab), α_1-antitrypsin, caeruloplasmin (Wilson's disease), iron studies: serum ferritin, iron, total iron binding capacity (haemochromatosis), antimitochondrial antibody (PBC), antinuclear antibodies (ANA), SMA (autoimmune hepatitis).
Ascitic tap: Microscopy, culture and sensitivity, biochemistry (protein, albumin, glucose, amylase) and cytology. If neutrophils >250/mm^3, this indicates spontaneous bacterial peritonitis (SBP).
Liver biopsy: Percutaneous or transjugular if clotting deranged or ascites present. Histopathology: Periportal fibrosis, loss of normal liver architecture and nodular appearance. Grade refers to the assessment of degree of inflammation, whereas stage refers to the degree of architectural distortion, ranging from mild portal fibrosis to cirrhosis.

Cirrhosis (continued)

Imaging: Ultrasound, CT or MRI (to detect complications of cirrhosis such as ascites, hepatocellular carcinoma, and hepatic or portal vein thrombosis, to exclude biliary obstruction), MRCP (if PSC suspected).

Endoscopy: Examine for varices, portal hypertensive gastropathy.

Child–Pugh grading: Class A is score 5–6, Class B is score 7–9, Class C is score 10–15.

Score	1	2	3
Albumin (g/L)	>35	28–35	<28
Bilirubin (mg/dL)	<2	2–3	>3
PT (s prolonged)	<4	4–6	>6
Ascites	None	Mild	Moderate or severe
Encephalopathy	None	Grade 1–2	Grade 3–4

MANAGEMENT   Treat the cause if possible, avoid alcohol, sedatives, opiates, NSAIDs and drugs that affect the liver. Nutrition is very important and if intake is poor, dietitian review and enteral supplements should be given; nasogastric feeding may be indicated.

Treat the complications:

Encephalopathy: Treat infections. Exclude a GI bleed. Lactulose, phosphate enemas and avoid sedation.

Ascites: Diuretics (spironolactone ± furosemide), dietary sodium restriction (88 meq or 2 g/day), therapeutic paracentesis (with human albumin replacement IV). Monitor weight daily. Fluid restriction in patients with plasma sodium <120 mmol/L. Avoid alcohol and NSAIDs.

SBP: Antibiotic treatment (e.g. cefuroxime and metronidazole), prophylaxis against recurrent SBP with ciprofloxacin.

Surgical: Consider insertion of TIPS to relieve portal hypertension (if recurrent variceal bleeds or diuretic-resistant ascites) although it may precipitate encephalopathy. Liver transplantation is the only curative measure.

COMPLICATIONS   Portal hypertension with ascites, encephalopathy or variceal haemorrhage, SBP, hepatocellular carcinoma. Renal failure (hepatorenal syndrome). Pulmonary hypertension (hepatopulmonary syndrome).

PROGNOSIS   Depends on the aetiology and complications. Generally poor; overall 5-year survival is ~50%. In the presence of ascites, 2-year survival of ~50%.

Hepatitis, autoimmune

DEFINITION   Chronic hepatitis of unknown aetiology, characterized by autoimmune features, hyperglobulinaemia and the presence of circulating autoantibodies.

AETIOLOGY   In a genetically predisposed individual, an environmental agent (e.g. viruses or drugs) may lead to hepatocyte expression of HLA antigens which then become the focus of a principally T-cell-mediated autoimmune attack. The raised titres of ANA, ASM and anti-liver/kidney microsomes (anti-LKM) are not thought to directly injure the liver. The chronic inflammatory changes are similar to those seen in chronic viral hepatitis with lymphoid infiltration of the portal tracts and hepatocyte necrosis, leading to fibrosis and, eventually, cirrhosis. Two major forms:

Type I (classic): ANA, anti-smooth muscle antibodies (ASMA), anti-actin antibodies (AAA), anti-soluble liver antigen (anti-SLA).

Type 2: Antibodies to liver/kidney microsomes (ALKM-1, directed at an epitope of CYP2D6), antibodies to a liver cytosol antigen (ALC-1).

Patients with variant forms of autoimmune hepatitis have clinical and serologic findings of autoimmune hepatitis plus features of PBC or PSC.

EPIDEMIOLOGY   Type 1 autoimmune hepatitis occurs in all age groups (although mainly in young women). Type 2 is generally a disease of girls and young women.

HISTORY   May be asymptomatic and discovered incidentally by abnormal LFT.

Insidious onset: Malaise, fatigue, anorexia, weight loss, nausea, jaundice, amenorrhoea, epistaxis.

Acute hepatitis (25%): Fever, anorexia, jaundice, nausea, vomiting, diarrhoea, RUQ pain. Some may also present with serum sickness (e.g. arthralgia, polyarthritis, maculopapular rash).

May be associated with keratoconjuctivitis sicca.

Personal or family history of autoimmune disease, e.g. type 1 diabetes mellitus and vitiligo. It is important to take a full history to rule out other potential causes of liver disease (e.g. alcohol, drugs).

EXAMINATION   Stigmata of chronic liver disease, e.g. spider naevi (*see* Cirrhosis).

Ascites, oedema and encephalopathy are late features.

Cushingoid features (e.g. rounded face, cutaneous striae, acne, hirsuitism) may be present even before the administration of steroids.

INVESTIGATIONS

Blood: *LFT:* $\uparrow\uparrow$ AST and ALT, $\uparrow\uparrow$ GGT, $\uparrow$ AlkPhos, $\uparrow$ bilirubin, $\downarrow$ albumin in severe disease. *Clotting:* $\uparrow$ PT in severe disease. *FBC:* Mild $\downarrow$ Hb, also $\downarrow$ platelets and WCC from hypersplenism if portal hypertension present.

Hypergammaglobulinaemia is typical (polyclonal gammopathy) with the presence of ANA, ASMA or anti-LKM autoantibodies.

Liver biopsy: Needed to establish the diagnosis. Shows interface hepatitis or cirrhosis.

Other investigations: To rule out other causes of liver disease, e.g. viral serology (hepatitis B and C) caeruloplasmin and urinary copper (Wilson's disease), ferritin and transferrin saturation (haemochromatosis), α_1-antitrypsin (α_1-antitrypsin deficiency) and antimitochondrial antibodies (PBC).

Ultrasound, CT or MRI of liver and abdomen: To visualize structural lesions.

ERCP: To rule out PSC.

MANAGEMENT

Indications: Aminotransferases $>10\times$ the upper limit of normal, symptomatic, histology: significant interface hepatitis, bridging necrosis or multiacinar necrosis.

Hepatitis, autoimmune (continued)

Immunosuppression with steroids (e.g. prednisolone), followed by maintenance treatment with gradual reduction in dose (treatment is often long term). Azathioprine or 6-mercaptopurine (6-MP) may be used in the maintenance phase as a steroid-sparing agent with frequent monitoring of LFT and FBC. (Test for TMPT[1] activity before starting azathioprine or 6-MP.)

Monitor: Ultrasound and α-fetoprotein level every 6–12 months in patients with cirrhosis (to detect hepatocellular carcinoma). Repeat liver biopsies for evidence of disease progression (<2 years).

Hepatitis A and B vaccinations.

Liver transplant: For patients who are refractory to or intolerant of immunosuppressive therapy and those with end-stage disease.

COMPLICATIONS   Fulminant hepatic failure. Cirrhosis and complications of portal hypertension (e.g. varices, ascites). Hepatocellular carcinoma. Side-effects of corticosteroid treatment.

PROGNOSIS   Older patients with type 1 autoimmune hepatitis are more likely to have cirrhosis at presentation but may be more likely to respond to treatment. Approximately 80% achieve remission by 3 years. Thirty five to 50% remain in remission when immunosuppression is withdrawn. Fifty percent require lifelong maintenance. Five-year survival rate is 85% if treated and 50% if untreated. Five-year survival after liver transplantation is >80%.

---

[1] TMPT: Thiopurine methyltransferase is the enzyme that metabolizes azathioprine.

Hepatitis, viral: A and E

DEFINITION Hepatitis caused by infection with the RNA viruses, hepatitis A (HAV) or hepatitis E virus (HEV), that follow an acute course without progression to chronic carriage.

AETIOLOGY HAV is a picornavirus and HEV is a calicivirus. Both are small non-enveloped single-stranded linear RNA viruses of ~7500 nucleotides, with transmission by the faecal–oral route.

Both viruses replicate in hepatocytes and are secreted into bile. Liver inflammation and hepatocyte necrosis is caused by the immune response, with targeting of infected cells by CD8 + T cells and natural killer cells. Histology shows inflammatory cell infiltration (neutrophils, macrophages, eosinophils and lymphocytes) of the portal tracts, zone 3 necrosis and bile duct proliferation.

EPIDEMIOLOGY HAV is endemic in the developing world, infection often occurs sub-clinically. In the developed world, better sanitation means that seroprevalence is lower, age of exposure ↑ and hence is more likely to be symptomatic. Annual UK incidence is 5000 cases (seroprevalence ~5%).

HEV is endemic in Asia, Africa and Central America.

HISTORY Incubation period for HAV or HEV is 3–6 weeks.

Prodromal period: Malaise, anorexia (distaste for cigarettes in smokers), fever, nausea and vomiting.

Hepatitis: Prodrome followed by dark urine, pale stools and jaundice lasting ~3 weeks. Occasionally, itching and jaundice last several weeks in HAV infection (owing to cholestatic hepatitis).

EXAMINATION Pyrexia, jaundice, tender hepatomegaly, spleen may be palpable (20%). Absence of stigmata of chronic liver disease, although a few spider naevi may appear, transiently.

INVESTIGATIONS

Blood: LFT (↑↑ AST and ALT, ↑ bilirubin, ↑ AlkPhos), ↑ ESR. In severe cases, ↓ albumin and ↑ platelets.

Viral serology:

Hepatitis A: Anti-HAV IgM (during acute illness, disappearing after 3–5 months), anti-HAV IgG (recovery phase and lifelong persistence).

Hepatitis E: Anti-HEV IgM (↑ 1–4 weeks after onset of illness), anti-HEV IgG. Hepatitis B and C viral serology is also necessary to rule out these infections.

Urinalysis: Positive for bilirubin, ↑ urobilinogen.

MANAGEMENT No specific management. Bed rest and symptomatic treatment (e.g. antipyretics, antiemetics). Colestyramine for severe pruritus.

Prevention and control:

Public health: Safe water, sanitation, food hygiene standards. Both are notifiable diseases. Personal hygiene and sensible dietary precautions when travelling.

Immunization (HAV only): Passive immunization with IM human immunoglobulin is only effective for a short period. Active immunization with attenuated HAV vaccine offers safe and effective immunity for those travelling to endemic areas, high-risk individuals (e.g. residents of institutions).

COMPLICATIONS Fulminant hepatic failure develops in 0.1% cases of HAV, 1–2% of HEV but up to 20% in pregnant women. Cholestatic hepatitis with prolonged jaundice and pruritus may develop after HAV infection.

Hepatitis, viral: A and E (continued)

Post-hepatitis syndrome: Continued malaise for weeks to months.

PROGNOSIS Recovery is usual within 3–6 weeks. Occasionally, a relapse during recovery. There are no chronic sequelae. Fulminant hepatic failure carries an 80% mortality.

Hepatitis, viral: B and D

DEFINITION   Hepatitis caused by infection with hepatitis B virus (HBV), which may follow an acute or chronic (defined as viraemia and hepatic inflammation continuing >6 months) course.
Hepatitis D virus (HDV), a defective virus, may only co-infect with HBV or superinfect persons who are already carriers of HBV.

AETIOLOGY   HBV is an enveloped, partially double-stranded DNA virus. Transmission is by sexual contact, blood and vertical transmission. Various viral proteins are produced, including core antigen (HBcAg), surface antigen (HBsAg) and e antigen (HBeAg). HBeAg is a marker of ↑ infectivity.
HDV is a single-stranded RNA virus coated with HBsAg.
Antibody- and cell-mediated immune responses to viral replication lead to liver inflammation and hepatocyte necrosis. Histology can be variable, from mild to severe inflammation and changes of cirrhosis.

ASSOCIATIONS/RISK FACTORS   Hepatitis B infection is associated with IV drug abuse, unscreened blood and blood products, infants of HbeAg-positive mothers and sexual contact with HBV carriers. Risk of persistant HBV infection varies with age, with younger individuals, especially babies, more likely to develop chronic carriage. Genetic factors are associated with ↑ rates of viral clearance.

EPIDEMIOLOGY   Common. 350 million worldwide infected with HBV; 1–2 million deaths annually. Common in Southeast Asia, Africa and Mediterranean countries. HDV also found worldwide. HBV is relatively uncommon in the UK.

HISTORY
Incubation period 3–6 months; 1- to 2-week *prodrome* of malaise, headache, anorexia, nausea, vomiting, diarrhoea and RUQ pain.
May experience serum-sickness-type illness (e.g. fever, arthralgia, polyarthritis, urticaria, maculopapular rash).
Jaundice then develops with dark urine and pale stools.
Recovery is usual within 4–8 weeks. One per cent may develop fulminant liver failure.
Chronic carriage may be diagnosed after routine LFT testing or if cirrhosis or decompensation develops.

EXAMINATION
Acute: Jaundice, pyrexia, tender hepatomegaly, splenomegaly and cervical lymphadenopathy in 10–20%. Occasionally, urticaria/maculopapular rash.
Chronic: May have no findings; signs of chronic liver disease or decompensation.

INVESTIGATIONS
Viral serology:
Acute HBV: HbsAg positive, IgM anti-HbcAg.
Chronic HBV: HbsAg positive, IgG anti-HBcAg, HbeAg positive or negative (latter in precore mutant variant).
HBV cleared or immunity: Anti-HBsAg positive, IgG anti-HBcAg.
HDV infection: Detected by IgM or IgG against HDV.
PCR: For detection of HBV DNA is the most sensitive measure of ongoing viral replication.
LFT: ↑↑ AST and ALT. ↑ Bilirubin. ↑ AlkPhos.
Clotting: ↑ PT in severe disease.
Liver biopsy: Percutaneous, or transjugular if clotting is deranged or ascites is present.

MANAGEMENT
Prevention: Blood screening, instrument sterilization, safe sex practices.

Hepatitis, viral: B and D (continued)

Passive immunization: Hepatitis B immunoglobulin (HBIG) following acute exposure and to neonates born to HbeAg-positive mothers (in addition to active immunization).

Active immunization: Recombinant HbsAg vaccine for individuals at risk and neonates born to HBV-positive mothers. Immunization against HBV protects against HDV.

Acute HBV hepatitis: Symptomatic treatment with bed rest, antiemetics, antipyretics and cholestyramine for pruritus. Notification to the consultant in communicable disease control.

Chronic HBV:

Indications for treatment with antivirals: HbeAg-positive or HbeAg-negative chronic hepatitis (depending on ALT and HBV DNA levels), compensated cirrhosis and HBV DNA >2,000 IU/mL, decompensated cirrhosis and detectable HBV DNA by PCR.

Patients may be treated with interferon alpha (standard or pegylated, which has ↑ half-life), or nucleos/tide analogues (adefovir, entecavir, telbivudine, tenofovir, lamivudine). The role of lamivudine as primary therapy has diminished due to high rates of drug resistance.

Interferon alpha is a cytokine which augments natural antiviral mechanisms. Side-effects include flu-like symptoms, fever, chills, myalgia, headaches, bone marrow suppression and depression, necessitating discontinuation in 5–10% of patients.

COMPLICATIONS Fulminant hepatic failure (1%), chronic HBV infection (∼10% adults, much higher in neonates), cirrhosis and hepatocellular carcinoma, extrahepatic immune complex disorders including glomerulonephritis, polyarteritis nodosa. Superinfection with HDV may lead to acute liver failure or more rapidly progressive disease.

PROGNOSIS In adults, 10% infections become chronic, and of these, 20–30% will develop cirrhosis. Factors predictive of a good response to interferon include high serum transaminases, low HBV DNA, active histological changes and the absence of complicating diseases.

Hepatitis, Viral: C

DEFINITION   Hepatitis caused by infection with hepatitis C virus (HCV), often following a chronic course (~80% cases).

AETIOLOGY   HCV is a small, enveloped, single-stranded RNA virus of the flavivirus family. As it is an RNA virus, fidelity of replication is poor and mutation rates are high, resulting in different HCV genotypes, and even in a single patient, many viral quasi-species may be present.

Transmission: Occurs via the parenteral route, and at-risk groups include recipients of blood and blood products prior to blood screening, IV drug users, non-sterile acupuncture and tattooing, those on haemodialysis and health care workers. Sexual and vertical transmission is uncommon (1–5%, ↑ risk in those co-infected with HIV).

Pathology/Pathogenesis: Although HCV is hepatotropic, it is not thought that the virus is directly hepatotoxic, rather that the humoral and cell-mediated response leads to hepatic inflammation and necrosis. On liver biopsy, chronic hepatitis is seen and a characteristic feature is lymphoid follicles in the portal tracts. Fatty change is also common and features of cirrhosis may be present.

EPIDEMIOLOGY   Common. Prevalence is 0.5–2% in developed countries, with higher rates in certain areas (e.g. Middle East) because of poor sterilisation practices. Different HCV genotypes have different geographical prevalence.

HISTORY
Ninety per cent of acute infections are asymptomatic with <10% becoming jaundiced with a mild 'flu-like' illness.
May be diagnosed after incidental abnormal LFT or in older individuals with complications of cirrhosis.

EXAMINATION
There may be no signs or may be signs of chronic liver disease in long-standing infection. Less common extra-hepatic manifestations include:
- skin rash, caused by mixed cryoglobulinaemia causing a small-vessel vasculitis; and
- renal dysfunction, caused by glomerulonephritis.

INVESTIGATIONS

Blood:
HCV serology: Anti-HCV antibodies, either IgM (acute) or IgG (past exposure or chronic).
Reverse-transcriptase PCR: Detection and genotyping of HCV RNA. Used to confirm antibody testing; also recommended in patients with clinically suspected HCV infection but negative serology.
LFT: Acute infection causes ↑ AST and ALT, mild ↑ bilirubin. Chronic infection causes 2–8 times elevation of AST and ALT, often fluctuating over time. Sometimes normal.
Liver biopsy: To assess degree of inflammation and liver damage as transaminase levels bear little correlation to histological changes. Also useful in diagnosing cirrhosis as patients with cirrhosis will require monitoring for hepatocellular carcinoma.

MANAGEMENT
Prevention: Screening of blood, blood products and organ donors, needle exchange schemes for IV drug abusers, instrument sterilization. No vaccine available at present.
Medical:
Acute: No specific management and mainly supportive (e.g. antipyretics, antiemetics, cholestyramine). Specific antiviral treatment can be delayed for 3–6 months.

Hepatitis, Viral: C (continued)

Chronic: Combined treatment with pegylated interferon-α (cytokine which augments natural antiviral mechanisms) and ribavirin (guanosine nucleotide analogue) is the treatment strategy of choice:

- HCV genotype 1 or 4: 24–48 weeks
- HCV genotype 2 or 3: 12–24 weeks

Monitoring of HCV viral load is recommended after 12 weeks of treatment to determine efficacy of treatment. Regular ultrasound of liver may be necessary if the patient has cirrhosis.

COMPLICATIONS   Fulminant hepatic failure in acute phase (0.5%), chronic HCV carriage, cirrhosis and hepatocellular carcinoma. Less common are porphyria cutanea tarda, cryoglobulinaemia and glomerulonephritis.

PROGNOSIS   Approximately eighty per cent of exposed progress to chronic HCV infection, and of these, 20–30% develop cirrhosis over 10–20 years.

Hepatocellular carcinoma

DEFINITION   Primary malignancy of hepatocytes, usually occurring in a cirrhotic liver.

AETIOLOGY
- Chronic liver damage (e.g. alcoholic liver disease, hepatitis B, hepatitis C, autoimmune disease),
- metabolic disease (e.g. haemochromatosis), and
- aflatoxins (*Aspergillus flavus* fungal toxin found on stored grains or biological weapons).

EPIDEMIOLOGY   Common making up ~1–2% of all malignancies, but less common than secondary liver malignancies. Rare in West (1–2 in 100 000/year). Very common malignancy in areas where Hepatitis B and C are endemic, i.e. Asia and sub-Saharan Africa (~500 in 100 000/year).

HISTORY
Symptoms of malignancy: Malaise, weight loss, loss of appetite.
Symptoms of chronic liver disease: Abdominal distension, jaundice.
History of carcinogen exposure: High alcohol intake, Hepatitis B or C, aflatoxins.

EXAMINATION
Signs of malignancy: Cachexia, lymphadenopathy.
Hepatomegaly: Nodular (but may be smooth). Deep palpation may elicit tenderness. There may be bruit heard over the liver.
Signs of chronic liver disease: Jaundice, ascite (*see* Cirrhosis).

INVESTIGATIONS
Blood: ↑ AFP (tumour marker with high sensitivity), Vitamin B12-binding protein is a marker of fibrolamellar hepatocellular carcinoma. LFT has poor specificity and sensitivity but may show biliary obstruction.
Abdominal ultrasound: Not sensitive for tumours <1 cm.
Duplex scan of liver: May be used to demonstrate large vessel invasion (e.g. into hepatic or portal veins).
CT (thorax, abdomen, pelvis): To define structural lesion and spread.
Hepatic angiography: Using lipiodol (an iodized oil).
Liver biopsy: Confirms histology of tumour but there is small risk of tumour seeding along biopsy tract.
Staging: CXR, CT (thorax, abdomen, pelvis), radionuclide bone scan.
Screening: AFP and abdominal ultrasound in at-risk individuals.

MANAGEMENT
Surgery: Surgical resection possible in <10% (40–50% of fibrolamellar hepatocellular carcinoma), tumours must be small and localized to a single lobe. Liver transplantation may be considered if disease is small and localized to the liver.
Local therapy: Percutaneous ethanol injection, cryoablation and radiofrequency ablation are approaches used.
Interventional radiography (e.g. embolization): Using microspheres, chemotherapy agents or radio-labelled $_{131}$I in lipiodol. Usually palliative.
Chemotherapy: Tumours tend to be chemoresistant to traditional agents (only 10% respond to doxorubicin, cisplatin and carboplatin).
Biological agents: Bevacizumab (anti-angiogenic monoclonal) can be used in adjunct to traditional chemotherapeutic agents.
Tyrosine kinase inhibitors (Sorafenib and Sunitinib): Small molecules which inhibit cellular signalling of a number of growth factor pathways. Some effectiveness in prolonging survival.

Hepatocellular carcinoma (continued)

COMPLICATIONS   Biliary tree compression, liver decompensation, cachexia, tumour necrosis and pain; more rarely, rupture and intraperitoneal bleeding, paraneoplastic syndromes.

PROGNOSIS   Poor (mean survival is months from diagnosis). After liver transplantation, 5-year survival rate is ~20%.

Hereditary haemochromatosis

DEFINITION   Body iron overload resulting from excessive intestinal iron absorption which may lead to organ damage (particularly liver, joints, pancreas, pituitary and heart).

AETIOLOGY   Hereditary haemochromatosis (HH) is caused by a mutation in the *HFE* gene on chromosome 6p. Most common mutation (90%) is C282Y, less common is H63D.
Two models for the pathogenesis of HH have been suggested:

Liver model: HFE deficiency causes ↓ expression of the hepatic hormone 'hepcidin' which causes ↑ duodenal iron absorption through a lack of the inhibitory effect of hepcidin on ferroportin (the protein which exports iron from enterocytes into circulation).

Crypt cell model: The HFE protein interacts with the transferrin receptor 1 in duodenal crypt cells. Mutations in HFE may impair uptake of transferrin-bound iron into crypt cells, resulting in upregulation of the iron transporter DMT1 in the crypt cells as they migrate up the villus and mature into enterocytes. This leads to ↑ iron absorption.

EPIDEMIOLOGY   Carrier frequency is up to 1 in 10 but not all express disease. Prevalence of those affected: ~1 in 400 (in white people). Typical age of presentation: 40–60 years. Females have a later onset and less severe presentation as a result of iron loss through menstruation.

HISTORY   May be asymptomatic.
Non-specific symptoms of weakness, fatigue, lethargy, abdominal pain.
Later features include small/large joint pains (most commonly second/third metacarpophalangeal joints), symptoms of liver disease, diabetes mellitus, hypogonadism, cardiac failure.
Exclude causes of secondary iron overload (e.g. multiple transfusions).

EXAMINATION   May be normal, but with severe iron overload:
Skin: Pigmentation ('slate-grey') resulting from ↑ melanin deposits.
Liver: Hepatosplenomegaly.
Heart: Signs of heart failure, arrhythmias.
Hypogonadism: Testicular atrophy, loss of hair, gynaecomastia.

INVESTIGATIONS
Blood: ↑ Iron, ↓ TIBC, ↑ ferritin and transferrin saturation (false-positives in alcoholic liver disease or in any inflammation).
Gene typing of HFE.
Tests for complications in various organs:
Liver: LFTs may be normal or deranged. Liver biopsy to assess tissue damage. Iron accumulation is visualized using Perls' stain. MRI may be used to estimate the degree of iron loading.
Pancreas: Fasting or random blood glucose to test for diabetes mellitus.
Pituitary function test: ↓ Testosterone (in men), ↓ or inappropriately normal LH, FSH (i.e. secondary hypogonadism), 9 am cortisol, TFTs, IGF-1.
Heart: ECG, echocardiography.
Joint X-ray: Linear calcification (chondrocalcinosis).

MANAGEMENT
If no symptoms or evidence of end-organ damage: Annual examination and measurement of the serum iron, ferritin and transferrin saturation.
If symptomatic or presence of end-organ damage (liver, endocrine organs, heart): Weekly/twice weekly phlebotomy (~450 mL) until ferritin concentration <50 ng/mL or transferrin saturation <50%.
Maintenance phlebotomy: Every 2–4 months 500 mL (target serum ferritin: ≤50 ng/mL).
If unable to tolerate phlebotomy therapy, then chelation therapy.
Advice: Limit alcohol intake, avoid iron, Vitamin C supplements and uncooked seafood.

Hereditary haemochromatosis (continued)

Screening of first-degree family members: Fasting transferrin saturation, ferritin and testing for mutations in the *HFE* gene, when they are between the ages of 18 and 30 years. Screen for hepatocellular carcinoma on a continuing basis in patients with cirrhosis.

COMPLICATIONS   Arthritis. Cirrhosis, ↑ risk of hepatocellular carcinoma. Diabetes. Dilated cardiomyopathy, cardiac failure and arrhythmias. Hypogonadism.

PROGNOSIS   Reducing iron overload decreases mortality from cardiac and liver failure and returns the life expectancy of non-cirrhotic non-diabetic patients to normal. Treatment may improve diabetes, cardiac function, hepatic fibrosis, secondary hypogonadism, varices and prevent the development of hepatocellular carcinoma. Hypogonadism and arthritis may not be reversed by venesection.

Liver abscesses and cysts

DEFINITION   Liver infection resulting in a walled off collection of pus or cyst fluid.

AETIOLOGY
Pyogenic: *Escherichia coli*, *Klebsiella*, enterococcus, bacteroides, streptococci, staphylococci. Sixty percent caused by biliary tract disease (gallstones, strictures, congenital cysts), cryptogenic (15%).
Amoebic: Entamoeba histolytica.
Hydatid cyst: Tapeworm *Echinococcus granulosis*.
Other: Tuberculosis.

EPIDEMIOLOGY
Pyogenic: Incidence 0.8 in 100 000, mean age 60 years, most common liver abscess in industrialized world.
Amoebic: Most common type worldwide (10% of world's population has been infected).
Hydatid disease: Common in sheep-rearing countries.

HISTORY   Fever, malaise, nausea, anorexia, night sweats, weight loss.
RUQ or epigastric pain, which may be referred to shoulder (diaphragmatic irritation). Jaundice, diarrhoea, pyrexia of unknown origin.
Ask about foreign travel.

EXAMINATION   Fever (continuous or spiking), jaundice.
Tender hepatomegaly, right lobe affected more commonly than left.
Dullness to percussion and ↓ breath sounds at right base of lung, caused by reactive pleural effusion.

INVESTIGATIONS
Blood: FBC (mild anaemia, leukocytosis, ↑ eosinophils in hydatid disease), LFTs (↑ AlkPhos, ↑ bilirubin), ↑ ESR, ↑ CRP, blood cultures, amoebic and hydatid serology.
Stool microscopy, cultures: For *E. histolytica* or tapeworm eggs.
Liver ultrasound or CT/MRI: Localizes structure of mass.
CXR: Right pleural effusion or atelectasis, raised hemidiaphragm.
Aspiration and culture of the abscess material: Most pyogenic liver abscesses are polymicrobial. Amoebic abscesses contain 'anchovy sauce' fluid of necrotic hepatocytes and trophozoites.

MANAGEMENT
Pyogenic: Needle aspiration (under ultrasound or CT guidance) if ≤5 cm or percutaneous catheter drainage if >5 cm.
Surgical drainage: For multiple/loculated abscesses, abscesses with viscous contents, inadequate response to percutaneous drainage within 7 days.
IV broad-spectrum antibiotics (e.g. ceftriaxone and metronidazole) until sensitivities are known. Switch to oral antibiotics when there is a clinical response (complete a 4–6 weeks course). Treatment of underlying cause.
Amoebic: Metronidazole and diloxanide furoate.
Hydatid: Surgical removal (pericystectomy) with mebendazole or albendazole to reduce risk of recurrence.

COMPLICATIONS   Septic shock, rupture and dissemination (e.g. into biliary tract causing acute cholangitis, intrathoracic rupture or peritonitis), allergic sequelae or anaphylaxis on rupture hydatid cyst.

PROGNOSIS   Untreated pyogenic liver abscesses are often fatal. Complications have high mortality. Amoebic abscesses have a better prognosis and usually have a quick response to therapy. Hydatid cysts may recur after surgery (10%).

Liver failure

DIAGNOSIS   Severe liver dysfunction leading to jaundice, encephalopathy and coagulopathy.

Hyperacute liver failure: Jaundice with encephalopathy occurring in <7 days.

Acute: Jaundice with encephalopathy occurring from 1 to 4 weeks of onset.

Subacute: Jaundice with encephalopathy occurring within 4–12 weeks of onset.

Acute-on-chronic: Acute deterioration (decompensation) in patients with chronic liver disease (see Cirrhosis).

AETIOLOGY

Viral: Hepatitis A, B, D, E, 'non-A-E hepatitis'.

Drugs: Paracetamol overdose (see Paracetamol overdose), idiosyncratic drug reactions (e.g. anti-TB therapy).

Less commonly: Autoimmune hepatitis, Budd–Chiari syndrome, pregnancy-related, malignancy (e.g. lymphoma), haemochromatosis, mushroom poisoning (Amanita phalloides), Wilson's disease.

Pathogenesis of manifestations:

- Jaundice: ↓ Secretion of conjugated bilirubin.
- Encephalopathy: ↑ Delivery of gut-derived products into the systemic circulation and brain from ↓ extraction of nitrogenous products by liver and portal systemic shunting. Ammonia may play a part.
- Coagulopathy: ↓ Synthesis of clotting factors, ↓ platelets (hypersplenism if chronic portal hypertension) or platelet functional abnormalities associated with jaundice or renal failure.

EPIDEMIOLOGY   Paracetamol overdose accounts for 50% of acute liver failure in the UK.

HISTORY   May be asymptomatic. Fever, nausea and possibly jaundice.

EXAMINATION   Jaundice, encephalopathy, liver asterixis (negative myoclonus), fetor hepaticus (smell of 'pear drops').

Ascites and splenomegaly (less common in acute or hyperacute).

Bruising or bleeding from puncture sites or GI tract.

Look for secondary causes (e.g. bronze skin colour, Kayser–Fleischer rings).

Pyrexia may reflect infection or liver necrosis.

INVESTIGATIONS

Identify the cause: Viral serology, paracetamol levels, autoantibodies (e.g. ASM, LKM antibody, immunoglobulins), ferritin, caeruloplasmin and urinary copper (↓ and ↑, respectively in Wilson's disease).

Blood (in addition to above): FBC: ↓ Hb if GI bleed, ↑ WCC if infection. U&E: May show renal failure (hepatorenal failure). Glucose, LFT (↑ bilirubin, transaminases, AlkPhos, GGT, ↓ albumin), ESR/CRP (inflammatory markers), coagulation screen (↑ PT, INR), ABG (to determine pH), group and save.

Ultrasound liver, CT scan: To image liver.

Ascitic fluid: Tap ascites and send for microscopy, culture, biochemistry (glucose, protein), cytology, >250 neutrophil/mm^3 indicates SBP.

Doppler scanning of hepatic or portal veins: To exclude Budd–Chiari syndrome.

Electroencephalogram: To monitor encephalopathy.

MANAGEMENT

Resuscitation (according to airway, breathing, circulation): ITU care and specialist unit support essential.

Treat the cause if possible: N-acetylcysteine for paracetamol overdose.

Treatment/prevention of complications: Invasive ventilatory and cardiovascular support often required.

- Monitor: Vital signs, PT, pH, creatinine, urine output and encephalopathy.
- Manage encephalopathy: Lactulose and phosphate enemas.
- Antibiotic and antifungal prophylaxis.
- Hypoglycaemia treatment.
- Coagulopathy treatment: IV Vitamin K, FFP, platelet infusions if required.
- Gastric mucosa protection: Proton pump inhibitors or sulcralfate.
- Avoid: Sedatives or drugs metabolized by the liver.
- Cerebral oedema: Nurse patient at 30 °C, ↓ intracranial pressure by IV mannitol, hyperventilate.

Renal failure: Haemofiltration, nutritional support.

Surgical: King's College Hospital criteria for liver transplantation:

If due to paracetamol overdose:
- arterial pH $<$ 7.3, or
- PT $>$ 100 s, creatinine $>$ 300 and severe encephalopathy.

For other causes (three out of five):
- age $<$ 10 or $>$ 40 years,
- bilirubin $>$ 300 μM,
- caused by non-A, non-E viral hepatitis or drugs,
- interval from jaundice onset to encephalopathy $>$7 days, or
- PT $>$ 100 s.

COMPLICATIONS Infection, coagulopathy, hypoglycaemia, disturbances of electrolyte, acid–base and cardiovascular system, hepatorenal syndrome (concurrent hepatic and renal failure), cerebral oedema, ↑ intracranial pressure, respiratory failure.

PROGNOSIS Depends on the severity and aetiology of the liver failure, poor prognostic indicators are shown above under surgical management. The traditional prognostic score for surgical mortality is the Childs–Pugh score. *See* Cirrhosis.

Primary biliary cirrhosis

DEFINITION   PBC is a chronic inflammatory liver disease involving progressive destruction of intrahepatic bile ducts, leading to cholestasis and, ultimately, cirrhosis.

AETIOLOGY   Unknown. Autoimmune aetiology is likely. Genetic and environmental factors have also been proposed. An environmental trigger (possibly infection, chemical or toxin) may cause bile duct epithelial injury. In susceptible individuals, this leads to a T-cell mediated autoimmune response directed against bile duct epithelial cells.

EPIDEMIOLOGY   Prevalence is 10–20 in 100 000 in UK. Usually affects middle-aged women ($\female : \male$ ratio is 9 : 1).

HISTORY   May be an incidental finding on blood tests (e.g. ↑ AlkPhos, ↑ cholesterol). Insidious onset. Fatigue, weight loss and pruritus.
Discomfort in the RUQ of the abdomen (rarely).
May present with a complication of liver decompensation (e.g. jaundice, ascites, variceal haemorrhage).
Symptoms of associated conditions, e.g. Sjögren's syndrome (dry eyes and mouth), arthritis, Raynaud phenomenon.

EXAMINATION
Early: May be no signs.
Late: Jaundice, skin pigmentation, scratch marks, xanthomas (secondary to hypercholesterolaemia), hepatomegaly, ascites and other signs of liver disease may be present.
Signs of chronic liver disease, e.g. palmar erythema, clubbing and spider naevi.

INVESTIGATIONS
Blood: LFT (↑ AlkPhos, ↑ GGT; bilirubin may be normal or ↑ in later stages; transaminases initially normal, ↑ with disease progression and development of cirrhosis), clotting (prolongation of PT). Antimitochondrial antibodies (AMA), ↑ IgM and ↑ cholesterol are typical. TFTs (PBC is associated with autoimmune thyroid disease), plasma calcium, phosphate, 25-hydroxyvitamin D.
Ultrasound: To exclude extrahepatic biliary obstruction (e.g. by gallstones or strictures).
Liver biopsy: Chronic inflammatory cells and granulomas around the intrahepatic bile ducts, destruction of bile ducts, fibrosis and regenerating nodules of hepatocytes. Repeat liver biopsies while on treatment.

MANAGEMENT
Ursodeoxycholic acid (UDCA): A hydrophilic bile acid which may ↓ the toxicity or improve elimination of retained bile acids. UDCA improves the biochemical markers and may improve symptoms and survival. Colchicine and then methotrexate may be added in non-responding patients.
Treatment of symptoms/complications:
Pruritus: Colestyramine (binds bile acids in the GI tract), rifampicin (may work by upregulating liver enzymes that metabolize factors which cause pruritus), naltrexone (opioid receptor antagonist) in patients who do not respond to rifampin.
Metabolic bone disease: Calcium and Vitamin D supplementation. Bisphosphonates (alendronate/risedronate) for osteoporosis, exercise programme, periodic DXA scans.
Vitamin replacement: Vitamin D, Vitamin A. Vitamins E and K may be required in those with advanced disease/liver failure awaiting liver transplantation.
Portal hypertension: β-Blockers and endoscopic banding of varices if present. Transjugular intrahepatic portosystemic shunt (TIPS): A radiological procedure whereby a vascular tract is created in the liver from hepatic to portal veins allowing decompression of the portal hypertension. TIPS ↑ risk of hepatic encephalopathy.

Liver transplantation: For intractable symptoms or end-stage liver disease. Prioritized using the Model for End-stage Liver Disease (MELD) score (validated chronic liver disease severity scoring system that uses serum bilirubin, creatinine and the INR to predict survival).

COMPLICATIONS Cirrhosis and associated complications: Jaundice, encephalopathy, ascites, variceal bleeding, hepatocellular carcinoma, osteoporosis, hyperlipidaemia and malabsorption of fat-soluble vitamins.

PROGNOSIS Rate of disease progression can be variable. Poor prognostic factors are ↑ serum bilirubin, ↓ serum albumin, significant interface hepatitis at the time of diagnosis and poor response to UDCA after 6 months of treatment. Median survival time from diagnosis ∼10 years. The 5-year survival rate after liver transplantation is >70%. PBC can recur in the transplanted liver.

Primary sclerosing cholangitis

DEFINITION   Chronic cholestatic liver disease characterized by progressive inflammatory fibrosis and obliteration of intrahepatic and extrahepatic bile ducts.

AETIOLOGY   Unknown. Postulated immune and genetic predisposition and toxic or infective triggers. Close association with IBD, especially UC (present in 70%). About 5% of those with UC will develop PSC.

EPIDEMIOLOGY   Prevalence 2–7 in 100 000. Usually presents between 25 and 40 years.

HISTORY   May be asymptomatic and diagnosed after persistently ↑ AlkPhos.
May present with intermittent jaundice, pruritus, RUQ pain, weight loss and fatigue.
Episodes of fever and rigors caused by acute cholangitis are less common.
History of ulcerative colitis.
Symptoms of complications.

EXAMINATION   May have no signs or have evidence of jaundice, hepatosplenomegaly, spider naevi, palmar erythema or ascites.

PATHOLOGY/PATHOGENESIS   Periductal inflammation with periductal concentric fibrosis ('onion skin'), portal oedema, bile duct proliferation and expansion of portal tracts, progressive fibrosis and development of biliary cirrhosis.

INVESTIGATIONS
Blood: LFT (↑ AlkPhos, ↑ GGT, mild ↑ transaminases). In later stages, ↓ albumin and ↑ bilirubin.
Serology: Immunoglobulin levels (↑ IgG in children, ↑ IgM in adults), ASM and ANA (present in ~30%), AMA (usually absent), pANCA (present in ~70%).
ERCP: Stricturing and interspersed dilation (beading) of intrahepatic and, occasionally, extrahepatic bile ducts, small diverticula on the common bile duct may be seen.
MRCP: Enables non-invasive imaging of the biliary tree.
Liver biopsy: Confirms diagnosis and allows staging of disease.

MANAGEMENT
Acute cholangitis: Resuscitation (particularly fluid), antibiotics (e.g. cephalosporin and metronidazole).
Medical: No curative treatment with management concentrating on symptom control. Cholestyramine or phototherapy for pruritus (UDCA has unproven efficacy at present), fat-soluble vitamins for deficiency, adequate dietary calcium. Endoscopic or percutaneous transhepatic stenting or balloon dilation of major extrahepatic bile duct strictures to relieve biliary obstruction.
Surgical: Liver transplantation for end-stage disease; a few recurrences in transplanted liver reported. Surgery for any co-existing ulcerative colitis has no effect on the course.

COMPLICATIONS   Recurrent cholangitis, biliary cirrhosis, cholangiocarcinoma (bile duct carcinoma, ~15% of cases), portal hypertension (encephalopathy, ascites/oedema, variceal bleeding), metabolic bone disease.

PROGNOSIS   Variable. Prognostic factors at presentation (Mayo model): Age, bilirubin, biopsy stage (histology), enlarged spleen. Median survival from presentation to liver transplantation or death is about 10 years. Four-year survival after liver transplantation is about 85%.

Wilson's disease

DEFINITION   An autosomal recessive disorder characterized by ↓ biliary excretion of copper and accumulation in the liver and brain, especially in the basal ganglia. Also known as hepatolenticular degeneration.

AETIOLOGY   The gene responsible is on chromosome 13, and codes for a copper-transporting ATPase (ATP7B) in hepatocytes. Mutations interfere with transport of copper into the intracellular compartments for incorporation into caeruloplasmin (and secretion into plasma) or excretion in the bile. Excess copper damages hepatocyte mitochondria, causing cell death and release of free copper into plasma, which is subsequently deposited in other tissues.

EPIDEMIOLOGY   Prevalence ~1 in 30 000, carrier frequency ~1 in 100. Liver disease may present in children (>5 years). Neurological disease usually presents in young adults.

HISTORY
Liver: May present with hepatitis, liver failure or cirrhosis. Jaundice, easy bruising, variceal bleeding, encephalopathy.
Neurological: Dyskinesia, rigidity, tremor, dystonia, dysarthria, dysphagia, drooling, dementia, ataxia.
Psychiatric: Conduct disorder, personality change, psychosis.

EXAMINATION
Liver: Hepatosplenomegaly, jaundice, ascites/oedema, gynaecomastia.
Neurological: As above.
Eyes: Green or brown Kayser–Fleischer ring at the corneal limbus, sunflower cataract (copper accumulation in the lens, seen with slit lamp).

INVESTIGATIONS
Blood: LFT (↑ AST, ALT and AlkPhos), serum caeruloplasmin and copper (low but may provide false-negatives as caeruloplasmin is an acute phase protein).
Twenty-four-hour urinary copper levels: Increased.
Liver biopsy: ↑ Copper content.
Genetic analysis: Wide variety of mutations in the gene cause the disease, so there is no simple genetic test and sequencing requires specialist genetic advice.

MANAGEMENT
Medical: Best managed by a specialist unit. Treat with copper chelators (e.g. D-penicillamine or trientine). Oral zinc (induces intestinal cell metallothionein which binds copper impairing absorption). Monitor urinary copper. General care for liver and neurological disease.
Genetic: Counselling and offer screening for relatives.
Surgery: Liver transplantation may be necessary.

COMPLICATIONS   Cirrhosis, permanent CNS damage, gallstones (caused by haemolysis), copper-induced renal tubular damage causing hypercalciuria, phosphaturia and osteomalacia, renal tubular acidosis.

PROGNOSIS   Severe liver disease and neurological damage have poor outcome. Early detection and treatment improves prognosis.

Glomerulonephritis

DEFINITION   Glomerulonephritis is immunologically mediated inflammation of renal glomeruli.

AETIOLOGY   There are many different types of glomerulonephritis with differing aetiologies. Some types of glomerulonephritis are ascribed to deposition of antigen–antibody immune complexes in the glomeruli that lead to inflammation and activation of complement and coagulation cascades. The immune complexes may either form within the glomerulus (more commonly) or be deposited from the circulation. The antigens in the immune complexes are often unknown but may occasionally be associated with the following:

Infection: *Bacterial*: *Streptococcus viridans*, group A β-haemolytic streptococci, staphylococci, gonococci, *Salmonella*, syphilis.

Viral: Hepatitis B/C, HIV, measles, mumps, EBV, VZV, coxsackie.

Protozoal: *Plasmodium malariae*, schistosomiasis, filariasis.

Inflammatory/systemic diseases: SLE, systemic vasculitis, cryoglobulinaemia.[1]

Drugs: Gold, penicillamine.

Tumours:

Classified based on the site of nephron pathology and its distribution.

Minimal-change glomerulonephritis: Normal appearance on light microscopy. Electron microscopy: Loss of epithelial foot processes.

Membranous glomerulonephritis: Thickening of GBM from immune complex deposition. Associated with Goodpasture's syndrome.[2]

Membranoproliferative glomerulonephritis (MPGN): Thickening of GBM, mesangial cell proliferation and interposition.

Type 1: Subendothelial immune complex deposits and reduplication of GBM.

Type 2: Dense intramembranous deposits (stain only for C3).

Focal segmental glomerulosclerosis: Glomerular scarring. Associated with HIV.

Focal segmental proliferative glomerulonephritis: Mesangial and endothelial cell proliferation. 'Focal' refers to involvement of some of the glomeruli, 'segmental' refers to involvement of parts of individual glomeruli.

Diffuse proliferative glomerulonephritis: Same as above but affects all glomeruli.

IgA nephropathy: Mesangial cell proliferation and mesangial IgA and C3 deposits.

Crescentric glomerulonephritis: Crescent formation by macrophages and epithelial cells, which fills up Bowman's space.

Focal segmental necrotizing glomerulonephritis: Peripheral capillary loop necrosis (e.g. in Wegener's granulomatosis, microscopic polyarteritis and other vasculitides). Often evolves into crescentric glomerulonephritis.

EPIDEMIOLOGY   Makes up to 25% of cases of chronic renal failure.

HISTORY   Haematuria, subcutaneous oedema, polyuria or oliguria, proteinuria. History of recent infection.

Symptoms of uraemia or renal failure (acute and chronic).

---

[1]Cryoglobulins are immunoglobulins that precipitate in cold, and may be monoclonal or polyclonal. They can cause cutaneous vasculitis.

[2]Goodpasture's syndrome result from anti-GBM antibody that binds to an antigen in the basement membrane. The antibody also reacts with pulmonary capillary basement membrane and can cause pulmonary haemorrhage.

Glomerulonephritis (continued)

EXAMINATION   May present with the signs of the following:

- hypertension;
- proteinuria (<3 g/24 h);
- haematuria (microscopic or macroscopic, especially IgA nephropathy);
- nephrotic syndrome (usually for minimal-change glomerulonephritis in children and membranous glomerulonephritis in adults; see nephrotic syndrome);
- nephritic syndrome (haematuria, proteinuria, subcutaneous oedema, oliguria, hypertension, uraemia);
- renal failure (acute or chronic); and
- partial lipodystrophy (loss of subcutaneous fat in MPGN type II).

INVESTIGATIONS   *Blood*: FBC, U&E and creatinine, LFT (albumin), lipid profile, complement studies (C3, C4, C3 nephritic factor in MPGN), ANA, anti-double stranded DNA, ANCA, anti-GBM antibody, cryoglobulins if appropriate.
Urine: Microscopy (dysmorphic RBCs, red-cell casts), 24-h collection: creatinine clearance, protein.
Imaging: Renal tract ultrasound (to exclude other pathology).
Renal biopsy: Light microscopy, electron microscopy, immunofluorescence microscopy.
Investigations for associated infections: e.g. hepatitis B, hepatitis C or HIV serology.

MANAGEMENT   *Fluid balance*: Monitor input/output and weight changes, avoid added salt and restrict fluid if there are signs of fluid overload or ↑ BP.
Treatment of complications: (*see* hypertension; renal failure, acute; renal failure, chronic; nephrotic syndrome).
Focal necrotizing glomerulonephritis, rapidly progressive crescentric glomerulonephritis, glomerulonephritis associated with SLE, primary vasculitides: Steroids, azathioprine, ciclosporin A, cyclophosphamide.
Consider plasma exchange, especially for severe disease affecting the basement membrane.

COMPLICATIONS   Pulmonary oedema: ↑ Risk of hypertension, hypertensive encephalopathy. Renal failure. Complications of nephrotic syndrome. Pre-eclampsia in pregnancy.

PROGNOSIS   Minimal-change glomerulonephritis and post-infective diffuse proliferative glomerulonephritis mostly resolve.
Risk of CRF: Focal segmental sclerosis 50–75%; focal proliferative glomerulonephritis 25%; membranous glomerulonephritis ~30%; MPGN >75%.
Poor prognostic factors: ↑ Creatinine when first seen, ↑ BP, persistent proteinuria.

Nephrotic syndrome

DEFINITION   Characterized by proteinuria (>3 g/24 h), hypoalbuminaemia (<30 g/L), oedema and hypercholesterolaemia.

AETIOLOGY   Commonest cause is minimal change glomerulonephritis in children, but all forms of glomerulonephritis can cause nephrotic syndrome.
Other causes: Diabetes mellitus, sickle cell disease, amyloidosis, malignancies (lung and GI adenocarcinomas), drugs (NSAIDs), Alport's syndrome, HIV infection.

EPIDEMIOLOGY   Most common cause of nephrotic syndrome in children (90%): minimal change glomerulonephritis (usually seen in boys <5 years, rare in black populations).
Most common causes of nephrotic syndrome in adults: diabetes mellitus, membranous glomerulonephritis.

HISTORY   Family history of atopy in those with minimal change glomerulonephritis, family history of renal disease.
Swelling of face, abdomen, limbs, genitalia.
Symptoms of the underlying cause (e.g. SLE).
Symptoms of complications (e.g. renal vein thrombosis: loin pain, haematuria).

EXAMINATION   *Oedema*: Periorbital, peripheral, genital.
Ascites: Fluid thrill, shifting dullness.

PATHOLOGY/PATHOGENESIS   Structural damage to the basement membrane or the reduction in the negatively charged components within it reduces the filtration of large protein molecules by the glomerulus, causing proteinuria and hypoalbuminaemia.

INVESTIGATIONS   *Blood*: FBC, U&E, LFT (↓ albumin), ESR/CRP, glucose, lipid profile (secondary hyperlipidaemia), immunoglobulins, complement (C3, C4).
Tests to identify the underlying cause of glomerulonephritis:
SLE: ANA, anti-dsDNA.
Infections: Group A β-haemolytic streptococcal infection (ASO titre), HBV infection (serology), plasmodium malariae (blood films).
Goodpasture's syndrome: Anti-glomerular basement membrane antibodies.
Vasculitides: e.g. Wegener's and microscopic polyarteritis (ANCA).
Urine: Urinalysis (protein, blood), microscopy, culture, sensitivity, 24-h collection (to calculate creatinine clearance and 24-h protein excretion).
Renal ultrasound: Excludes other renal diseases that may cause proteinuria, e.g. reflux nephropathy.
Renal biopsy: In all adults and in children who have unusual features or do not respond to steroids.
Other imaging: Doppler ultrasound, renal angiogram, CT or MRI are options if renal vein thrombosis is suspected.

MANAGEMENT   *Treat oedema:*
- Fluid restriction (~1 L/day),
- Na + restriction (~50 mmol/day),
- diuretics (e.g. oral furosemide ± metolazone or spironolactone),
- occasionally, IV diuretics and salt-poor albumin may be required for initiation of diuresis.

Treat the cause:
- *Minimal change glomerulonephritis*: High-dose steroids (60 mg for 2 months) and gradually ↓ the dose, treat relapses (~40% within 3 years) with steroids, immunosuppressants: cyclophosphamide or ciclosporin for steroid non-responders or those with relapses.
- *Membranous glomerulonephritis*: The benefit of steroids and immunosuppressants is uncertain.
- *SLE*: Corticoteroids, cyclophosphamide.

Nephrotic syndrome (continued)

Monitor:
- BP, U&E, weight, fluid balance.
- *Thromboprophylaxis*: Heparin.

COMPLICATIONS   Renal failure (caused by hypovolaemia especially following diuretics, renal vein thrombosis, progression of underlying renal disease), ↑ susceptibility to infection (e.g. peritonitis, pneumococcal because of loss of immunoglobulins and lipid content in the urine), thrombosis (e.g. renal vein and DVT caused by hypovolaemia and hypercoagulable state caused by loss of antithrombin in the urine and ↑ synthesis of fibrinogen in the liver), hyperlipidaemia (possibly caused by ↑ synthesis of trigylcerides and cholesterol along with albumin in the liver).

PROGNOSIS   Varies according to the underlying condition and presence of complications.

Polycystic kidney disease (PKD)

DEFINITION Autosomal dominant inherited disorder characterized by the development of multiple renal cysts that gradually expand and replace normal kidney substance, variably associated with extrarenal (liver and cardiovascular) abnormalities.

AETIOLOGY Eighty five percent are mutations in *PKD1* (polycystin-1) on chromosome 16, a membrane-bound multidomain protein involved in cell–cell and cell–matrix interactions; 15% are mutations in *PKD2* (polycystin-2) on chromosome 4, a Ca^{2+} permeable cation channel.

Pathological process is considered to be a proliferative/hyperplastic abnormality of the tubular epithelium. In early stages, cysts are connected to the tubules from which they arise and the fluid content is glomerular filtrate. When cyst diameter >2 mm, most detach from the patent tubule and the fluid content is derived from secretions of the lining epithelium. With time, cysts enlarge and cause progressive damage to adjacent functioning nephrons.

EPIDEMIOLOGY Most commonly inherited kidney disorder affecting one in 800, responsible for nearly 10% of end-stage renal failure in adults.

HISTORY Usually present at 30–40 years. Twenty percent have no family history.
May be asymptomatic.
Pain in flanks as a result of cyst enlargement/bleeding, stone, blood clot migration, infection.
Haematuria (may be gross).
Hypertension.
Associated with intracranial 'berry' aneurysms and may present with subarachnoid haemorrhage: sudden onset headache.

EXAMINATION Abdominal distension, enlarged cystic kidneys and liver palpable, hypertension. Signs of chronic renal failure at late stage.
Signs of associated aortic aneurysm or aortic valve disease.

INVESTIGATIONS *Ultrasound or CT imaging*: Multiple cysts observed bilaterally in enlarged kidneys, sensitivity of detection poor for those <20 years. Liver cysts may also be seen.

MANAGEMENT *Blood pressure control*: Slows the rate of decline in renal function and minimizes the risk of rupture of a cerebral aneurysm. ACE inhibitors can effectively ↓ blood pressure and minimize the degree of secondary glomerular injury by ↓ intraglomerular pressure.
Haematuria: Managed conservatively.
Infections: Prompt treatment with non-nephrotoxic antibiotics (ciprofloxacin or co-trimoxazole). Avoid the use of NSAIDs.
End-stage renal failure: (*see* renal failure, chronic).
Consider screening for intracranial aneurysm if family history of aneurysm.
Surgery: Cyst decompression reserved for selected cases. Liver cyst aspiration, marsupialization or resection if gives rise to pain.
Genetic counselling.

COMPLICATIONS Chronic renal failure, renal stones (20%).
1–2% suffer subarachnoid haemorrhage/intracerebral bleed.
Cysts develop in the liver (70%) and pancreas (10%) but these rarely cause organ dysfunction. Mitral valve prolapse, diverticulosis of the colon.

PROGNOSIS Fifty percent develop end-stage renal failure by age 60 years. Renal replacement therapy prolongs life by 15 years (mean). Patients with hypertension are much more likely to develop progressive renal failure.

Renal artery stenosis

DEFINITION   Stenosis of the renal artery.

AETIOLOGY   *Main cause:*
- Atherosclerosis (older patient): Widespread aortic disease involving the renal artery ostia.
- Fibromuscular dysplasia (younger patient): Fibromuscular dysplasia is of unknown aetiology but may be associated with collagen disorders, neurofibromatosis and Takayasu's disease. This may be associated with micro-aneurysms in the mid and distal renal arteries (resembling string of beads on angiography).

EPIDEMIOLOGY   Prevalence is unknown but believed to account for 1–5% of all hypertension; fibromuscular dysplasia occurs mainly in women with hypertension at <45 years.

HISTORY   History of hypertension in <50 years.
Hypertension refractory to treatment.
Accelerated hypertension and renal deterioration on starting ACE inhibitor.
History of flash pulmonary oedema.

EXAMINATION
Hypertension.
Signs of renal failure in advanced bilateral disease.
An abdominal bruit may be heard over the stenosed artery.

PATHOLOGY/PATHOGENESIS   Renal hypoperfusion stimulates the renin-angiotensin system leading to ↑ circulating angiotensin II and aldosterone, increasing BP, which in turn, with time, causes fibrosis, glomerosclerosis and renal failure.

INVESTIGATIONS   *Non-invasive*: Duplex ultrasound (technically difficult if obese). Ultrasound measurement of kidney size (predicts outcome after revascularization, kidneys <8 cm are unlikely to improve).
CT angiography or MRA: Often used now; risk of contrast nephrotoxicity.
Digital subtraction angiography: Gold standard assessment.
Renal scintigraphy: Uses the radio-agent ^{99}Tc-DTPA (excreted by glomerular filtration) or ^{99}Tc -MAG3 (excreted by tubules). Addition of an ACE inhibitor (captopril renography) causes delayed clearance by the affected kidney (may not be helpful if bilateral RAS).

MANAGEMENT   *Medical*: Pharmacological control of hypertension. In atherosclerotic cases, medical treatment is often preferred together with modulation of other cardiovascular risk factors. Avoidance of ACE inhibitors and other nephrotoxic agents.
Intervention: In cases of uncontrolled hypertension, progressive renal failure, flash pulmonary oedema, stenoses >60%.
Angioplasty +/– stenting: Treatment of choice for fibromuscular dysplasia, less effective in atherosclerotic cases.
Surgical revascularisation: Several approaches are used, e.g. aortorenal bypass using saphenous vein or synthetic grafts (PTFE or Dacron), aortic replacement and renal reconstruction, endarterectomy of atherosclerotic RAS, extra-anatomical bypass (hepatorenal on right, splenorenal on left).

COMPLICATIONS   Drug-refractory hypertension, renal failure.
Of angioplasty: Restenosis (occurs in up to 20%), rarely renal artery rupture or thrombotic occlusion may require emergency surgery (with high mortality ~40%).

PROGNOSIS   Untreated hypertension will progress to renal failure. With intervention 50–70% will have improvement in BP and renal function. Curative in 15%.

Renal calculi

DEFINITION   Different types include calcium oxalate (65%), calcium phosphate (15%) magnesium ammonium phosphate (10–15%), uric acid (2–5%), cystine (1%)[1].

AETIOLOGY   Commonly idiopathic or caused by dehydration or urinary tract infections. Other risk factors are:

Changes in urinary pH: Calcium oxalate, calcium phosphate and magnesium ammonium phosphate stones arise in alkaline urine, cystine and uric acid stones arise in acid urine.

Hypercalciuria: Usually idiopathic, drug (lithium, thiazides).

Hypercalcaemia: Malignancy, hyperparathyroidism, sarcoidosis, myeloma, ↑ calcium intake ('milk-alkali syndrome').

Hyperoxaluria: Causes: ↑ intake (in rhubarb, spinach, strawberries, tea, tomatoes, beetroots, beans, chocolate, nuts), ↑ colonic absorption in patients with small bowel disease or resection, autosomally recessive inherited enzyme deficiency → ↑ oxalate production and excretion.

Hyperuricaemia: Tumour lysis syndrome, high cell turnover states.

Cystinuria: Autosomal recessive, defect of renal tubular transport of cystine and dibasic amino acids.

Anatomical anomalies: e.g. horseshoe kidneys.

EPIDEMIOLOGY   UK prevalence 2%, lifetime incidence up to 12%. Peak age of presentation 20–50 years. ♂: ♀ ∼ 2:1.

HISTORY AND EXAMINATION   May be asymptomatic.

Pain: Loin pain (kidney stones). Renal colic radiating from loin → groin, scrotum, labium (ureteric stones). Dysuria, frequency, strangury, penile tip pain (bladder stones). Urinary retention and bladder distension (urethral stones).

Haematuria.

Symptoms of urinary tract infection and obstruction.

INVESTIGATIONS   *Blood*: U&E, calcium, phosphate, albumin.

PTH, vitamin D, urate, bicarbonate, serum ACE, thyroid function.

Urine: Urinalysis (blood, protein, nitrites), microscopy and culture. 24-h collection: creatinine clearance, calcium, phosphate, oxalate and urate. Random urine for cystine, glyoxolate, citrate.

Plain radiography ('KUB'): Shows radio-opaque stones (calcium oxalate stones are radio-opaque, cystine stones are semi-opaque, urate stones are radio-lucent).

Intravenous urograpm (IVU): IV contrast followed by radiographs may show a filling defect in the urinary outflow.

High resolution helical CT-abdomen: High diagnostic accuracy and can visualise radio-lucent calculi.

Renal ultrasound: To assess for hydronephrosis or hydroureter.

Chemical analysis of the stone: If passed.

---

[1]Appearances of renal calculi depend on composition:
Calcium oxalate: 'Mulberry' stones with spiky surface, dark (covered by blood from the mucosa of the renal pelvis injured by the sharp projections).
Calcium phosphate and magnesium ammonium phosphate: Smooth, may be large and take the shape of calyces. 'Staghorn' calculi, dirty white.
Uric acid: Hard, smooth, faceted, yellow/light brown. These are radiolucent.
Cystine: Translucent, white.

Renal calculi (continued)

MANAGEMENT *Medical Expulsive Treatment*: Suitable for <10 mm calculi.
Opiate and NSAID analgesics.
Rehydration (Oral or IV).
Treat exarcebtaing factors and UTI.
Calcium channel antagonists (e.g. nifedipine) reduce ureteric spasm.
Alpha-antagonists (e.g. tamsulosin) reduce ureteric spasm.

Extracorporeal shockwave lithotripsy (ESWL): Provides non-invasive outpatient treatment and usually combined with medical treatment. Usually suitable for smaller stones in the kidneys or ureter.

Cystoscopy: allows visualization of the stone and urinary tract as well as laser to break up the stone.

Percutaneous nephrolithotomy: May be necessary for calculi >2 cm or not suitable for other modalities.

Prevention: ↑ Fluid intake (e.g. >3 L/day avoiding high Ca^{2+} water).

Calcium stones: ↓ calcium and vitamin D intake.

Oxalate stones: ↓ oxalate-containing foods and vitamin C intake.

Uric acid stones: Allopurinol (inhibits xanthine oxidase and uric acid synthesis), urinary alkalization (oral sodium bicarbonate).

Cystine stones: D-penicillamine, urinary alkalinization.

COMPLICATIONS Obstruction and hydronephrosis, infection, complications of the cause, e.g. renal failure in primary hyperoxaluria.

PROGNOSIS Approximately 20% of calculi will not pass spontaneously. Up to 50% of patients may have recurrence within 5 years.

Renal failure (acute)

DEFINITION   Impairment of renal function over days or weeks, which often results in ↑ plasma urea/creatinine and oliguria (<400 mL/day) and is usually reversible. The term acute kidney injury (AKI) represents the full spectrum of acute kidney dysfunction.

AETIOLOGY   Pre-renal (↓ renal perfusion):
Shock (hypovolaemic, septic, cardiogenic), hepatorenal syndrome (liver failure).
Renal:
Acute tubular necrosis (ATN): Ischaemia, drugs and toxins (paracetamol, aminoglycosides, amphotericin B, NSAIDs, ACE-inhibtors, lithium).
Acute glomerulonephritis.
Acute interstitial nephritis: NSAIDs, penicillins, sulphonamides, leptospirosis.
Small or large vessel obstruction: Renal artery/vein thrombosis, cholesterol emboli, vasculitis, haemolytic microangipathy (e.g. HUS or TTP).
Others: Light-chain (myeloma), urate (lympho- or myeloproliferative disorders, particularly after chemotherapy/radiation induced cell lysis), pigment (haemolysis, rhabdomyolysis, malaria) nephropathy, accelerated phase hypertension (e.g. in pre-eclampsia).
Post-renal: Stone, tumour (pelvic, prostate, bladder), blood clots, retroperitoneal fibrosis.

EPIDEMIOLOGY   A population-based study estimates an incidence of 1800 per million.

HISTORY   Malaise, anorexia, nausea, vomiting, pruritus, drowsiness, convulsions, coma (caused by uraemia). Symptoms of the cause or complications usually dominate (see below).

EXAMINATION   Oedema, signs of the cause and complications (see below).

INVESTIGATIONS   Blood: ABG, FBC, U&E (urea, creatinine, Na^+, K^+), LFT, ESR/CRP, Ca^{2+}, clotting, culture, blood film: red cell fragmentation in HUS/TTP.
Other blood tests: CK (for rhabdomyolysis), urate, serum electrophoresis and autoantibodies.
Urine:*Stick testing*: Haematuria, proteinuria (e.g. glomerulonephritis).
Microscopy: Red cell casts (in glomerulonephritis). *Culture* and *sensitivity*. *Bence-Jones protein* (exclude myeloma). *Urine osmolality/Na$^+$*:
- *Renal ARF*: ↓ Urine osmolality/specific gravity (as a result of ↓ renal concentrating ability), ↑ urine Na^+ (as a result of ↓ reabsorptive ability), ↑ fractional excretion of Na^+ ($P_{Cr}U_{Na}/P_{Na}U_{Cr}$): >2%.
- *Pre-renal ARF*: ↑ Urine osmolality, ↓ urine Na^+, ↓ fractional excretion of Na^+ (<1%).
CXR: To monitor for fluid overload.
ECG: Check for hyperkalaemia (tented T waves).
Renal ultrasound: To exclude an obstructive cause.
Renal biopsy (e.g. acute tubulointerstitial nephritis: tubulitis and intense interstitial cellular infiltrate including eosinophils).

MANAGEMENT   *Assess hydration and fluid balance*: Pulse rate, lying and standing BP, JVP, skin turgor, chest auscultation, ?peripheral oedema, CVP, fluid and weight charts.
Treat the complications:
Hyperkalaemia (if ECG changes or $K^+ > 7$ mmol/L):
- 10 mL of 10% calcium gluconate IV (protect the myocardium) and ECG monitoring.
- 50 mL 50% dextrose with 5U actrapid insulin over 15 min (drive K^+ into cells).
- Nebulized salbutamol can also ↓ K^+.
- Ca^{2+}/Na^+ resonium PO/PR (↓ bowel absorption).
- Contact renal team and arrange for dialysis if appropriate (see below).

Metabolic acidosis (if pH < 7.2):
- 50–100 mL of 8.4% bicarbonate via central line over 15–30 min.

Pulmonary oedema:
- O_2, consider CPAP.
- IV GTN 2–10 mg/h.

Renal failure (acute) (continued)

- IV furosemide: 250 mg over 1 h, followed by infusion (5–10 mg/h).
- IV diamorphine (single dose of 2.5 mg) relieves anxiety and breathlessness.

Treat the cause:
- *IV fluids* if volume depleted: 500 mL colloid or 0.9% saline over 30 min, assess response (i.e. urine output/CVP), continue fluids until CVP ~5–10 cm. *Inotropes* if hypotension persists in spite of CVP of >10 cm.
- *Treatment of infection:* adjust the dose of antibiotics *in view of the renal im*pairment.
- *Stop the nephrotoxic drugs* (e.g. ACEI and NSAIDs) and non-essential drugs.
- *Identify intrinsic renal disease* and treat.
- *Relieve the obstruction* e.g. urinary catheter, nephrostomies.

Optimize nutritional support.
Identify and treat bleeding tendency: Prophylaxis with PPIs or H2 antagonist, transfuse if required, avoid aspirin.
Indications for haemofiltration/dialysis (see below): Persistent hyperkalaemia ($K^+ > 7$ mmol/L), fluid overload (e.g. refractory pulmonary oedema), pericarditis, acidosis (arterial pH < 7.1, bicarbonate <12 mmol/L), symptomatic uraemia (tremor, cognitive impairment, coma, fits, urea typically >45 mmol/L).

Haemofiltration (continuous arteriovenous or venous–venous): Filtration of plasma water across the membrane induced by the hydrostatic pressure gradient, and 'convective' transport of solutes in the same direction as water. Substitution fluid is required to prevent excessive fluid removal.
Dialysis: Intermittent haemodialysis (using central venous catheters or arteriovenous fistulae) or peritoneal dialysis (using a double cuff straight Tenckhoff catheter). Solutes passively diffuse down their concentration gradient (urea, creatinine and potassium move from blood to dialysate, calcium and bicarbonate, move from dialysate to blood).
Venesect ~250–500 mL if delay for dialysis.
The choice of modality depends upon: availability, expertise, haemodynamic stability, vascular access, and whether the primary need is for fluid and/or solute removal. Haemofiltration is preferred in hypotensive or haemodynamically unstable patients since the rate of fluid and solute removal is slow.

Treatment of pigment/light chain/urate nephropathy
Pigment nephropathy: Isotonic saline to maintain diuresis of ~200–300 mL/h. Careful monitoring for fluid overload. If a diuresis is established, switch to an alkaline solution (bicarbonate). ↑ Urine pH to >6.5 may ↓ release of free iron from myoglobin and intratubular pigment deposition and cast formation. If the desired diuresis is not established with adequate volume repletion alone: loop diuretics or mannitol (if mannitol is used, monitor plasma osmolality).
Myeloma cast nephropathy: Thalidomide and dexamethasone to ↓ light chain production. Isotonic fluids (aim urine output ≥3 L/day), careful monitoring for fluid overload.
Urate nephropathy: Allopurinol, loop diuretic and fluids (to wash out the obstructing uric acid crystals). Haemodialysis if diuresis cannot be induced.

COMPLICATIONS *Common and life-threatening:* Hyperkalaemia, sepsis, metabolic acidosis, pulmonary oedema, hypertension.
Less common: Gastric ulceration, bleeding (platelet dysfunction), muscle wasting (hypercatabolic state), uraemic pericarditis, uraemic encephalopathy, acute cortical necrosis.

PROGNOSIS ATN has biphasic recovery starting with oliguria then leading to polyuria (resulting from regeneration of the tubular cells). Prognosis depends on the number of other organs involved, e.g. heart, lung. Many of those with ATN recover. Acute cortical necrosis may cause hypertension and chronic renal failure.

Renal failure (chronic)

DEFINITION   Chronic renal failure or chronic kidney disease (CKD) is defined as either kidney damage or GFR $<60\,mL/min/1.73\,m^2$ for 3 months. Kidney damage is defined as pathologic abnormalities or markers of damage, including abnormalities in blood or urine tests or imaging studies.

Stage	GFR (mL/min/1.73 m²)
1	≥90
2	60–89
3	30–59
4	15–29
5	<15

AETIOLOGY   Diabetes mellitus and hypertension are the two most common causes.
Vascular disease: Hypertension, renal artery atheroma, vasculitis.
Glomerular disease: Glomerulonephritis, diabetes, amyloid, SLE.
Tubulointerstitial disease: Pyelonephritis/interstitial nephritis, nephrocalcinosis, tuberculosis.
Obstruction and others: Myeloma, HIV nephropathy, scleroderma, gout, renal tumour, inborn errors of metabolism (e.g. Fabry's disease).
Congenital/inherited: Polycystic kidney disease, Alport's syndrome, congenital hypoplasia.

EPIDEMIOLOGY   Incidence of end-stage CRF in England >110 per million population per year. Higher incidence in Asian immigrants than native British population.

HISTORY   Anorexia, nausea, malaise, pruritus. Later: diarrhoea, drowsiness, convulsions, coma.
Symptoms of the cause and other complications.

EXAMINATION   *Systemic*: Kussmaul's breathing (acidosis), signs of anaemia, oedema, pigmentation, scratch marks.
Hands: Leuconychia, brown line at distal end of nail.
There may be an arteriovenous fistula (buzzing lump in wrist or forearm).
Signs of complications (e.g. neuropathy, renal bone disease).

INVESTIGATIONS   *Blood*: FBC (↓ Hb: normochromic, normocytic), U&E (↓ urea and creatinine), eGFR (can be derived from creatinine and age using the MDRD calculator), ↓Ca^{2+}, ↑ phosphate, AlkPhos, PTH.
Investigate for suspected aetiology: e.g. ANCA, ANA, glucose.
24-h urine collection: Protein, creatinine clearance (which is a rough estimate of GFR).
Imaging: Signs of osteomalacia and hyperparathyroidism. CXR may show pericardial effusion or pulmonary oedema.
Renal ultrasound: Measure size, exclude obstruction and visualize structure.
Renal biopsy: For changes specific to the underlying disease, contraindicated for small kidneys.

MANAGEMENT   Treat the underlying cause: Control diabetes
Manage complications of chronic kidney disease:
- *Anaemia*: Correct iron stores. Regular IV or SC erythropoietin (usually monthly).
- *BP control*: ACE inhibitors and Angiotensin-II antagonists (caution with renal artery stenosis).
- *Hypocalcaemia*: Maintain serum levels with 1-hydroxylated vitamin D analogues, e.g. alfacalcidol. Consider bisphosphonates.
- *Diet*: High-energy intake, potassium intake restriction (in hyperkalaemia or acidosis, oral $NaHCO_3$ may be required), restriction of protein and phosphate intake (using phosphate binders, e.g. calcium bicarbonate or aluminium hydroxide to ↓ phosphate absorption).

Renal failure (chronic) (continued)

- *Drugs*: Avoid nephrotoxic drugs (e.g. NSAIDs). Dose adjustments for drugs excreted from kidneys.
- *Oedema*: Diuretics, e.g. furosemide (frusemide), metolazone.

Renal replacement therapy:
- *Peritoneal dialysis (CAPD)*: Dialysate is introduced and exchanged through a 'Tenkoff' catheter, inserted via a subcutaneous tunnel into the peritoneum.
- *Haemodialysis*: Blood is removed via an arteriovenous fistula surgically constructed in the wrist or forearm to provide high flow. Uraemic toxins are removed by diffusion across a semipermeable membrane in an extracorporeal circuit (this may activate coagulation so patients are heparinized).
- *Renal transplantation*: Requires long-term immunosuppressants to ↓ rejection (e.g. steroids, ciclosporin A, tacrolimus, azathioprine, daclizumab).

COMPLICATIONS *Haematological*: Anaemia (↓ erythropoietin production, ↓ marrow activity, ↓ RBC survival, ↓ dietary Fe/folate, ↑ blood loss: haemodialysis/sampling), abnormal platelet activity (bruising, epistaxis).
CVS: Accelerated atherosclerosis, ↑ BP, pericarditis.
Neuromuscular: Peripheral & autonomic neuropathy, myopathy.
Renal osteodystrophy: Osteoporosis, osteomalacia (↓ 1α-hydroxylation of vitamin D), secondary or tertiary hyperparathyroidism, adynamic bone disease (↓ bone turnover and fractures secondary to excessive suppression of the parathyroid gland with current therapies), osteosclerosis.
Endocrine: Amenorrhoea, erectile impotence, infertility.
Peritoneal dialysis: Peritonitis (e.g. staphylococcus epidermidis).
Haemodialysis:
- *Acute*: Hypotension (excessive removal of extracellular fluid).
- *Long-term*:
  - Atherosclerosis.
  - Sepsis (secondary to peritonitis, Staph. aureus infection).
  - Amyloidosis: Failure of removal of β2-microglobulin (component of HLA molecules) by dialysis membranes → periarticular deposition → arthralgia (e.g. shoulder) and carpal tunnel syndrome.
  - Aluminum toxicity: Accumulation of aluminum from the dialysis fluid and phosphate binders → dementia, osteodystrophy, microcytic anaemia (rare).

Transplantation/immunosuppression: ↑ BP, opportunistic infections (e.g. CMV), malignancies (lymphomas and skin), recurrence of renal disease (e.g. Goodpasture's syndrome), side-effects of drugs (e.g. steroids: features of iatrogenic Cushing's syndrome; ciclosporin: gum hyperplasia).

PROGNOSIS   Depends on complications. Timely dialysis and transplantation ↑ survival.

Renal tubular acidosis

DEFINITION Normal anion gap metabolic acidosis caused by impaired renal H^+ secretion or bicarbonate reabsorption.

Type 1: $\downarrow H^+$ secretion in distal renal tubules.

Autoimmune/hyperglobulinaemic conditions (Sjögren's syndrome, SLE, rheumatoid arthritis, PBC). Sickle cell disease. Obstructive uropathy. Renal transplantation. Toxic (amphotericin, lithium, ifosfamide). Familial (autosomal dominant/recessive).

Type 2: $\downarrow$ Bicarbonate reabsorption in proximal renal tubules.

Hereditary (part of Fanconi's syndrome along with glycosuria/phosphaturia/amino aciduria, fructose intolerance, cystinosis, Wilson's disease, tyrosinaemia). Myeloma. Amyloidosis. Vitamin D deficiency. Drugs/toxins (acetazolamide, ifosfamide, heavy metals). Hyperparathyroidism. Paroxysmal nocturnal haemoglobinuria.

Type 4: $\downarrow$ Renin and aldosterone or tubular resistance to the action of aldosterone. Metabolic acidosis is due to suppression of ammonia excretion by hyperkalemia.

Diabetic nephropathy, pyelonephritis (tubulo-interstitial disease). Drugs (potassium-sparing diuretics, NSAIDs, ACE inhibitors, ciclosporin, heparin). HIV infections.

EPIDEMIOLOGY Type 4 is the most common. Types 1 and 2 are rare.

HISTORY
Often asymptomatic.

Type 1: Symptoms of hypokalaemia (muscle weakness), renal stones (hypercalciuria occurs secondary to the effects of chronic acidosis on both bone resorption and the renal tubular reabsorption of calcium).

Type 2: Symptoms of hypokalaemia (muscle weakness), osteomalacia/rickets, failure to thrive/grow (children).

Type 4: Symptoms of the associated condition e.g. diabetes mellitus.

EXAMINATION
Types 1 and 2: Weakness.
Type 4: Signs of the underlying cause, e.g. diabetes mellitus.

INVESTIGATIONS ABG: Normal anion gap (hyperchloraemic) metabolic acidosis: $\downarrow$ pH, $\downarrow HCO3^-$, $\uparrow Cl^-$, $\downarrow Pco_2$. (anion gap $= [Na^+ + K^+] - [Cl^- + HCO3^-]$). In normal anion gap metabolic acidosis, $\downarrow HCO3^-$ is accompanied by an $\uparrow Cl^-$.

$\downarrow$ Plasma renin activity and aldosterone levels in type 4.

U&Es: $\downarrow K^+$ (type 1 and 2). $\uparrow K^+$ in type 4.

Urine pH: >5.5 in type 1. Variable in type 2. <5.3 in type 4.

IV sodium bicarbonate infusion:

Type 1: Fractional excretion of bicarbonate[1] <3%, urine pH will remain relatively stable.

Type 2: Fractional excretion of bicarbonate >15%, urine pH will be >7.5.

Imaging: Abdominal film of kidney–ureters–bladder (may show calculi/nephrocalcinosis).

Determine the underlying cause.

MANAGEMENT Treat the underlying condition, e.g. stop causative drug.

Type 1 and 2: Potassium citrate (or sodium bicarbonate). Higher doses of alkali are required in type 2. Thiazide diuretics may be given to $\downarrow$ alkali requirements (mild volume depletion $\uparrow$ proximal reabsorption of sodium and secondarily that of bicarbonate).

Phosphate and vitamin D supplementation (type 2).

Type 4: Most patients respond to restriction of dietary potassium and, if necessary, diuretics. Fludrocortisone is not often used because hypertension, heart failure, and oedema may be exacerbated in patients with renal insufficiency.

---

[1](Urine bicarbonate x plasma creatinine)/(plasma bicarbonate x urine plasma creatinine).

Renal tubular acidosis (continued)

COMPLICATIONS   Nephrocalcinosis, nephrolithiasis, UTI (type 1). Osteomalacia/rickets in type 2 (hypophosphataemia due to ↓ proximal phosphate reabsorption may contribute to this). Complications of the associated disease (e.g. diabetes mellitus in type 4).

PROGNOSIS   Depends on the associated conditions. Type 1 renal tubular acidosis may progress to renal failure.

Ankylosing spondylitis

DEFINITION   Seronegative inflammatory arthropathy affecting preferentially the axial skeleton and large proximal joints.

AETIOLOGY
Unknown. Strong linkage with HLA-B27 gene (>90% HLA-B27 positive, general population frequency ~8%). Infective triggers and antigen cross-reactivity with self-peptides have been suggested.

Inflammation starts at the entheses (sites of attachment of ligaments to vertebral bodies). Persistent inflammation is followed by reactive new bone formation. Changes start in lumbar and progress to thoracic and cervical regions:

Squaring of the vertebral bodies. Formation of syndesmophytes (vertical ossifications bridging the margins of the adjacent vertebrae). Fusion of syndesmophytes and facet joints (ankylosis and spinal immobility). Calcification of anterior and lateral spinal ligaments.

EPIDEMIOLOGY   Common: Affects ~0.25–1% of UK population. Earlier presentation in ♂ (♂: ♀ ~ 6 : 1 at 16 years and ~2 : 1 at 30 years).

HISTORY
Low back and sacroiliac (SI) pain disturbing sleep (worse in morning, improves on activity, returning with rest). Progressive loss of spinal movement. Symptoms of asymmetrical peripheral arthritis.

Pleuritic chest pain (caused by costovertebral joint involvement). Heel pain (caused by plantar fasciitis). Non-specific symptoms malaise, fatigue.

EXAMINATION
↓ Range of spinal movements (particularly hip rotation).

↓ Lateral spinal flexion and occiput–wall distance (with the patient standing next to the wall).

Schober's test: A mark is made on the skin of the back in the middle of a line drawn between the posterior iliac spines. A mark 10 cm above this is made. The patient is asked to bend forward and the distance between the two marks should ↑ by >5 cm on forward flexion. This is reduced in ankylosing spondylitis.

There may be tenderness over SI joints.

In later stages, thoracic kyphosis and spinal fusion, question-mark posture.

Signs of extra-articular disease: Anterior uveitis (red eye); apical lung fibrosis, reduced chest expansion (fusion of costovertebral joints); aortic regurgitation (cardiac diastolic murmur).

INVESTIGATIONS
Blood: FBC (anaemia of chronic disease), rheumatoid factor (negative), ↑ ESR/CRP.

Radiographs: Anteroposterior and lateral radiographs of spine: 'Bamboo spine' may be seen. Anteroposterior radiographs of the SI joints: Symmetrical blurring of joint margins. Later there are erosions, sclerosis and SI joint fusion.[1] CXR: To look for association with apical fibrosis.

Lung function tests: Assesses mechanical ventilatory impairment from kyphosis.

MANAGEMENT
NSAIDs can provide symptomatic relief. Sulfasalazine and other immunosuppressants may be useful as second-line treatment.

Intra-articular injections of corticosteroids help acutely inflamed joints, especially with peripheral joint involvement. TNF-α inhibitors (adalimumab and etanercept, but not infliximab) also effective disease-modifying agents but are often reserved for severe disease.

---

[1] Sacroiliitis also occurs in other seronegative arthropathies: Reiter's syndrome (reactive arthritis), entero-pathic arthropathy (inflammatory bowel disease), psoriatic arthropathy.

Ankylosing spondylitis (continued)

Physiotherapy: Educate on proper exercise and posture to maintain maximum range of back movements.

COMPLICATIONS   Apical lung fibrosis, Achilles tendonitis, aortitis, aortic regurgitation, systemic amyloidosis, respiratory failure, cauda equina syndrome (rare).

PROGNOSIS   Most lead a normal life with intensive physiotherapy and surveillance for complications but 10% progress to crippling disease.

Gout

DEFINITION   A disorder of uric acid metabolism causing recurrent bouts of acute arthritis caused by deposition of monosodium urate crystals in joints, and also soft tissues and kidneys.

AETIOLOGY
The underlying metabolic disturbance is hyperuricaemia which may be caused by the following:

Increased urate intake or production: ↑ Dietary intake, ↑ nucleic acid (purine) turnover (e.g. lymphoma, leukaemia, polycythaemia vera, psoriasis) or, rarely, caused by ↑ synthesis (e.g. Lesch–Nyhan syndrome[1]).

Decreased renal excretion: Idiopathic, drugs (e.g. 'CANT LEAP': ciclosporin, alcohol, nicotinic acid, thiazides, loop diuretics, ethambutol, aspirin, pyrizinamide), renal dysfunction.

EPIDEMIOLOGY   Prevalence 0.2 %. ♂: ♀ ~ 10 : 1. Very rare in pre-puberty and in pre-menopausal women. More common in higher social classes.

HISTORY
Acute attack: May be precipitated by trauma, infection, alcohol, starvation, introduction or withdrawal of hypouricaemic agents. Sudden excruciating monoarticular pain, usually the metatarsophalangeal joint of the great toe. The symptoms peak at 24 h and resolve in 7–10 days. Occasionally, acute attacks present with cellulitis, polyarticular or periarticular involvement. Attacks are often recurrent, but the patient is symptom free between attacks.

Intercritical gout: Asymptomatic period between acute attacks.

Chronic tophaceous gout: Follows repeated acute attacks. Persistent low-grade fever, polyarticular pain with painful tophi (urate deposits), best seen on tendons and the pinna of the ear.

Symptoms of urate urolithiasis: (*see* renal calculi).

INVESTIGATIONS
Synovial fluid aspirate: Diagnosis depends on the presence of monosodium urate crystals which are needle-shaped and negatively birefingent under polarized light. Microscopy and culture (to exclude septic arthritis).

Blood: FBC (↑ WCC), U&E, ↑ urate (but may be normal in acute gout), ↑ ESR.

AXR/KUB film: Uric acid renal stones are often radiolucent.

MANAGEMENT
Acute attack: NSAIDs. Colchicine if NSAIDs contraindicated. Intra-articular corticosteroids. Intramuscular ACTH for difficult cases.

Surgery: May be necessary for large or ulcerating tophus.

Prophylaxis: Allopurinol (xanthine oxidase inhibitor) provides prophylaxis against acute attacks. Alternative prophylaxis agents include long-term colchicine (risk of neuromyopathy), probenecid or sulfinpyrazone (uricosurics). Encourage ↑ fluid intake to lower risk of renal calculi.

Advice: Reduce meat and alcohol intake.

COMPLICATIONS   Renal failure, urate urolithiasis, urate nephropathy. Secondary infection or ulceration of tophi.

PROGNOSIS   Seventy five percent have a second attack within 2 years. Prophylactic treatment often necessary in long term.

---

[1] Lesch–Nyhan syndrome is a result of hypoxanthine–guanine phosphoribosyl transferase deficiency, and presents with chorea, ↓ IQ and self-mutilation. Prevention: Treat associated features (e.g. obesity) with lifestyle changes and drugs.

Osteoarthritis

DEFINITION

Age-related degenerative synovial joint disease when cartilage destruction exceeds repair, causing pain and disability.

AETIOLOGY

Can be classified according to distribution of affected joints.

Pathogenesis: Synovial joint cartilage fissuring and fibrillation. Eventually, there is loss of joint volume as a result of altered chondrocyte activity, subchondral sclerosis, bone cysts, osteophyte formation, patchy chronic synovial inflammation and fibrotic thickening of the joint capsules.

Primary: Aetiology unknown. Likely to be multifactorial; 'wear and tear' concept proposed in the past.

Secondary: Other diseases can cause altered joint architecture and stability. Commonly associated diseases include:

1. Developmental abnormalities (e.g. hip dysplasia, Perthes' disease, slipped femoral epiphysis).
2. Trauma (e.g. previous fractures).
3. Inflammatory (e.g. rheumatoid arthritis, gout, septic arthritis).
4. Metabolic (e.g. alkaptonuria, haemochromatosis, acromegaly).

EPIDEMIOLOGY Common, with 25% of those >60 years symptomatic (70% have radiographical changes). More common in females, Caucasians and Asians.

HISTORY

Joint pain or discomfort, usually use-related, stiffness or gelling after inactivity.

Difficulty with certain movements or feelings of instability.

Restriction walking, climbing stairs, manual tasks.

Systemic features are typically absent.

EXAMINATION

Local joint tenderness.

Bony swellings along joint margins, e.g. Heberden's nodes (at distal interphalangeal joints).

Bouchard's nodes (at proximal interphalangeal joints).

Crepitus and pain during joint movement, joint effusion.

Restriction of range of joint movement.

INVESTIGATIONS

Joint X-ray: Radiographs of involved joints typically show four classic features:

1. Joint space narrowing (resulting from cartilage loss).
2. Subchondral cysts.
3. Subchondral sclerosis.
4. Osteophytes.

The severity of radiological changes is not a good indicator of symptom severity.

Synovial fluid analysis: Clear synovial fluid, viscous with low cell count and cartilage fragments.

MANAGEMENT

Treatment goals include symptom relief, optimizing joint function, minimizing disease progression and limiting disability.

Medical: Analgesia with paracetamol, codeine, NSAIDs, COX-2 inhibitors, quinine and glucosamine. Topical NSAIDs or capsaicin provide benefit in some. Intra-articular injection of steroids and hyaluronic acid provides good symptomatic relief. Tidal irrigation (intra-articular instillation of normal saline) is not very effective.

Supportive: Patient education. Encourage lifestyle changes (e.g. weight loss, exercise). Physiotherapy, occupational therapy and psychosocial support.

Surgical: Various techniques can provide benefit, such as arthroscopic irrigation, osteophyte removal, joint replacement (arthroplasty) and joint fusion (arthrodesis).

COMPLICATIONS   Pain and disability, nerve entrapment syndromes, falls and fractures caused by reduced mobility.

PROGNOSIS   Although symptoms may improve or worsen in phases, disease evolution is usually slow, with the natural history depending on the joint site involved.

Pseudogout

DEFINITION   Arthritis associated with deposition of calcium pyrophosphate dihydrate (CPPD) crystals in joint cartilage.

AETIOLOGY
CPPD crystal formation is initiated in cartilage located near the surface of chondrocytes. The disorder is associated with excessive cartilage pyrophosphate production leading to local calcium pyrophosphate supersaturation and CPPD crystal formation/deposition. Shedding of crystals into the joint cavity precipitates acute arthritis.

Most causes of joint damage predispose to pseudogout (e.g. osteoarthritis, trauma), More rarely, conditions such as haemochromatosis, hyperparathyroidism, hypomagnesaemia, hypophosphatasia[1] can predispose to pseudogout. Familial cases and associations with metabolic diseases have been described.

Provoking factors: Intercurrent illness, surgery, local trauma.

EPIDEMIOLOGY   ♀: ♂ ratio is ~2 : 1. More common in elderly (>60 years).

HISTORY
Acute arthritis: Painful, swollen joint (e.g. knee, ankle, shoulder, elbow, wrist).
Chronic arthropathy: Pain, stiffness, functional impairment.
Uncommon presentations: Tendonitis (e.g. achilles), tenosynovitis (tendons of the hand), bursitis (e.g. olecranon bursitis).

EXAMINATION
Acute arthritis: Red, hot, tender, restricted range of movement, fever.
Chronic arthropathy (similar to osteoarthritis): Bony swelling, crepitus, deformity, e.g. varus in knees, restriction of movement.

INVESTIGATIONS
Blood: FBC (may show ↑ WCC in acute attack), ESR (may be ↑), blood culture (excludes infective arthritis).
Joint aspiration: Microscopy shows short rhomboid brick-shaped crystals, with weak positive birefringence under polarized light. Culture or Gram staining (exclude infective arthritis).
Plain radiograph of the joint: Chondrocalcinosis (linear calcification of cartilage), or signs of osteoarthritis: loss of joint space, osteophytes, subchondral cysts, sclerosis.

MANAGEMENT   *Acute*: Joint aspiration, intra-articular steroids (e.g. for large joints: triamcinolone acetonide mixed with 1% procaine) Analgesia: NSAIDs (with caution in elderly) or oral colchicine. Rest and mobilization after acute attack has settled.
Chronic: Similar to osteoarthritis (e.g. lose weight, walking aids), physiotherapy, simple analgesics (e.g. paracetamol). Oral daily colchicine for patients with ≥3 attacks of pseudogout annually.
Surgery may be necessary for severe cases.

COMPLICATIONS   Chronic pyrophosphate arthropathy, GI haemorrhage (secondary to NSAID use).

PROGNOSIS   Acute attacks resolve in 1–3 weeks. Chronic pyrophosphate arthropathy has good outcome. Rarely, a destructive arthropathy (with Charcot's joint features), recurrent haemarthrosis and joint capsular rupture occur in very elderly women.

---

[1] Hypophosphatasia is an autosomal recessive disease, characterized by reduced bone mineralization, ↓ serum alkaline phosphatase, which can lead to rickets and recurrent fractures.

Reactive arthritis

DEFINITION Characterized by a sterile arthritis occurring after an extra-articular infection (commonly gastrointestinal or urogenital). Reiter's syndrome is defined by a triad of reactive arthritis, urethritis and conjunctivitis.

AETIOLOGY Associated with infections of gastrointestinal tract (e.g. Salmonella, Shigella, Yersinia, Campylobacter) and urogenital origin (*Chlamydia trachomatis* in ~60%). Initial activation of the immune system by a microbial antigen may be followed by an autoimmune reaction that involves the skin, eyes, and joints. *HLA-B27* identified in 70–80% of patients. *HLA-B27* may share molecular characteristics with bacterial epitopes, facilitating an auto-immune cross reaction.

EPIDEMIOLOGY

♂: ♀ ratio is about 20 : 1. Age of onset 20–40 years. Seen in 2% of patients with non-specific urethritis and 0.2% of those with dysentery.
Prevalence ~30–40/100 000 adults.

HISTORY

Symptoms may develop 3–30 days after the infection.
Symptoms of burning or stinging on passing water (urethritis), arthritis, low back pain (sacroiliitis), painful heels (enthesitis, plantar fasciitis), conjunctivitis.

EXAMINATION

Signs of arthritis: Asymmetric oligoarthritis (often affecting the lower extremities, sausage-shaped digits).
Signs of conjunctivitis: red eye. *Anterior uveitis* (10 % of patients): painful red eye.
Oral ulceration: Usually painless.
Circinate balanitis: Scaling red patches, which may evolve, encircling the glans penis.
Keratoderma blenorrhagica (10% of patients): Brownish-red macules, vesicopustules and yellowish brown scales on soles or palms.
Other: Fever. Nail dystrophy, hyperkeratosis or onycholysis.

INVESTIGATIONS

Blood: FBC (anaemia may be an indication of severity and extent of systemic illness), ↑ ESR or CRP, *HLA-B27* testing in patients with an intermediated likelihood of reactive arthritis.
Stool or urethral swabs and cultures: May be negative by the time arthritis develops.
Urine: Screening for *Chlamydia trachomatis*.
Plain X-ray radiographs (chronic cases): Erosions at insertions of tendons (entheses) e.g. Achilles tendon, plantar spurs, sacroiliitis, spinal disease with asymmetrical syndesmo-phytes. *Joint aspiration*: To exclude septic or crystal associated arthritis.

MANAGEMENT

Arthritis: Initially rest. NSAIDs e.g. indomethacin. Aspiration of effusions.
When intra-articular infection has been excluded, intra-articular injections of steroids may be used in those who do not respond to NSAIDs.
Mobilize/exercise. If NSAIDs (2 week course) and intraarticular steroids do not control symptoms, sulfasalazine may be used. A therapeutic trial of etanercept may be given to patients with contraindications to, or with intolerance of, sulfasalazine.
Conjunctivitis: Antibiotic for secondary infection, artificial tear substitute, management of anterior uveitis by ophthalmologists (*see* uveitis, anterior).
Treatment of active gastrointestinal or chlamydial infection
Oral ulcers: Antiseptics, local anaesthetic mouthwash.
Balanitis: One percent hydrocortisone ointment, local hygiene.

COMPLICATIONS Chronic inflammatory joint disease, cardiac complications similar to ankylosing spondylitis.

PROGNOSIS Most remit completely or have little active disease 6 months after presen-tation. After entering remission, pain is occasionally noted in the joints, at entheses, or in the spine. Chronic arthritis, lasting >6 months, occurs in a small proportion of patients. Some develop ankylosing spondylitis.

Rheumatoid arthritis

DEFINITION   Chronic inflammatory systemic disease characterized by symmetrical deforming polyarthritis and extra-articular manifestations.

AETIOLOGY   Autoimmune disease of unknown cause. Associated with other autoimmune phenomenon (e.g. Raynaud's phenomenon, Sjögren's syndrome) and HLA DR-1 and DR-4 haplotypes.

EPIDEMIOLOGY   Common. Prevalence is 1% of general population. Three times more common in females, peak incidence at 30–50 years.

HISTORY

Gradual (occasionally rapid) onset.
Joint pain, swelling, morning stiffness, impaired function.
Usually affects peripheral joints symmetrically (occasionally monoarticular involvement, e.g. knee).
Systemic: Fatigue, fever, weight loss.

EXAMINATION   *Arthritis*: Most common sites are in the hands.
Early:
- Spindling of fingers.
- Swelling at MCP and PIP joints.
- Warm, tender joints.
- Reduction in range of movement.

Late:
- Symmetrical deforming arthropathy.
- Ulnar deviation of fingers as a result of subluxation (partial dislocation) at MCP joints.
- Radial deviation of the wrist.
- Swan neck deformity (MCP and DIP fixed flexion, PIP extension).
- Boutonnière deformity (MCP and DIP joint extension, PIP flexion).
- Z deformity of the thumb.
- Trigger finger (unable to straighten finger, tendon sheath nodule palpable), tendon rupture.
- Wasting of the small muscles of the hand, palmar erythema.

Rheumatoid nodules: Firm subcutaneous nodules (e.g. on elbows, palms, over extensor tendons).
Signs of complications: See COMPLICATIONS.

INVESTIGATIONS

Blood: FBC ($\downarrow$Hb, $\uparrow$platelets), $\uparrow$ ESR and CRP, rheumatoid factor (monoclonal IgM against Fc portion of IgG, present in 70% of patients and 5% normal population, associated with subcutaneous nodules and extra-articular manifestations), antinuclear antibodies (30%).
Acutely: Consider joint aspiration to exclude septic arthritis.
Joint X-ray radiography: Soft tissue swelling, angular deformity, periarticular erosions and osteoporosis.

MANAGEMENT   *Medical*: A variety of agents are used for treating disease with immunosuppressants and biological agents conferring long-lasting benefits (disease-modifying):
- *Immunosuppressants*: Disease-modifying drugs such as methotrexate (a first-line agent combined with folic acid), sulfasalazine, penicillamine, azathioprine, gold, hydroxychloroquine and cyclophosphamide. May take months to work, reduce complications and slow the disease progression. Careful monitoring is needed for side effects, e.g. FBC (for bone marrow suppression), LFT (for hepatitis), U&E (for renal failure), urinalysis (for nephrotic syndrome), eye examination (for retinopathy and corneal deposits).

- *Biological agents*: Monoclonals against TNF-α (Etanercept, Infliximab) and CD20 on the surface of B-cells (Rituximab) have proven efficacy. Very expensive and used as second-line agents.
- *NSAIDs*: For treating pain and stiffness.
- *Steroids*: Use limited by side effects. Only used in severe extra-articular disease or with rapid or widespread arthritis. Intra-articular long-acting steroids into large joints (e.g. knee, shoulder) may ↓ pain and joint effusions.

Disease monitoring: Annual reviews are recommended for measuring disease activity using functional rating scales, clinical examination, radiological appearances and biochemical markers (ESR, CRP); also useful for detecting complications of rheumatoid disease (e.g. cervical myelopathy).

Physiotherapy and occupational therapy: Essential to maintain joint function and quality of life.

Surgery: Synovectomy, arthrodesis, arthroplasty, tendon repair or joint replacement.

COMPLICATIONS

Numerous organs can be involved.

Vasculitis (of skin): Nail-fold infarcts, digital gangrene, ulcers, pyoderma gangrenosum, purpuric rash.

Lung: Pleural effusion, fibrosis, rheumatoid nodules in parenchyma, obliterative bronchioloitis.

Heart: Pericarditis, pericardial rub, myocarditis, conduction abnormalities, valvular regurgitation.

Haematological:
- Anaemia of chronic disease.
- Megaloblastic anaemia (↑ demand for folic acid).
- Aplastic anaemia (from drugs).
- Haemolytic anaemia (in Felty's syndrome).

Neuromuscular: Mononeuritis multiplex, peripheral neuropathy, carpal tunnel syndrome, atlantoaxial subluxation and spinal cord compression.

Renal: Analgesic nephropathy, amyloidosis.

Eyes: Scleritis, episcleritis, scleromalacia and scleromalacia perforans.

PROGNOSIS Variable. 10% severely affected after 10 years and ~20% have minimal disease. Poor prognostic factors are ♀, persistent ↑ inflammatory markers, high-titre rheumatoid factor, extra-articular manifestations.

---

[1] **Felty's syndrome** is the combination of rheumatoid arthritis, splenomegaly, neutropenia and lower limb pigmentation.

Sarcoidosis

DEFINITION   Multisystem granulomatous inflammatory disorder.

AETIOLOGY   Unknown. Transmissible agents (e.g. viruses, atypical mycobacterium, *Propionibacterium acnes*), environmental triggers and genetic factors have all been suggested.

EPIDEMIOLOGY   Uncommon. More common in 20–40 year olds, Africans and females. The prevalence is variable worldwide. Prevalence in UK is 16 in 100 000 (highest in Irish women).

HISTORY AND EXAMINATION
General: Fever, malaise, weight loss, bilateral parotid swelling, lymphadenopathy, hepatosplenomegaly.
Lungs: Breathlessness, cough (usually unproductive), chest discomfort. Minimal clinical signs (e.g. fine inspiratory crepitations).
Musculoskeletal: Bone cysts (e.g. 'dactylitis' in phalanges), polyarthralgia, myopathy.
Eyes: Keratoconjunctivitis sicca (dry eyes), uveitis, papilloedema.
Skin: Lupus pernio (red–blue infiltrations of nose, cheek, ears, terminal phalanges), erythema nodosum, maculopapular eruptions.
Neurological: Lymphocytic meningitis, space-occupying lesions, pituitary infiltration, cerebellar ataxia, cranial nerve palsies (e.g. bilateral facial nerve palsy), peripheral neuropathy.
Heart: Arrhythmia, bundle branch block, percarditis, cardiomyopathy, congestive cardiac failure.

PATHOLOGY/PATHOGENESIS   The unknown antigen is presented on the MHC Class II complex of macrophages to CD4 (Th1) lymphocytes, which accumulate and release cytokines (e.g. IL-1/IL-2). This results in formation of non-caseating granulomas in a variety of organs.

INVESTIGATIONS
Blood: $\uparrow$ Serum ACE, $\uparrow$ Ca^{2+}, $\uparrow$ ESR, FBC (WCC may be $\downarrow$ because of lymphocyte sequestration in the lungs), immunoglobulins (polyclonal hyperglobulinaemia), LFT ($\uparrow$ alkaline phosphatase and GGT).
24-h urine collection: Hypercalciuria.
CXR: *Stage 0*: May be clear. *Stage 1*: Bilateral hilar lymphadenopathy. *Stage 2*: Stage 1 with pulmonary infiltration and paratracheal node enlargement. *Stage 3*: Pulmonary infiltration and fibrosis.
High-resolution CT scan: For diffuse lung involvement.
[67]Gallium scan: Shows areas of inflammation (classically parotids and around eyes).
Pulmonary function tests: $\downarrow$ FEV_1, FVC and gas transfer (showing restrictive picture).
Bronchoscopy and bronchoalveolar lavage: $\uparrow$ Lymphocytes with $\uparrow$CD4: CD8 ratio.
Transbronchial lung biopsy (or lymph node biopsy): Non-caseating granulomas composed of epithelioid cells (activated macrophages), multinucleate Langhans cells and mononuclear cells (lymphocytes).

MANAGEMENT   Corticosteroids (e.g. oral prednisolone reducing slowly) for symptomatic pulmonary, cardiac and neurologic sarcoidosis.
Musculoskeletal: NSAIDs. If no relief: colchicine, hydroxychloroquine, or prednisolone. For refractory arthritis/patients who require high doses of glucocorticoids: methotrexate with folic acid supplementation. If steroids and other immunosuppressants are ineffective, not tolerated or contraindicated: consider infliximab (anti-tumour necrosis factor alpha agent).
Ocular sarcoid: Topical corticosteroids and a mydriatic (atropine).
Skin: Chloroquine or methotrexate may be used for lupus pernio.
Arrhythmias: Pacemakers, automatic implantable cardioverter-defibrillator.

COMPLICATIONS   Multiple organ involvement (see above), nephrocalcinosis and interstitial nephritis.

PROGNOSIS   Acute arthritis (often involving the lower extremities) associated with hilar adenopathy and erythema nodosum (Lofgren's syndrome) usually resolves spontaneously. Two-thirds of Caucasian patients and one-third of black patients remit without treatment. Mortality (e.g. as a result of respiratory failure) is up to 10 % in Afro-Caribbean and <5% in white people. Best prognosis is in Caucasians with Stage 1 disease.

Sjögren's syndrome

DEFINITION   Characterized by inflammation and destruction of exocrine glands (usually salivary and lacrimal glands). When associated with other autoimmune diseases, Sjögren's syndrome is termed secondary.

AETIOLOGY

Unknown. linked to HLA-B8, DR3.

Associated with rheumatoid arthritis, scleroderma, SLE, polymyositis and organ-specific autoimmune diseases (e.g. primary biliary cirrhosis, autoimmune hepatitis, autoimmune thyroid disease, myasthenia gravis).

EPIDEMIOLOGY   Onset usually between 15 and 65 years. ♂: ♀ ~ 1 : 9.

HISTORY

General: Fatigue, fever, weight loss, depression.
Dry eyes (keratoconjunctivitis sicca): Gritty, sore eyes.
Dry mouth (xerostomia): Dysphagia may result secondarily.
Dry upper airways: Dry cough, recurrent sinusitis.
Dry skin or hair (uncommon).
Dry vagina (uncommon): May cause dyspareunia.
↓ Gastrointestinal mucus secretion causing symptoms of reflux oesophagitis, gastritis, constipation.

EXAMINATION

Parotid or salivary gland enlargement.
Dry eyes.
Dry mouth or tongue.
Signs of the associated conditions.

INVESTIGATIONS

Blood: ↑ ESR, ↑ amylase if salivary glands involved.
Auto-antibodies: Rheumatoid factor, ANA (present in 60%), Anti-ENA (anti-La, anti-Ro).
Schirmer's test: Filter paper strip under eyelid. Positive if <10 mm of the strip is wet in 5 min.
Fluorescein/rose bengal stains: May show punctate or filamentary keratitis (clumps of mucus on the cornea).
Others: ↓ Parotid salivary flow rate, ↓ uptake or clearance on isotope scan.
Biopsy: Salivary or labial glands (lower lip).

MANAGEMENT

Dry mouth: Saliva substitutes, good oral hygiene, treatment of oral candidiasis.
Dry eyes: Shielded spectacles, artificial tears (hypromellose eye drops), simple ointment (at night), topical acetylcysteine (mucolytic), treatment of secondary bacterial conjunctivitis. Lacrimal punctol occlusion (temporary/permanent) or tarsorrhaphy may rarely be required.
Systemic disease: Steroids or immunosuppressants. Rituximab has been shown to be effective.

COMPLICATIONS

Mouth: Chronic oral candidiasis, caries.
Eyes: Conjunctivitis, corneal epithelial, thinning, filamentary keratitis.
Vasculitis: Occurs in <10% of patients. Associated with myositis, mononeuritis multiplex, axonal neuropathy, immune complex glomerulonephritis, purpura and cerebral vasculitis.
Kidney: Interstitial nephritis.
Lymphoma: Forty times increased risk. Usually B-cell non-Hodgkin type.
Pregnancy: Anti-Ro and anti-La (can cross placenta and cause congenital heart block, 1% risk).

PROGNOSIS   Good for primary Sjögren's. Depends on accompanying autoimmune disorder in secondary Sjögren's.

Systemic lupus erythematosus (SLE)

DEFINITION   Multi-system inflammatory autoimmune disorder.
4 out of 11 diagnostic criteria of the American College of Rheumatology provides 95% specificity and 85% sensitivity for SLE:

(1) Malar rash
(2) Photosensitivity
(3) Non-erosive arthritis
(4) Renal disease (urine casts/proteinuria)
(5) Neurological disease (psychosis/seizures)
(6) Haematological (haemolytic anaemia/leukopenia/thrombocytopenia)
(7) Immunological disorder (anti-dsDNA/anti-Sm/anti-phospholipid)
(8) Antinuclear antibodies (ANA)
(9) Discoid rash
(10) Oral ulcers
(11) Pleuritis or pericarditis (serositis)

AETIOLOGY   Unknown. Tissue damage may be mediated by vascular immune complex deposition related to the auto-antibodies. Combination of hormonal, genetic (HLA clustering) and exogenous factors (e.g. drugs such as hydralazine and procainamide can cause a reversible SLE-like disorder).

EPIDEMIOLOGY   Common. Prevalence is 1–2 in 1000. More common in young (20–40-year-olds. 15% cases >60 years), Afro-Caribbean and Chinese. Nine times more common in females.

HISTORY AND EXAMINATION
General: Fever, fatigue, weight loss, lymphadenopathy, splenomegaly.
Raynaud's phenomenon: Common, seen in 30%.
Oral ulcers.
Skin rash:
- *Malar (butterfly) rash*: Primarily affects the cheeks and the bridge of the nose.
- *Discoid lupus*: Red and scaly patches (e.g. face), which later heal with scarring and pigmentation.
- *Atypical rashes*: Photosensitivity, vasculitic (digital infarcts), urticaria, purpura, bullae, livedo reticularis, atypical erythema multiforme-like rash (Rowell's syndrome), hair loss.

Systemic involvement:
- *Musculoskeletal*: Arthritis, tendonitis, myopathy, avascular necrosis of femoral head.
- *Heart*: Pericarditis, myocarditis, arrhythmias, Libman–Sacks endocarditis (non-infective mitral valve disease), aortic valve lesions.
- *Lung*: Symptoms of pleuritis, pleural effusions, basal atelectasis, restrictive lung defects.
- *Neurological*: Headache, stroke, cranial nerve palsies, confusion, chorea, fits, peripheral neuropathy.
- *Psychiatric*: Depression, psychosis.
- *Renal*: Symptoms of glomerulonephritis.

INVESTIGATIONS
Blood: FBC, U&E, LFT, ↑ ESR with normal CRP, clotting, complement (↓ C3 levels).
Autoantibodies:
Anti-dsDNA: : 60% of cases.
Rheumatoid factor: 30–50% of cases.
Anti-ENA:
Anti-RNP: 30% of cases.
Anti-Sm: 30% of cases.
Anti-Ro (SSA): 30% of cases.
Anti-La (SSB): 15% of cases.

Systemic lupus erythematosus (SLE) (continued)

Anti-histone: In drug-induced lupus.
Anti-phospholipid/Anti-cardiolipin: See anti-phospholipid syndrome.

Urine: Haematuria, proteinuria, microscopy (for casts).
Joints: Plain radiographs.
Heart and lung: CXR, ECG, echocardiogram, CT scan.
Kidney: Renal biopsy (if glomerulonephritis suspected).
CNS: MRI scan, lumbar puncture.

MANAGEMENT
Mild disease: Topical corticosteroids and sun-avoidance. Simple analgesia or intra-articular joint injections for musculoskeletal pain. Consider hydroxychloroquine (with ophthalmic monitoring).
Moderate disease: Oral corticosteroids or systemic immunosuppressants (e.g. cyclophosphamide, azathioprine, cyclosporine, mycophenolate), particularly in renal or cerebral disease.
Resistant disease: For resistant thrombocytopenia, various options include oral danazol, IV immunoglobulins or plasmapharesis. Rituximab (anti-CD20 against B-cells) have been used off-label, but clear evidence of efficacy is lacking.

COMPLICATIONS   Vasculitis affecting any organ. Large vessel thrombosis. Anti-Ro can cross the placenta and cause congenital heart block in the foetus.

PROGNOSIS   Ten-year survival rate is 80–90%. Mortality is usually a result of infection (e.g. streptococcal sepsis) or renal failure. Prognosis worse if onset with renal involvement during pregnancy.

Systemic sclerosis

DEFINITION   Rare connective tissue disease characterized by widespread small blood vessel damage and fibrosis in skin and internal organs. Also known as scleroderma. Spectrum of disease includes the following.

Pre-scleroderma: Raynaud's phenomenon, nail-fold capillary changes and antinuclear antibodies.

Diffuse cutaneous systemic sclerosis (~40%): Raynaud's phenomenon followed by skin changes with truncal involvement, tendon friction and joint contractures, early lung, heart, GI and renal disease, nail-fold capillary dilation.

Limited cutaneous systemic sclerosis (~60%): Previously known as CREST (calcinosis, Raynaud's, oesophageal dysmotility, sclerodactyly, telangiecstasia).

Scleroderma sine scleroderma (~1%): Internal organ disease with no skin changes.

AETIOLOGY   Unknown. Genetic and environmental factors (e.g. vinyl chloride, epoxy resins) have been suggested. Exact pathogenesis unclear, but specific antibodies (humoral immunity) and activated monocytes, macrophages and lymphocytes (cellular immunity) may interact with:
- Endothelial cells → endothelial cell damage, platelet activation, myointimal cell proliferation and narrowing of blood vessels.
- Fibroblasts → lay down collagen in the dermis.

EPIDEMIOLOGY   Age of onset 30–60 years. Three times more common in females. Annual incidence is one in 10 000.

HISTORY AND EXAMINATION

Skin: *Raynaud's phenomenon*[1]. *Hands*: Initially swollen oedematous painful fingers. Later they become thickened, tight, shiny and bound to underlying structures. Changes in pigmentation and finger ulcers. *Face*: Microstomia (puckering and furrowing of perioral skin), telangiecstasia.

Lung: Pulmonary fibrosis leading to pulmonary hypertension.

Heart: Pericarditis or pericardial effusion, myocardial fibrosis, heart failure or arrhythmias.

GI: Dry mouth, oesophageal dysmotility (dysphagia), reflux oesophagitis, gastric paresis (nausea, vomiting, anorexia), watermelon stomach, bacterial overgrowth, small bowel pseudo-obstruction, colonic hypomotility (constipation), anal incontinence, angiodysplasia.

Kidney: Hypertensive renal crisis, chronic renal failure.

Neuromuscular: Trigeminal neuralgia, muscular wasting or weakness.

Other: Hypothyroidism, impotence, dryness of mucus membranes can cause dyspareunia. Overlap syndromes with polymyositis and SLE.

INVESTIGATIONS

Blood: *Antinuclear antibodies*:

Anti-centromere: 70% positive in limited cutaneous systemic sclerosis.

Anti-topoisomerase (anti-Scl-70): 30% positive in diffuse cutaneous systemic sclerosis.

Anti-nucleolar antibodies. PmScl (associated with myositis).

Anti-RNA-polymerase (associated with renal crisis).

Nail-fold capillary ophthalmoscopy or microscopy: To detect fine nail-fold changes.

Investigations for complications:

Lung: CXR, pulmonary function tests, high-resolution CT scan.

---

[1] Raynaud phenomenon is an exaggerated vascular response to cold temperature or emotional stress (abnormal vasoconstriction of digital arteries and cutaneous arterioles). Presents with colour changes of the skin of the digits: white → blue (cyanosis) → crimson (reactive hyperemia). May be primary (without any associated disorder) or secondary (associated with a related illness, such as SLE or systemic sclerosis).

Systemic sclerosis (continued)

Heart: ECG, echocardiography.
GI: Endoscopy, barium studies, gastric/oesophageal scintigraphy.
Kidney: U&E and measurement of creatinine clearance.
Neuromuscular: Electromyography, nerve conduction studies, biopsy.
Joints: Radiography (for subcutaneous calcification, acro-osteolysis, flexion deformities).
Skin: Biopsy (to exclude fasciitis, rarely necessary), muscle biopsy for associated myositis.

MANAGEMENT
Skin: Moisturizers and anti-thymocyte globulin may be used for skin sclerosis. Laser therapy for telangiectasia. Calcinosis: Diltiazem, surgical removal using a dental drill.
Raynaud's phenomenon: Avoid cold temperatures, stress, nicotine, caffeine and vasoconstrictor drugs. Warm clothing. Long acting calcium channel blocker (nifedipine or amlodipine). If ineffective, add transdermal nitroglycerin or a phosphodiesterase inhibitor (sildenafil). Pain control. In severe cases: IV infusion of the prostacyclin analogue iloprost (potent vasodilator, also inhibits platelet aggregation and adhesion). Bosentan (*see* below) may have a beneficial effect upon digital ischaemia. Surgical therapy for patients who do not respond to medical management (digital sympathectomy, lumbar sympathectomy for feet problems).
Lung: Pulmonary hypertension: Bosentan (endothelin-receptor antagonist), sildenafil (phosphodiesterase-5 inhibitor), IV prostacyclin analogue (prolongs life expectancy) and warfarin. Patients with alveolitis who have yet to develop advanced fibrotic lung disease: corticosteroids and cyclophosphamide.
GI: Proton pump inhibitors for reflux disease, promotility drugs, pancreatic supplements, PEG feeding or parenteral nutrition may all be necessary at some stage.
Renal: ACE-inhibitors ↓ incidence of renal crisis. In renal crisis, IV prostacyclin analogue or peritoneal dialysis may be used.
Myositis: Corticosteroids and methotrexate.

COMPLICATIONS   *See* History and Examination above.

PROGNOSIS   Variable (5-year survival rate is 35–75%). Poor prognostic factors: male sex, age, ↑ extent of skin involvement, heart, lung and renal disease. More severe in non-white patients. Lung (both pulmonary hypertension and pulmonary fibrosis) is the primary cause of scleroderma-related deaths today.

Vasculitides (primary)

DEFINITION Vasculitis is the inflammation and necrosis of blood vessels. Primary vasculitides[1] are classified according to the main vessel size affected.

Large: Giant cell arteritis (GCA), Takayasu's aortitis (TA).

Medium: Polyarteritis nodosa (PAN), Kawasaki's disease (KD).

Small: Churg–Strauss syndrome (CSS), microscopic polyangiitis (MP), Henoch–Schönlein purpura (HSP), Wegener's granulomatosis (WG), mixed essential cryoglobulinaemia (MEC), relapsing polychondritis (RP).

AETIOLOGY Unknown. Postulated to be of autoimmune origin. Immune complex deposition in vessel walls triggers classical complement activation and inflammation.

ASSOCIATIONS/RISK FACTORS PAN is associated with hepatitis B infection. MEC is associated with hepatitis C infection. MP is associated with presence of pANCA. WG is associated with presence of c-ANCA.

EPIDEMIOLOGY Annual incidence of small vessel vasculitis is ~1 in 10000. TA is more common in Japanese young females, PAN may affect any age ($\male$: $\female$ = 2 : 1).

HISTORY AND EXAMINATION

The large vessel vasculitides have classical clinical patterns resulting from the vessels affected. Medium and small vessel vasculitides are characterized by multiorgan involvement with less specific clinical features.

Possible features of all diseases:

General: Fever, night sweats, malaise, weight loss.

Skin: Rash (vasculitic, purpuric, maculopapular, livedo reticularis).

Joint: Arthralgia or arthritis.

GI: Abdominal pain, haemorrhage from mucosal ulceration, diarrhoea.

Kidney: Glomerulonephritis, renal failure.

Lung: Dyspnoea, cough, chest pain, haemoptysis, lung haemorrhage.

CVS: Pericarditis, coronary arteritis, myocarditis, heart failure, arrhythmias.

CNS: Mononeuritis multiplex, infarctions, meningeal involvement.

Eyes: Retinal haemorrhage, cotton wool spots.

Features characteristic of specific subtypes:

GCA: (*see* giant cell arteritis).

TA: Constitutional upset, head or neck pain, tenderness over affected arteries (aorta and the major branches), dizziness, fainting, ↓ peripheral pulses, hypertension.

PAN: Microaneurysms, thrombosis, infarctions (e.g. causing GI perforations), hypertension, testicular pain.

KD: Age <5 years, fever of >5 days, fissured lips, red swollen palms and soles followed by desquamation, skin rash, inflamed oral cavity, conjunctival congestion, lymphadenopathy, coronary artery aneurysm.

CSS: Asthma, eosinophilia.

HSP: Purpura (leg and buttocks), arthritis, gut symptoms, glomerulonephritis with IgA deposition.

MP: Non-specific with multiple organs affected. Glomerulonephritis with no glomerular Ig deposits.

WG: Granulomatous vasculitis of upper and lower repiratory tract, nasal discharge, ulceration and deformity, haemoptysis, sinusitis, corneal thinning, glomerulonephritis.

RP: Affecting cartilage (e.g. ear pinna, nose, larynx) causing swelling, hoarse voice, tenderness, cartilage destruction and deformity (e.g. saddle nose).

MEC: Arthritis, splenomegaly, skin vasculitis, renal disease, cryoglobulins (IgG and IgM mix).

---

[1] Vasculitis may also occur secondary to infections, abscesses, malignancies and connective tissue diseases (e.g. rheumatoid arthritis, SLE).

Vasculitides (primary) (continued)

PATHOLOGY/PATHOGENESIS Acute and chronic inflammatory cells in vessel wall. Some subtypes (GCA, WG, CS and PAN) have evidence of granulomatous inflammation.

INVESTIGATIONS
Blood: FBC (normocytic anaemia, ↑ platelets, ↑ neutrophils), ↑ ESR/CRP.
Autoantibodies: *c-ANCA*: Anti-proteinase 3, associated with WG. *p-ANCA*: Anti-myeloperoxidase seen in MP and CSS but also IBD, primary biliary cirrhosis and chronic active hepatitis. *ANA*, anti-dsDNA may suggest SLE. *Rheumatoid factor*: Positive in 50%. *Cryoglobulins* (immunoglobulins and complement components that precipitate at temperatures <37 °C).
Urine: Haematuria, proteinuria. Red cell casts
CXR: Diffuse, nodular or flitting shadows. Atelectasia.
Biopsy: Renal, lung (transbronchial), temporal artery (in GCA).
Angiography: To identify aneurysms (in PAN).

MANAGEMENT
Steroids (e.g. prednisolone, hydrocortisone) and immunosuppressants usually cyclophosphamide (oral or pulse cyclophosphamide based upon physician experience & disease severity). The steroid dose may be reduced after 1–2 months of combined therapy. Therapy is usually continued for 6–12 months to ↓ the risk of relapse. Azathioprine and methotrexate may be used for less severe forms of vasculitis and as maintenance therapy after remission has been achieved with cyclophosphamide.
In fulminating vasculitis, plasma exchange and intravenous immunoglobulins may be warranted. In KD, aspirin is used in addition to the above therapies.
Prolonged monitoring is indicated.

COMPLICATIONS *See* History and Examination. Relapse. Vascular injury during the acute phase → scarring and narrowing of the vessels, leading to signs of ischaemia.
Complications of the therapy: infection or malignancy.

PROGNOSIS Most remit on treatment or spontaneously (e.g. HSP), but up to 50% of small vessel vasculitides may relapse. 5-year survival 60% in PAN and 70% in Wegener granulomatosis treated with cyclophosphamide. Most deaths are related to cardiovascular, renal and treatment complications.

Acoustic Neuroma

DEFINITION Schwann cell-derived tumours that commonly arise from the vestibular portion of the eight cranial nerve. More than 90% of cases are unilateral. Bilateral cases are seen in neurofibromatosis type 2.

AETIOLOGY Risk factors include:
- Neurofibromatosis type 2.
- Exposure to loud noise.
- Childhood exposure to low-dose radiation for benign conditions of the head and neck.

EPIDEMIOLOGY Incidence is one in 100 000 per year. The median age at diagnosis is approximately 50 years. Account for 8% of all intracranial tumours in adults and 80–90% of cerebellopontine angle tumours.

HISTORY Symptoms of cranial nerve compression by the tumour:
VIII nerve: Hearing loss (95%), tinnitus and unsteadiness while walking.
V nerve: Facial numbness, paraesthesia and pain (17%).
VII nerve: Facial weakness (6%).
With tumour progression (expansion into the cerebellopontine angle):
Compression of the cerebellum resulting in ataxia.
Compression of the lower cranial nerves (IX, X and XI) resulting in dysarthria and dysphagia.

EXAMINATION Abnormal cranial nerve examination:
VIII nerve: Hearing loss, the Weber and Rinne tests suggest asymmetric sensorineural hearing impairment, nystagmus (beating away from tumour).
V nerve: Loss of corneal reflex, facial numbness.
VII nerve: Lower motor neuron facial palsy.
Cerebellar compression: Ipsilateral ataxia and nystagmus.
Look for signs of neurofibromatosis.

INVESTIGATIONS *Audiometry*: Asymmetric sensorineural hearing loss.
Brainstem-evoked response audiometry: Delay in nerve conduction time on the affected side.
MRI with gadolinium contrast: Sshows acoustic neuromas in the region of the internal auditory canal with variable extension into the cerebellopontine angle.

MANAGEMENT *Surgery* is aimed to prevent further disability and does not restore hearing. There are three operative approaches: retromastoid suboccipital, translabyrinthine and middle fossa.
Radiation therapy: Stereotactic radiosurgery (using multiple convergent beams to deliver a high single dose of radiation) may be considered for neuromas <3 cm and in patients unfit for surgery. Stereotactic radiotherapy (using focused doses of radiation given over a series of treatment sessions) and proton beam therapy may also be used. The choice of therapy depends upon the availability of the appropriate expertise and patient preferences.

COMPLICATIONS Compression of brainstem and the fourth ventricle resulting in hydrocephalus, increased intracranial pressure and death can occur in untreated cases.

PROGNOSIS Hearing loss is often permanent. Treatment merely prevents further damage.

Alzheimer's disease

DEFINITION   Primary chronic progressive neurodegenerative dementia[1] characterized by extracellular deposition of β-amyloid protein[2] and intracellular neurofibrillary tangles.

Mild cognitive impairment: Impairment in some cognitive domains but insufficient to qualify for diagnosis of dementia or to affect quality of life.

AETIOLOGY   Unknown cause. Majority of cases are idiopathic with rare monogenic cases. Risk factors include age, prior intellectual level and family history.

Pathophysiology: Characterised by extracellular deposition of amyloid plaques containing β-42 peptides and intracellular accumulation of neurofibrillary tangles containing hyperphosphorylated tau protein (microtubule protein). It remains unclear which is the causative pathology. Neurone count is reduced particularly in hippocampus, mesial temporal and precuneate cortex.

EPIDEMIOLOGY   Very common, affecting 5% of those >65 years and accounts for 60–80% of all dementias. Diagnosis before age 60 years is exceptional. The incidence ↑ exponentially with age.

HISTORY   Reliable history is best obtained from relative.

Gradual deterioration of cognitive functions:
- Initially, anterograde amnesia, change of personality, apathy, loss of concentration and disorientation. May be accompanied with psychiatric manifestations (hallucinations and delusions).
- Language is typically spared until late.
- In late stages, cognitive impairment in all cognitive domains (memory, language, visuospatial), myoclonus, seizures, behavioural disturbances, incontinence and loss of independence.

EXAMINATION   Mini-Mental State Exam (MMSE) is a useful screening tool (<27 qualifies for dementia) but premorbid intellectual function needs to be taken into account. Typically, in amnestic Alzheimer's, delayed recall is impaired even with prompting.

INVESTIGATIONS   Investigations are aimed at excluding treatable causes of dementia.

Blood: FBC, U&E, LFT, ESR, CRP, TFT (exclude hypothyroidism), folate, ANA, ANCA, vitamin B12, treponemal serology. Consider HIV serology.

CT/MRI-brain: May show cerebral or hippocampal atrophy. Useful for excluding tumours, infarction, inflammatory causes, subdural haematoma.

Psychometric testing: Useful for defining domains of impairment. May be helpful for distinguishing depressive pseudo-dementia.

Electroencephalography: Not diagnostic, but may be useful to exclude non-convulsive status epilepticus as a cause.

Lumbar puncture: Not usually necessary except if disease is relatively subacute onset or rapid to exclude other causes (e.g. encephalitis, prion disease). Tau and β-42 peptide levels can also be measured.

Nuclear imaging: Primarily research tools. ^{11}C-PIB PET can image amyloid distribution in brain and ^{99m}Tc-HMPAO-SPECT shows regional hypoperfusion of affected cerebral regions.

MANAGEMENT   Best provided by multidisciplinary team composing of psychiatrist, social worker, neuropsychologist.

---

[1] Dementia is the significant impairment of memory and one or more other domain of cognition (language, visuospatial skills and praxis) in a setting of clear consciousness and interfering with work, social activities or relationships.

[2] β-amyloid deposition can also occur in the cerebral arteries causing cerebral amyloid angiopathy. This is typified by lobar haemorrhages and can be detected by MRI-gradient echo sequences.

Treatment of intercurrent illness or exarcebating factors: Avoid sedative drugs, antimuscarinic agents and alcohol, environmental management.

Adaptations: Medicalert bracelet, memory aids (diaries, labels).

Pharmacological: Anticholinesterase inhibitors (e.g. rivastigminem donepezil, galantamine) are only licensed for mild to moderate disease and provide only modest benefit.

Social: Manage psychological impact of disease on carer and patient. Initiate social support systems early before advanced disease requires institutional care. Early discussion of end-of-life care may be helpful.

COMPLLICATIONS Poor quality of life, loss of independence, devastating effect on family.

PROGNOSIS The average life expectancy from diagnosis is between 3 and 8 years.

Bell's palsy

DEFINITION   Idiopathic lower motor neurone facial (VII) nerve palsy.

AETIOLOGY   Idiopathic. Sixty percent are preceded by an upper respiratory tract infection, suggesting a viral or post-viral aetiology.

EPIDEMIOLOGY   Annual incidence is 15–40 in 100 000. Most cases: 20–50 year.

HISTORY   Prodrome of pre-auricular pain in some cases followed by acute (hours/days) onset unilateral facial weakness and droop. Maximum severity within 1–2 days.
Fifty percent experience facial, neck or ear pain or numbness.
Hypersensitivity to sound (hyperacusis caused by stapedius paralysis).
Loss of taste sense (uncommon).
Tearing or drying of exposed eye.

EXAMINATION   Lower motor neurone weakness of facial muscles (affects all the ipsilateral muscles of facial expression and does not spare the muscles of the upper part of the face as seen in UMN facial nerve palsy).
Bell's phenomenon: Eyeball rolls up but eye remains open when trying to close the eyes. Although patient may report unilateral facial numbness, clinical testing of sensation is normal. The ear should be examined to exclude other causes (e.g. otitis media, herpes zoster infection).

INVESTIGATIONS   Usually unnecessary except to exclude other causes, e.g. Lyme serology, herpes zoster serology.
EMG: May show local axonal conduction block in facial canal. Only useful >1 week after onset.

MANAGEMENT   Protection of cornea with protective glasses/patches and artificial tears. High-dose corticosteroids (prednisolone) is beneficial within 72 h (given only if Ramsay Hunt's syndrome is excluded). Little evidence for aciclovir.
Surgery: Lateral tarsorrhaphy (suturing the lateral parts of the eyelids together) if imminent or established corneal damage.

COMPLICATIONS   Corneal ulcers, eye infection. Aberrant reinnervation may occur, e.g. blinking may cause contraction of the angle of the mouth as a result of simultaneous innervation of obicularis oculi and ori. Parasympathetic fibres may also aberrantly reinnervate causing 'crocodile tears' when salivating.

PROGNOSIS   Most (85–90%) recover function within 2–12 weeks with or without treatment.

Carotid artery disease

DEFINITION   Narrowing of the carotid artery by atherosclerosis; a common cause of stroke.

AETIOLOGY   Atheromatous plaque at the common carotid bifurcation or any of the carotid branches can cause stroke or blindness by distal embolization, thrombosis or low flow. The carotid artery bifurcation is an area of the vascular tree where atherosclerosis is common. In combination with systemic risk factors, local haemodynamics, including low shear stress and ↑ turbulence affecting the outer walls opposite the flow divider pre-dispose to atheroma development, luminal narrowing and risk of plaque rupture, thrombosis or embolism.

EPIDEMIOLOGY   Common, third leading cause of death in UK and major cause of long-term disability, ↑incidence with age, more common in men.

HISTORY
Often *asymptomatic*.
Amaurosis fugax: Transient unilateral vision loss—'like a curtain coming down' caused by embolism into the ophthalmic artery (internal carotid artery branch).
Transient ischaemic attacks (TIAs): Focal symptoms lasting <24 h may be a precursor of a stroke. (*see* Transient ischaemic attack).
Crescendo TIAs: TIAs that increase in duration, severity or frequency. This is associated with a critical stenosis of the internal carotid artery, carotid dissection and may require anti-coagulation or carotid endarterectomy.
Stroke: Persistant neurological deficit (dependent on region affected by infarct). (*see* Stroke).

EXAMINATION   If asymptomatic, often no abnormality on examination.
A carotid bruit, if present, does not reflect the degree of stenosis.
Signs of TIA or CVA (e.g. dysarthria, dysphasia, weakness in limbs).

INVESTIGATIONS   *Duplex Doppler carotid ultrasound*: Non-invasive imaging to assess degree of stenosis. There are two criteria of assessing degree of stenosis (NASCET or ECST), and the method of evaluation needs to be noted.
CT, CTA, MRI and MRA: Brain and carotid imaging.
Angiography: Invasive (risk of precipitating stroke ~1%), enables very accurate assessment of stenosis severity.

MANAGEMENT   The EXPRESS study (Early use of eXisting PREventive Strategies for Stroke, Lancet 2007) showed that urgent assessment and treatment reduced the 90-day risk of recurrent stroke by 80%. All patients should be seen in a TIA clinic (urgency determined by ABCD2 scoring).
Medical treatment: Low-dose aspirin, stopping smoking and treatment of other risk factors, hypercholesterolaemia, hypertension and diabetes, for:
- asymptomatic stenosis,
- <70% internal carotid artery stenosis (ECST criteria),
- <50% (NASCET criteria), or
Surgical treatment: Carotid endarterectomy within 2 weeks of stroke or TIA reduces risk of further stroke in ECST and NASCET trials, although carries a significant peri-operative risk. May be considered in:
- symptomatic stenosis of 70–99% (ECST criteria),
- symptomatic stenosis of 50–99% (NASCET criteria) or
- crescendo TIAs not responding to medical treatment.
The role of surgical treatment in asymptomatic disease is controversial.
Angioplasty +/− stenting: Under evaluation compared to carotid endarterectomy for symptomatic disease. The SPACE and EVA-3S trials failed to show non-inferiority of

Carotid artery disease (continued)

carotid stenting vs. endarterectomy. The ICSS trial showed that carotid endarterectomy is superior to stenting at 30-day follow-up, longer follow-up results are pending. The CREST trial is underway but unlikely to overturn existing evidence.

COMPLICATIONS *Complications of disease*: Stroke (thromboembolic or watershed).
Complications from surgery: Cardiac ischaemia or infarction (3%), nerve injury (2–7%, mandibular branch of facial nerve, recurrent laryngeal nerve or hypoglossal nerves), haematoma, peri-operative stroke (1–5%). The peri-operative mortality rate is 0.5–1.8%.

PROGNOSIS For carotid artery stenosis of >70%, annual stroke rate is 10–20%. If untreated, asymptomatic stenosis of <50% has an annual stroke risk of 1%.
If surgically corrected: 6–8 fold relative risk reduction of stroke in 1 year.

Carotid artery dissection is the formation of a false lumen via a tear in the carotid intima which pre-disposes to TIAs and strokes. Often idiopathic, or may be associated with minor neck strain or iatrogenic (from angiography). Managed with either anti-coagulation or anti-platelet agents (no evidence which is better).

Carpal tunnel syndrome

DEFINITION   Carpal tunnel syndrome (CTS) refers to the symptom complex brought on by compression of the median nerve in the carpal tunnel.

AETIOLOGY   Compression of the median nerve within the carpal tunnel (formed by the flexor retinaculum superiorly and the carpal bones inferiorly). Usually idiopathic (43%) but may be secondary to:
Tenosynovitis: Overuse, rheumatoid arthritis, other inflammatory rheumatic disease.
Infiltrative diseases of the canal/increased soft tissue: Amyloidosis, myeloma myxoedema, acromegaly.
Bone involvement in the wrist: Osteoarthritis, fracture, tumour.
Fluid retention states: Pregnancy, nephrotic syndrome.
Other: Obesity, menopause, diabetes, end-stage renal disease

EPIDEMIOLOGY   Overall prevalence 2.7%. Incidence in adults 0.1% per year. Lifetime risk 10%.

HISTORY   Tingling and pain in the hand and fingers (patients may be woken up at night). Weakness and clumsiness of hand.

EXAMINATION   Sensory impairment in median nerve distribution (first $3\frac{1}{2}$ fingers). Weakness and wasting of the thenar eminence (abductor pollicis brevis and opponens)
Tinel's sign: Tapping carpal tunnel triggers symptoms.
Phalen's test: Maximal flexion of the wrist for 1 min may cause symptoms. Signs of the underlying cause, e.g. hypothyroidism or acromegaly.

INVESTIGATIONS   *Blood*: TFTs, ESR.
Nerve conduction study: Not always necessary. Shows impaired median nerve conduction across the carpal tunnel in the context of normal conduction elsewhere.

MANAGEMENT   *Mild to moderate CTS*: Nocturnal wrist splinting in the neutral position. If there is inadequate response: a single injection of methylprednisolone into the carpal tunnel.
Referral to an occupational therapist/carpal bone mobilization.
Moderate to severe CTS refractory to conservative measures: Surgical decompression.

COMPLICATIONS   Permanent motor and sensory impairment of the hand.

PROGNOSIS   Good. Majority of cases wax and wane over years. Secondary cases are more likely to progress further.

Cervical spondylosis

DEFINITION   Progressive degenerative process affecting the cervical vertebral bodies and intervertebral discs, and causing compression of the spinal cord and/or nerve roots.

AETIOLOGY   Osteoarthritic degeneration of vertebral bodies produces osteophytes, which protrude on to the exit foramina and spinal canal, and compress nerve roots (radiculopathy) or the anterior spinal cord (myelopathy).

EPIDEMIOLOGY   The mean age at diagnosis is 48 years. Annual incidence: 107 per 100 000 in men and 64 per 100 000 in women.

HISTORY   Neck pain or stiffness. Arm pain (stabbing or dull ache).
Paraesthesia, weakness, clumsiness in hands.
Weak and stiff legs, gait disturbance.
Atypical chest pain, breast pain or pain in the face.

EXAMINATION
Arms:
- Atrophy of forearm or hand muscles may be seen.
- Segmental muscle weakness in a nerve root distribution: C5: Shoulder abduction and elbow flexion weaknesses. C6: Elbow flexion and wrist extension weaknesses. C7: Elbow extension, wrist extension and finger extension weaknesses. C8: Wrist flexion and finger flexion weaknesses.
- Hyporeflexia. In C5 and C6 lesions, 'inverted' reflexes may be seen as a result of LMN impairment at the level of compression and UMN impairment below the level. Hoffmann's sign (flexion of the terminal thumb phalanx when rapidly extending the terminal phalanx of the 3nd or 3rd finger).
- Sensory loss (mainly pain and temperature).
- Pseudoathetosis (writhing finger motions when hands are outstretched, fingers spread and eyes closed).
Legs (seen in those with cervical cord compressions):
- ↑ Tone, weakness, hyper-reflexia and extensor plantars.
- ↓ Vibration and joint position sense (spinothalamic loss is less common) with a sensory level (few segments below the level of cord compression).
Lhermitte's sign: Neck flexion produces crepitus and/or paraesthesia down the spine.

INVESTIGATIONS

Spinal X-ray (lateral): May detect osteoarthritic change in the cervical spine. Rarely diagnostic in non-traumatic cervical radiculopathy. Flexion and extension films are important in the setting of trauma, and are helpful to evaluate for possible subluxation of one vertebral over another.
MRI: Assessment of root and cord compression and to exclude spinal cord tumour, and nerve root infiltration by tumour or granulomatous tissue. Many elderly people have some degree of cervical spondylosis and this may not be the cause of the symptoms.
Needle electromyography (EMG): May reveal a myotomal pattern of denervation.

MANAGEMENT

Conservative: Physiotherapy. Intermittent neck immobilization (soft neck collar), pain management (e.g. NSAIDs) and restriction of high-risk or aggravating activities. Close neurologic follow-up should assess for deterioration when surgery is deferred.
Acute deterioration is a neurologic emergency. Confirm the diagnosis with MRI. Seek surgical consultation. IV methylprednisolone within 8 h of acute deterioration.
Surgery (for more severe myelopathy or progressing deficits): Spinal decompression, facetectomy, laminectomy (only about 50% improve after surgery).

COMPLICATIONS   Lower cervical roots, particularly C7, are more frequently affected. Acute spinal cord compression. Bladder and sphincter dysfunction.

PROGNOSIS   If untreated, there can be a high quality of life impairment. Surgical treatment may only partially alleviate the impairment.

CNS tumours

DEFINITION   Primary tumours arising from any of the brain tissue types.

AETIOLOGY   In children, it probably reflects embryonic errors in development. In adults, the aetiology is unknown.

EPIDEMIOLOGY   Annual incidence of primary tumours 5–9 in 100 000. Two peaks of incidence (children and the elderly).

HISTORY   Headache or vomiting (↑ intracranial pressure), epilepsy (focal or generalized), focal neurological deficits (dysphagia, hemiparesis, ataxia, visual field defects, cognitive impairment), personality change.

EXAMINATION   Papilloedema/false localizing signs (↑ intracranial pressure).
Focal neurological deficits (visual field defects, dysphasia, agnosia, hemianopia, hemiparesis, ataxia, personality change).
Some localizing syndromes:

Location	Features
Olfactory groove	Anosmia, frontal lobe dysfunction
Cavernous sinus	Opthalmoplegia (III, IV, VI nerve palsies), V1 and V2 sensory loss
Foster Kennedy syndrome	Sphenoid wing meningioma compresses II nerve causing ipsilateral optic atrophy and contralateral papilloedema
Pituitary fossa	Bitemporal hemianopia (suprasellar expansion and optic chiasm compression), hypopituitarism or hypersecretion of specific hormones (e.g. acromegaly, hyperprolactinaemia, Cushing's disease)
Parinaud's syndrome (pineal region)	Impairing upgaze (superior midbrain lesion) or obstructive hydrocephalus (at the level of third ventricle)
Para-sagittal region	Spastic paraparesis (mimicking cord compression)
Cerebellopontine angle	Unilateral deafness, facial weakness, then unilateral ataxia and hemifacial sensory impairment

PATHOLOGY/PATHOGENESIS
- *Meningioma*: Benign and most common primary CNS tumour.
- *Fibrilliary astrocytoma*: Most common form, usually in cerebrum.
- *Pilocytic astrocytoma*: Cystic, in cerebellum and brainstem.
- *Glioblastoma multiforme*: High-grade invasive tumour.
- *Haemangioblastoma*: Vascular tumours, often in the cerebellum.
- *Pituitary adenoma*: Benign. Space-occupying and endocrine effects.
- *Oligodendroglioma*: Ten percent of gliomas. Epileptogenic.
- *Medulloblastoma*: Invasive midline cerebellar tumour in children.
- *Ependymoma*: Benign, in spinal cord and fourth ventricle.
- *Lymphoma*: In immunosuppressed patients, highly malignant.

INVESTIGATIONS   *CT-head*: Usual initial investigation.
MRI-brain: Higher sensitivity. Diffusion-weighted-imaging and MR spectroscopy can be helpful in characterizing lesion without biopsy. Functional MRI may be necessary if the lesion is located in dominant hemisphere for surgical planning.
Chest X-ray or CT (thorax, abdomen, pelvis): To determine if the lesion is secondary or primary.
Blood: CRP, ESR, consider HIV screen, toxoplasma serology.
Brain biopsy: Type and grading (degree of differentiation of tumour).
Lumbar puncture: Lumbar puncture is a relative contraindication if there is evidence of raised intracranial pressure, may cause coning (herniation).

CNS tumours (continued)

MANAGEMENT

Medical: Anticonvulsants for epilepsy. Dexamethasone to reduce brain oedema. Chemotherapy (e.g. temozolomide), radiotherapy and gamma-knife surgery to reduce tumour size.

Surgery: Debulking or total resection of the tumour (especially for benign tumours). Not preferred if on dominant hemisphere or near speech centres. In pituitary adenomas, trans-sphenoidal resection is possible. Intraventricular shunts for hydrocephalus. Surgery may be inappropriate for low-grade glioma causing epilepsy only or for multiple metastases.

COMPLICATIONS Pressure effect on surrounding tissue; herniation (falcine, tentorial, tonsillar); cerebrovascular accident (haemorrhage; *see* Stroke); focal or generalized fits (*see* Epilepsy).

PROGNOSIS Generally good for benign tumours, that are extra-axial (originate from meninges or cranial nerves). Malignant tumours that are intra-axial are generally incurable. Median survival is good in low-grade tumours (>5 year) but very poor in glioblastomas (about 9 months).

Encephalitis

DEFINITION Inflammation of the brain parenchyma.

AETIOLOGY In the majority of cases encephalitis is the result of a viral infection.

Virus: Most common in the UK is HSV. Other viruses are herpes zoster, mumps, adenovirus, coxsackie, echovirus, enteroviruses, measles, EBV, HIV, rabies (Asia), Nipah (Malaysia) and arboviruses transmitted by mosquitoes, e.g. Japanese B encephalitis (Asia), St. Louis and West Nile encephalitis (USA).

Non-viral: (rare) e.g. syphilis, Staphylococcus aureus.

Immunocompromised: CMV, toxoplasmosis, Listeria.

Autoimmune or paraneoplastic: May be associated with antibodies e.g. anti-NMDA or anti-VGKC.

EPIDEMIOLOGY Annual UK incidence is 7.4 in 100 000.

HISTORY In many cases, encephalitis is a mild self-limiting illness.

Subacute onset (hours to days) headache, fever, vomiting, neck stiffness, photophobia, i.e. symptoms of meningism (meningoencephalitis) with behavioural changes, drowsiness and confusion.

There is often a history of seizures.

Focal neurological symptoms (e.g. dysphasia and hemiplegia) may be present.

It is important to obtain a detailed travel history.

EXAMINATION ↓ level of consciousness with deteriorating GCS, seizures, pyrexia.

Signs of meningism: Neck stiffness, photophobia, Kernig's test positive. Signs of raised intracranial pressure: hypertension, bradycardia, papilloedema.

Focal neurological signs.

Minimental examination may reveal cognitive or psychiatric disturbances.

INVESTIGATIONS *Blood*: FBC (↑ lymphocytes), U&E (SIADH may occur), glucose (compare with CSF glucose), viral serology, ABG.

MRI/CT: Excludes mass lesion. HSV produces characteristic oedema of the temporal lobe on MRI.

Lumbar puncture: ↑ Lymphocytes, ↑ monocytes, ↑ protein, glucose usually normal. CSF culture is difficult, viral PCR is now first line.

EEG: May show epileptiform activity, e.g. spiking activity in temporal lobes.

Brain biopsy: Now very rarely performed.

MANAGEMENT Resuscitate and consider ITU.

Start empirical IV aciclovir (± antibiotics) immediately.

Mechanical ventilation if respiratory failure.

Monitor vital signs closely.

Manage fluid balance closely (risk of cerebral oedema), consider dexamethasone.

Anticonvulsants. Antipyretics. Antiemetics. Analgesia for headache.

COMPLICATIONS Post-encephalitic neurological sequalae, particularly epilepsy and cognitive impairment in 10–30% with variation according to viral aetiology.

PROGNOSIS Treated mortality is 20%. Survivors may have epilepsy or cognitive impairment. Increased chance of sequelae in age >30 years, GCS <6 on initiation of treatment.

Epilepsy

DEFINITION[1]   Epilepsy: >2 seizures.

Seizure (Ictus): Paroxysmal synchronised cortical electrical discharges.

- *Focal seizure*: Seizure localised to specific cortical regions, such as temporal lobe seizures, frontal lobe seizures, occipital seizures, complex partial seizures. Older nomenclature divided into simple partial (does not affect consciousness) and complex partial seizures (affects consciousness).
- *Generalised seizure*: Seizures which affect consciousness typically tonic-clonic, absence attacks, myoclonic, atonic (drop attacks) or tonic seizures.

AETIOLOGY   The majority of cases are idiopathic.

- Primary epilepsy syndromes (e.g. idiopathic generalised epilepsy, temporal lobe epilepsy, juvenile myoclonic epilepsy)
- Secondary seizures (symptomatic epilepsy)
  - Tumour.
  - Infection (e.g. meningitis, encephalitis, abscess).
  - Inflammation (vasculitis, rarely multiple sclerosis).
  - Toxic/metabolic (sodium imbalance, hyper- or hypoglycaemia, hypocalcaemia, hypoxia, porphyria, liver failure,
  - Drugs (e.g. including withdrawal e.g.alcohol, benzodiazepines).
  - Vascular (haemorrhage, infarction).
  - Congenital anomalies (e.g. cortical dysplasia)
  - Neurodegenerative disease (e.g. Alzheimer's disease).
  - Malignant hypertension or eclampsia.
  - Trauma.
- Common seizure mimics
  - Syncope
  - Migraine
  - Non-epileptiform seizure disorder (e.g. dissociative disorder)

Pathophysiology: Seizures result from an imbalance in the inhibitory and excitatory currents (e.g. Na^+ or K^+ ion channels) or neurotransmission (i.e. glutamate or GABA neurotransmitters) in the brain. Precipitants include any trigger which promotes excitation of the cerebral cortex (e.g. flashing lights, drugs, sleep deprivation, metabolic), but often cryptogenic.

EPIDEMIOLOGY: Common. Prevalence in 1% of general population. Peak age of onset is in early childhood or in the elderly.

HISTORY   Obtain history from a witness as well as the patient.

Key features from history to determine seizure semiology:

1) Rapidity of onset?
2) Duration of episode
3) Any alteration of consciousness?
4) Any tongue-biting or incontinence?
5) Any rhythmic synchronous limb jerking?
6) Any post-ictal period?
7) Drug history (alcohol, recreational drugs)

Focal seizures:

- *Frontal lobe focal motor seizures*: Motor convulsions. May demonstrate Jacksonian march (spasm spreading from mouth or digit). There may be post-ictal flaccid weakness (Todd's paralysis).

---

[1] Refer to the International League Against Epilepsy (ILAE) website for detailed classification and definitions.

- *Temporal lobe seizures*: Aura (visceral and psychic symptoms: fear or deja-vu sensation), hallucinations (olfactory, gustatory)
- *Frontal lobe complex partial seizures*: Loss of consciousness with associated automatisms and rapid recovery.

Generalised seizures:
- *Tonic-clonic (grand mal)*: Vague symptoms before an attack (e.g. irritability), followed by tonic phase (generalised muscle spasm), followed by a clonic phase (repetitive synchronous jerks), and associated faecal or urinary incontinence, tongue biting. After a seizure, there is often impaired consciousness, lethargy, confusion, headache, back pain, stiffness.
- *Absence (petit mal)*: Usual onset in childhood. Characterized by loss of consciousness but maintained posture (patient stops talking and stares into space for seconds), blinking or rolling up of eyes with other repetitive motor actions (e.g. chewing). No postictal phase.
- *Non-convulsive status epilepticus*: Acute confusional state. Often fluctuating. Difficult to distinguish from dementia.

EXAMINATION Depends on aetiology, usually normal between seizures.
Look for focal abnormalities indicative of brain lesions.

INVESTIGATIONS
Blood: FBC, U&E, LFTs, glucose, Ca^{2+}, Mg^{2+}, ABG, toxicology screen, prolactin (transient increase shortly after a 'true' seizure).
EEG: Helps confirm or refute the diagnosis; assists in classifying the epileptic syndrome. Usually performed inter-ictally and often normal and does not rule out epilepsy. Ictal EEGs combined with video telemetry are more useful but requires adequate facilities.
CT/MRI: For structural, space-occupying and vascular lesions.
Other investigations: Particularly for secondary seizures according to suspected aetiology e.g. lumbar puncture, HIV serology.

MANAGEMENT

Status epilepticus (seizure >30 min, failure to regain consciousness): Although defined as >30 min or repeated seizures with failure to regain consciousness, treatment is often initiated in 5–10 minutes as early treatment has higher treatment success.
- Resuscitate and protect airway, breathing and circulation.
- Check glucose and give if hypoglycaemic. Consider thiamine.
- IV lorazepam or IV or PR diazepam (repeat once after 15 min if needed). If seizures recur or fail to respond, IV phenytoin (15mg/kg) under ECG monitoring. Alternative IV agents include phenobarbitone, levetiracetam or sodium valproate.
- If these measures fail, consider general anaesthesia. This requires intubation and mechanical ventilation.
- Treat the cause: e.g. correct hypoglycaemia or hyponatraemia.
- Check plasma levels of all anticonvulsants.

Pharmacological treatment: Only start anti-convulsant therapy after >2 unprovoked seizures. There are numerous anti-convulsant agents, but the SANAD trial suggests that lamotrigine or carbamazepine as first line treatment for focal seizures, and sodium valproate for generalised seizures. Other commonly used agents include phenytoin, levetiracetam, clobazam, topiramate, gabapentin, vigabatrin, ethosuximide (absence).Start treatment with single anti-epileptic drug (AED).

Patient education: Patient education, avoid triggers (e.g. alcohol), encourage seizure diaries. Recommend supervision for swimming or climbing, driving is only permitted if seizure free for 6 months. Women of childbearing age should be counseled regarding possible teratogenic effects of AEDs and should consider taking supplemental folate to limit the risk.

Epilepsy (continued)

Drug interactions e.g. enzyme-inducing AEDs can limit the effectiveness of oral contraception.

Surgery for refractory epilepsy: Removal of definable epileptogenic focus (determined from detailed EEG, intracortical recordings, ictal SPECT, neuropsychometry). Alternatively, vagus nerve stimulator.

COMPLICATIONS Fractures with tonic-clonic seizures, behavioural problems, sudden death in epilepsy (SUDEP).

Complications of AEDs (e.g. gingivial hypertrophy with phenytoin, neutropenia or osteoperosis with carbamazepine, Stevens-Johnson syndrome with lamotrigine).

PROGNOSIS Fifty percent remission at 1 year. Mortality 2 in 100 000/year, directly related to seizure or secondary to injury.

Giant cell arteritis (Temporal arteritis)

DEFINITION   Granulomatous inflammation of large arteries, particularly branches of the external carotid artery, most commonly the temporal artery.

AETIOLOGY   Unknown. Increasing age, genetic and ethnic background, and infection may have causative roles. Associated with *HLA-DR4* and *HLA-DRB1*.
Both the humoral and cellular immune systems have been implicated in the pathogenesis of GCA.

EPIDEMIOLOGY   Annual incidence is 18 in 100 000. $♀:♂ = 2–4 : 1$. Peak age onset 65–70 years.

HISTORY   Subacute onset, usually over a few weeks.
Headache: Scalp and temporal tenderness (pain on combing hair). Jaw and tongue claudication.
Visual disturbances: Blurred vision, sudden blindness in one eye (amaurosis fugax[1]).
Systemic features: Malaise, low-grade fever, lethargy, weight loss, depression.
Symptoms of polymyalgia rhuematica (PMR): Early morning pain and stiffness of the muscles of the shoulder and pelvic girdle (40–60% of cases are associated with PMR).

EXAMINATION   Swelling and erythema overlying the temporal artery. Scalp and temporal tenderness.
Thickened non-pulsatile temporal artery.
↓Visual acuity.
Blood: ↑ ESR, FBC (normocytic anaemia of chronic disease).
Temporal artery biopsy: Within 48 h of starting corticosteroids. Note that a negative biopsy does not exclude the diagnosis, because skip lesions occur.

MANAGEMENT   Start on high dose oral prednisolone (40–60 mg/day) immediately to prevent visual loss. The majority of patients experience immense symptomatic relief within 48 h of commencing steroid therapy. ↓ Dose of prednisolone gradually (according to symptoms and ESR) to a maintenance dose of 7.5–10 mg/day. Many patients require prednisolone for 1–2 years.
Low dose aspirin (plus PPIs for gastroprotection) to ↓ the risk of visual loss, TIAs or stroke. Osteoporosis prevention (adequate dietary calcium and vitamin D intake, bisphosphonates).
If GCA is complicated by visual loss: IV pulse methylprednisolone (1 g for 3 days) followed by oral prednisolone (60 mg/day, as above).
Annual CXR for up to 10 years to identify thoracic aortic aneurysms. If detected, monitor with CT every 6–12 months.

COMPLICATIONS   Carotid artery or aortic aneurysms. Thrombosis may occur followed by recanalization or embolism to the ophthalmic artery leading to visual disturbances, amaurosis fugax or sudden monocular blindness.

PROGNOSIS   In most cases the condition lasts for ∼2 years before complete remission.

---

[1] Amaurosis fugax is a gradual descending mono-ocular 'curtain' of vision loss.

Guillain–Barre syndrome

DEFINITION   Acute inflammatory demyelinating polyneuropathy.

AETIOLOGY   An inflammatory process where antibodies after a recent infection reacts with self-antigen on myelin or neurons. There are rare axonal variants with no demyelination. Often no aetiological trigger is identified (idiopathic in about 40%), in other cases:
- Post-infection (1–3 weeks): bacterial (e.g. *Campylobacter jejuni*), HIV, herpes viruses (e.g. zoster, CMV).
- Malignancy (lymphoma, Hodgkin's disease).
- Post-vaccination.

EPIDEMIOLOGY   Annual UK incidence is 1–2 in 100 000. Affects all age groups.

HISTORY   Progressive symptoms of ≤1 month duration of:
- Ascending symmetrical limb weakness (lower > upper).
- Ascending paraesthesia.

Cranial nerve involvement (e.g. dysphagia, dysarthria and facial weakness).
In severe cases, the respiratory muscles may be affected.
Miller–Fisher variant (rare): Opthalmoplegia, ataxia and arreflexia.

EXAMINATION   *General motor examination*: Hypotonia, flaccid paralysis, arreflexia (typically ascending upwards from feet to head).
General sensory examination: Impairment of sensation in multiple modalities (typically ascending upwards from feet to head).
Cranial nerve palsies (less frequently): Facial nerve weakness (lower motor neurone pattern), abnormality of external ocular movements, signs of bulbar palsy. If pupil constriction is affected, consider botulism[1].
Type II respiratory failure: Important to identify early (e.g. CO_2 flap, bounding pulse, drowsiness). This can be insidious, and needs regular assessment.
Autonomic function: Assess for postural BP change and arrhythmias.

INVESTIGATIONS

Lumbar puncture: ↑ CSF protein, cell count and glucose normal.
Nerve conduction study: ↓ Conduction velocity or conduction block, but can be normal in the early phase of the disease.
Blood: Anti-ganglioside antibodies are positive in Miller–Fisher variant and 25% of Guillain–Barré syndrome cases; consider *C. jejuni* serology.
Spirometry: ↓ Fixed vital capacity indicates ventilatory weakness.
ECG: Arrhythmias may develop.

MANAGEMENT

Acute: High-dose IV immunoglobulin or plasmapheresis may reduce duration or severity of disease.
Supportive: Actively monitor vital capacity and ECG, as patients may require intubation. DVT prophylaxis, regular physiotherapy with care of pressure areas. Dysphagia may warrant nasogastric feeding.

COMPLICATIONS   Respiratory failure, cardiac arrhythmias, sepsis (e.g. aspiration pneumonia, UTIs), pulmonary embolus, incomplete recovery, relapse, death.

PROGNOSIS   Eighty five percent complete recovery, usually within 3–6 months. Ten percent have residual neurological disability. Mortality rate of 5%. Poorer outcome in axonal-variants.

---

[1] Botulism is caused by the botulinum toxin produced by the *Clostridium botulinum* anaerobe. Typically toxins are ingested from improperly cooked meat, but can also be iatrogenic (e.g. botox IM injections) or via wounds. Typically presents with descending paralysis affecting bulbar and ocular muscles first and causing bilateral fixed pupils. Treatment consists of supportive airway management and antitoxin (does not reverse the weakness).

Huntington's disease

DEFINITION   Autosomal dominant trinucleotide repeat disease characterized by progressive chorea and dementia, typically commencing in middle age.

AETIOLOGY   The huntingtin gene is located on chromosome 4p and codes for the protein huntingtin. In the huntingtin gene there is an extended trinucleotide repeat expansion (CAG) resulting in a toxic gain of function. The disease is inherited in an autosomal dominant pattern and exhibits anticipation (earlier age of onset in each successive generation).

EPIDEMIOLOGY   Worldwide prevalence eight in 100 000. Average age onset 30–50 years. Rare in East Asian populations (particularly Japan).

HISTORY   Family history of Huntington's disease.
Insidious onset in middle-age of progressive fidgeting and clumsiness, developing into involuntary, jerky, dyskinetic movements often accompanied by grunting and dysarthria.
In late disease, the patient may become rigid, akinetic and bed-bound.
Early cognitive, emotional and behavioural changes are dominated by lability, dysphoria, mental inflexibility, anxiety, leading on to dementia.
Inquire about drug history (especially cocaine, anti-psychotics).

EXAMINATION   Classically, patient presents with chorea and dysarthria.
Slow voluntary saccades and supranuclear gaze restriction.
Other presentations include parkinsonism and dystonia (especially in juvenile-onset disease).
Mental state examination reveals cognitive and emotional deficits.

INVESTIGATIONS   *Genetic analysis*: Diagnostic if >39 CAG repeats in the HD gene. Intermediate repeat lengths (27–39) exist with reduced penetrance.
Imaging: Brain MRI or CT may show symmetrical atrophy of the striatum (particularly the caudate nuclei) and butterfly dilation of the lateral ventricles.
Bloods: May be necessary to exclude other pathology: caeruloplasmin, anti-nuclear antibodies blood film (acanthocytes), TFT, ESR.

MANAGEMENT   Best managed by a specialist unit due to extensive ramifications to the patient and his/her family. Psychological support for patient and family.
Treatment of symptoms
• Antidepressants for depression.
• Dopamine-depleting drugs (reserpine, tetrabenazine) and benzodiazepines for chorea.
• Atypical anti-psychotics (for psychosis).

Multidisciplinary approach consisting of:
• Occupational therapy.
• Speech and language therapy.
• Dietician.

Genetic counselling of patient and relatives.

COMPLICATIONS   Fifty percent of offspring will carry the Huntington's disease gene. High risk of depression, attempted suicide (28%) and suicide (7%).

PROGNOSIS   Most patients die in 15–20 years after first onset of symptoms usually from respiratory tract infection.

Hydrocephalus

DEFINITION   Enlargement of the cerebral ventricular system. Subdivisible into obstructive and non-obstructive (or communicating or non-communicating). *Hydrocephalus ex vacuo* is a term used to describe apparent enlargement of ventricles but this is a compensatory change due to brain atrophy.

AETIOLOGY   Abnormal accumulation of CSF in the ventricles can be caused by:
(1) Impaired outflow of the CSF from the ventricular system (obstructive)
    - lesions of the third ventricle, fourth ventricle, cerebral aqueduct;
    - posterior fossa lesions (e.g. tumour, blood) compressing the fourth ventricle;
    - cerebral aqueduct stenosis.
(2) Impaired CSF resorption in the subarahnoid villi (non-obstructive)
    - tumours;
    - meningitis (typically tuberculosis);
    - Normal pressure hydrocephalus (NPH) is the idiopathic chronic ventricular enlargement. The long white matter tracts (corona radiata, anterior commisure) are damaged causing gait and cognitive decline.

EPIDEMIOLOGY   Bimodal age distribution. Congenital malformations and tumours in the young, tumours and strokes in the elderly.

HISTORY
Obstructive hydrocephalus: Acute drop in conscious level. Diplopia.
NPH: Chronic cognitive decline, falls, urinary incontinence.

EXAMINATION
Obstructive hydrocephalus: Impaired GCS, papilloedema, VI nerve palsy ('false localizing sign' of increased ICP). In neonates, the head circumference may enlarge, and 'sunset sign' (downward conjugate deviation of eyes).
NPH: Cognitive impairment. Gait apraxia (shuffling). Hyper-reflexia.

INVESTIGATIONS
CT head: First-line investigation to detect hydrocephalus. May also detect the cause (e.g. tumour in the brainstem).
CSF: Obtained from ventricular drains or lumbar puncture may indicate an underlying pathology (e.g. tuberculosis). Check for MC&S, protein, glucose (CSF and plasma).
Lumbar puncture: This is contra-indicated in obstructive hydrocephalus as it can cause tonsilar herniation and death. May be necessary in NPH as a therapeutic trial.

MANAGEMENT   *Emergency*: Airway, breathing and circulation. If GCS is impaired, protect and secure airway. Treat seizures. Obtain CT and liase with neurosurgery urgently.
External ventricular drain: Insertion of a catheter into the lateral ventricle to bypass any obstruction.
Ventriculo-peritoneal shunting: Implantation of a ventricular catheter into one or both lateral ventricles and connecting it to a subcutaneous drain which leads to the peritoneal cavity. Carries risk of shunt infection, block or malfunction (especially as some are electronic).
Lumbar-peritoneal shunting: Alternative procedure that may be suitable for communicating hydrocephalus.
Advanced neurosurgery: Endoscopic ventriculostomy and aqueductoplasty are other options used to bypass blockages or maintain patency for CSF flow.

COMPLICATIONS   Cerebral herniation, coning and death.

PROGNOSIS   Obstructive hydrocephalus is often fatal if untreated.
Cognitive and gait decline in NPH can improve with shunting.

Inflammatory myopathies

DEFINITION   Idiopathic primary inflammatory myopathies characterized by chronic inflammation of striated muscle (polymyositis and inclusion body myositis, IBM) and skin (dermatomyositis).

AETIOLOGY   Unknown. Proposed autoimmune aetiology, possibly infective or malignancy trigger in genetically pre-disposed individual.

ASSOCIATIONS/RISK FACTORS
- Polymyositis may be associated with autoimmune connective tissue diseases (e.g. scleroderma).
- Dermatomyositis may be associated with bronchial, stomach, testicular, breast and ovarian malignancy, and auto-antibodies anti-Jo-1, anti-Scl, anti-Mi2, HLA linkage to DRW52.

EPIDEMIOLOGY   Rare. Annual incidence is 0.2–1 in 100 000. Peaks at childhood (5–15 years) and adult (40–60 years).
Inclusion body myositis is the most common inflammatory myopathy in person of >50 years.

HISTORY

Polymyositis and dermatomyositis: Gradual onset (3–6 months) of progressive painless proximal muscle weakness (difficulty raising objects above head, rising from chair, climbing stairs).
Inclusion body myositis: Insidious onset (over months to years). Affects rising from chair, climbing stairs and dexterity of hands. There may be dysphagia and neck droop.
Fatigue, malaise, dyspnoea are typical general symptoms.
Myalgia and arthralgia may also occur.
Enquire about skin rash and Raynaurd's phenomenon.

EXAMINATION

Polymyositis and dermatomyositis: Proximal muscle weakness and atrophy affecting both upper and lower limbs.
Inclusion body myositis: Proximal and distal muscle weakness and atrophy (particularly wrist and deep finger flexors, quadriceps). Weakness of erector spinae and dysphagia is common.
Skin lesions in dermatomyositis: Macular 'lilac' heliotrope rash on upper eyelids with periorbital oedema, rash on chest wall, neck, elbows or knees. Gottren's papules (scaly erythematous raised plaques on finger joints, periungal telangiecstasia, ragged cuticles), 'mechanics' hands' (fissuring dermatitis of finger pads).

PATHOLOGY/PATHOGENESIS
- *Polymyositis*: Cytotoxic CD8+ T-cell infiltrate which appear to recognize an antigen on muscle fibre surface.
- *Dermatomyositis*: Probably humorally-mediated disorder with perivascular and perifascicular infiltrate in skeletal muscle.
- *Inclusion body myositis*: T-cell inflammatory infiltrate into the skeletal muscle suggests an immune basis. Non-inflamed skeletal muscle fibres may contain rimmed vacuoles and amyloid deposits suggesting a degenerative process.

INVESTIGATIONS   Careful evaluation for underlying malignancy.
Blood: FBC (↓ Hb of chronic disease), ↑ESR (normal in one-third), CK (↑ in 95% of cases), auto-antibody titres.
EMG: Shows ↑ insertional activity, ↑ spontaneous fibrillations; abnormal low-amplitude short-duration polyphasic motor potentials and bizarre high-frequency discharges indicative of myopathy.
Muscle biopsy: Required for definitive diagnosis. Inclusion body myositis has typical features of inflammation as well as vacuolated uninflamed muscle fibres and amyloid deposits.
CT or MRI: To look for malignancies.

Inflammatory myopathies (continued)

MANAGEMENT
Medical:
- *Polymyositis and dermatomyositis*: Corticosteroids are mainstay of therapy (e.g. prednisolone, monitoring response by CK levels). Steroid-sparing therapies (e.g. methotrexate, azathioprine, mycophenolate, IV immunoglobulin).
- *Inclusion body myositis*: Classically unresponsive to steroids and immunosuppression.

Other: Physiotherapy and occupational therapy aids.

COMPLICATIONS   Severe bulbar and respiratory muscle weakness may result in aspiration pneumonia or respiratory failure.
Dermatomyositis: Incidence of malignancy is highest in the 2 years after initial diagnosis of dermatomyositis. Interstitial pneumonitis and cardiac involvement can occur.
Inclusion body myositis: Slowly progressive and disabling but does not affect life span.

PROGNOSIS   Long remissions are possible, especially in children. The majority of patients experience multiple remissions and exacerbations.

Meningitis

DEFINITION Inflammation of the leptomeningeal (pia mater and arachnoid) coverings of the brain, most commonly caused by infection.

AETIOLOGY
Bacterial:
Neonates: Group B streptococci, *Escherichia coli, Listeria monocytogenes*.
Children: *Haemophilus influenzae, Neisseria meningitidis, Streptococcus pneumoniae*.
Adults: *Neisseria meningitidis* (meningococcus), *Streptococcus pneumoniae*, tuberculosis.
Elderly: *Streptococcus pneumoniae, Listeria monocytogenes*.
Viral: Enteroviruses, mumps, HSV, VZV, HIV.
Fungal: *Cryptococcus* (associated with HIV infection).
Others[1]: Aseptic meningitis[1], Mollaret's meningitis[2]
Risk factors: Close communities (e.g. dormitories), basal skull fractures, mastoiditis, sinusitis, inner ear infections, alcoholism, immunodeficiency, splenectomy, sickle cell anaemia, CSF shunts, intracranial surgery.

EPIDEMIOLOGY Variation according to geography, age, social conditions. UK Public Health Laboratory Service receives ~2500 notifications/year. More common in recent visitors to the Haj (meningococcal serogroup W135), epidemics occur in the meningitis belt of Africa (meningococcal serogroup A).

HISTORY Severe headache, photophobia, neck or backache, irritability, drowsiness, vomiting, high-pitched crying or fits (common in children), clouding of consciousness, fever.
Careful history should include travel and exposure history: exposure to rodents (Lymphocytic choriomeningitis virus), ticks (e.g. Lyme borrelia, Rocky Mountain spotted fever), mosquitoes (West Nile virus, St. Louis encephalitis virus), sexual activity (HSV-2, HIV, syphilis), travel (*C. immitis, A. cantonensis*) and contact with other individuals with viral exanthems (enteroviruses).

EXAMINATION *Signs of meningism*: Photophobia, neck stiffness (Kernig's sign: with hips flexed, pain/resistance on passive knee extension; Brudzinski's sign: flexion of hips on neck flexion). *Signs of infection*: Fever, tachycardia and hypotension, skin rash (petechiae with meningococcal septicaemia), altered mental state.

INVESTIGATIONS *Blood*: Two sets of blood cultures (do not delay antibiotics).
Imaging: CT scan to exclude a mass lesion or ↑ intracranial pressure before LP, (may lead to cerebral herniation during subsequent CSF removal). A CT scan of the head must be done before LP in patients with: immunodeficiency, history of CNS disease, ↓ consciousness, fit, focal neurologic deficit or papilloedema.
Lumbar puncture: Note opening CSF pressure. Send CSF for microscopy with, culture, sensitivity and Gram staining (*Streptococcus pneumoniae*: Gram-positive diplococcic, *Neisseria Meningitidis*: gram-negative diplococcic), biochemistry and cytology. *Bacterial*: Cloudy CSF, ↑ neutrophils, ↑ protein, ↓ glucose (CSF: serum glucose ratio of <0.5).
Viral: ↑ Lymphocytes, ↑ protein, normal glucose.
TB: Fibrinous CSF, ↑ lymphocytes, ↑ protein, ↓ glucose.

---

[1] *Aseptic meningitis* : Characterized by clinical and laboratory evidence for meningeal inflammation and negative routine bacterial cultures. May be secondary to:
- Enterovirus (most common cause), mycobacteria, fungi, spirochetes.
- Autoimmune e.g. Sarcoidosis, Behcet's disease, Systemic lupus erythematosus.
- Malignancy (lymphoma, leukaemia, metatstatic carcinomas).
- Medication (NSAIDs, trimethoprim, azathioprine).
[2] *Mollaret's meningitis*: Recurrent benign lymphocytic meningitis. Fifty percent exhibit transient neurological manifestations. The most common cause is HSV-2. CSF: large granular plasma cells on Papanicolaou's stain, PCR for HSV DNA. Treat with acyclovir.

Meningitis (continued)

Staining of petechiae scrapings may detect meningococcus in ~70%.

Additional studies e.g. viral PCR, staining/culture for mycobacteria and fungi, HIV test depending on the clinical presentation/CSF findings.

MANAGEMENT *Immediate IV/IM antibiotics* if meningitis suspected (before lumbar puncture or CT). Third-generation cephalosporin (cefotaxime 2 g qds or ceftriaxone 2 g bd). Benzylpenicillin may be given as initial 'blind' therapy and for sensitive meningococci and pneumococci. Amoxicillin + gentamicin for *Listeria*. For penicillin- and cephalosporin resistant pneumococci: add vancomycin and if necessary rifampicin. If there is history of anaphylaxis to penicillin or cephalosporins or if the organism is resistant to these, use chloramphenicol. Give rifampicin for 2 days to patients treated with benzylpenicillin or chloramphenicol (to eliminate nasopharyngeal carriage).

Dexamethasone IV (10 mg QDS for 4 days) given shortly before or with first dose of antibiotics. Continue in pneumococcal or *H. influenzae* meningitis: ↓ complications: death (*S. pneumoniae*) and hearing loss (*H. influenza*). Avoid dexamethasone if HIV is suspected.

Resuscitation: Patient is best managed in ITU. *Prevention* (only applicable to meningococcal meningitis): *Notify* public health services and consult a consultant in communicable disease control for advice regarding chemoprophylaxis (e.g. rifampicin for 2 days) and vaccination for close contacts. Vaccination against meningococcal serogroups A and C. (Note that there is no vaccine for serogroup B, the most common serological group isolated in UK.)

COMPLICATIONS Septicaemia, shock, DIC, renal failure, fits, peripheral gangrene, cerebral oedema, cranial nerve lesions, cerebral venous thrombosis, hydrocephalus, Waterhouse–Friderichsen syndrome (bilateral adrenal haemorrhage).

PROGNOSIS Mortality rate from bacterial meningitis is high (10–40% with meningococcal sepsis). In developing countries mortality rate often higher. Viral meningitis self-limiting.

Migraine

DEFINITION   Severe episodic headache that may have a prodrome of focal neurological symptoms (aura) and is associated with systemic disturbance. Can be subclassified as migraine with aura (classical migraine) or without aura (common migraine) and migraine variants (familial hemiplegic, opthalmoplegic and basilar).

AETIOLOGY   Precise pathophysiological mechanism poorly understood. Early aura of cortical spreading depression associated with intracranial vasoconstriction resulting in localized ischaemia. This is followed by meningeal and extracranial vasodilation mediated by 5-HT, bradykinin and the trigeminovascular system.
Familial hemiplegic migraine: Rare; mutations in the P/Q-type calcium channel are the cause of this rare form of migraine.

EPIDEMIOLOGY   Prevalence is 6% in males and 15–20% in females. $♀:♂ = 3:1$. Usual onset in adolescence or early adulthood, but can occur in middle age.

HISTORY   *Headache*: Pulsating. Bilateral (in 30–40%). Duration 4–72 h. Obtain a detailed history of headache frequency and pattern. Most migraine attacks are episodic and chronic daily headache lasting many weeks suggest either analgesia-overuse headache or secondary headaches.
Associated symptoms: Associated with nausea, vomiting, photophobia or phonophobia. May be preceded by *aura* that may include visual disturbance, flashing lights, spots, blurring, zigzag lines (fortification spectra), blindspots (scotomas) or other sensory symptoms such as tingling or numbness in limbs.
Triggers and risk factors: Obtain a detailed history of possible triggers including stress, exercise, lack of sleep, oral contraceptive pill, certain foods (e.g. caffeine, alcohol, cheese, chocolate) and the pattern of analgesia use.

EXAMINATION   Usually no specific physical findings. Examination of mental state, neurological examination, funduscopy, sinuses, cervical spine, general examination to exclude secondary causes. (e.g. meningoencephalitis, idiopathic intracranial hypertension, subarachnoid haemorrhage, space-occupying lesion, temporal arteritis).

INVESTIGATIONS   Diagnosis based on history. Investigations may be needed to exclude other diagnoses.
Blood: FBC, ESR.
CT/MRI: If suspicion of secondary headache disorders.
Lumbar puncture: If suspicion of meningitis. Do not perform until space-occupying lesion excluded.

MANAGEMENT   *Medical*: Beware of analgesia-overuse headaches as many patients use OTC preparations.
Acute: NSAID (e.g. naproxen), paracetamol, codeine and antiemetics (e.g. metoclopramide). A variety of 'triptans' (5-HT$_1$ agonists) are available but commonly used ones are sumatriptan and zolmitriptan (which can be given orally, nasally or subcutaneously). Ergotamine is rarely used due to complex dosing schedules.
Prophylaxis (if > 2/month, 50% patients benefit): β-blockers, amitriptyline, topiramate and sodium valproate, pizotifen (5-HT2 antagonist) and calcium-channel blocker (flunarizine). Menstrual migraine can be controlled by the oral contraceptive pill.
Advice: Encourage regular meals and sleep, caffeine restriction, measures to reduce stress, avoid triggers, symptom diary. Rest in quiet dark room during episode.

COMPLICATIONS   Disruption of daily activities. Can progress onto analgesia-overuse headache due to chronic use of analgesics.

PROGNOSIS   Usually chronic, but majority of cases can be managed well by preventative/early treatment measures.

Motor neuron disease

DEFINITION A progressive neurodegenerative disorder of cortical, brainstem and spinal motor neurons (lower and upper motor neuron). Various subtypes:

- Amyotrophic lateral sclerosis (ALS) or Lou Gehrig's disease: combined degeneration of upper and lower motor neurones producing a mix of UMN and LMN neurones.
- Progressive muscular atrophy variant: Only LMN signs, e.g. flail arm or flail foot syndrome. Better prognosis.
- Progressive bulbar palsy variant:[1] Dysarthria and dysphagia with wasted fasciculating tongue (LMN) and brisk jaw jerk (UMN).
- Primary lateral sclerosis variant: UMN pattern of weakness, brisk reflexes, extensor plantar responses, without LMN signs.

AETIOLOGY Unknown. Free radical damage and glutamate excitotoxicity have been Implicated as mutations in superoxide dismutase (SOD1 gene) affect 20% with familial motor neuron disease and 1–4% of 'sporadic' cases. SOD1 codes for a metalloenzyme for the conversion of free radicals.

Pathology: Progressive motor neuron degeneration and death with gliosis replacing lost neurons. Neurons may exhibit intracellular inclusions (neurofilaments or ubiquinated inclusions) containing the TAR-DNA binding protein 43 (TDP-43).

Association: Associated with frontotemporal lobar dementia (FTLD) from proganulin mutations.

EPIDEMIOLOGY Rare, annual incidence is 2 per 100 000. Mean age of onset is 55 years. 5–10% have family history with autosomal dominant inheritance.

HISTORY
Weakness of limbs (focal or asymmetrical).
Speech disturbance (slurring or reduction in volume).
Swallowing disturbance (e.g. choking on food, nasal regurgitation).
There may be behavioural changes (e.g. disinhibition, emotional lability).

EXAMINATION Combination of upper motor neuron (UMN) and lower motor neuron (LMN) signs often affecting several regions asymmetrically.

LMN features: Muscle wasting, fasciculations, flaccid weakness, depressed or absent reflexes.
UMN features: Spastic weakness, brisk reflexes, extensor plantars.
Sensory examinaiton: Should be normal.

INVESTIGATIONS Investigations aimed to confirm the diagnosis by providing evidence of combined UMN and LMN loss and excluding other causes.

Blood: CK (mild ↑), ESR. Consider testing for anti-GM1 ganglioside antibodies (present in multifocal motor neuropathy[2]).

Electromyography (EMG): Features of acute and chronic denervation with giant motor unit action potentials in more than 1 limb and/or paraspinals.

Nerve conduction studies: Most often normal.

MRI: To exclude cord or root compression, and brainstem lesion in progressive bulbar palsy variant. May show high signal in motor tracts on T2 imaging.

---

[1] Bulbar palsy: Any lesion affecting cranial nerves (IX–XII) at nuclear, nerve or muscle level, presenting with nasal speech, nasal regurgitation of food, especially fluids (palatal weakness), ↓ gag reflex, absent jaw jerk, wasted fasciculating tongue.

Pseudobulbar palsy: Any UMN (corticobulbar) lesion to the lower brainstem, presenting with monotonous or explosive speech, dysphagia, " ↑ gag reflex, brisk jaw reflex, shrunken immobile tongue, emotional lability, UMN limb spasticity and weakness.

[2] Multifocal motor neuropathy: Characterized by asymmetrical LMN signs. Important to distinguish from MND as treatable. Motor nerve conduction studies show evidence of conduction block, representing focal demyelination. Associated with GM1 autoantibodies. Treatable with intravenous immunoglobulin, steroids or immunosuppression.

Spirometry: To assess respiratory muscle weakness (FVC)

MANAGEMENT Mainstay of treatment is supportive and symptomatic.

Pharmacological: Riluzole (inactivator of voltage-gated sodium channels and indirect inhibitor of glutamate release) has a modest effect on prolonging survival. Monitor LFTs.

Symptomatic treatment: Spasticity (e.g. baclofen), salivation (anti-cholinergics), dyspnoea and anxiety (opiates, benzodiazepines)

Multidisciplinary management: Psychological support, physiotherapy, walking aids, home adaptations, speech and language therapy, communication aids, swallowing assessment, dietician input.

End of life management: Consider percutaneous endoscopic gastrostomy (PEG) and non-invasive ventilation if appropriate and compatible with patient's wishes. Consider hospice care in terminal stages.

COMPLICATIONS Depression, emotional lability, frontal type dementia. Weight loss and malnutrition (resulting from dysphagia). Immobility-related problems: DVT, aspiration pneumonia.

Respiratory failure because of weakness of ventilatory muscles (usual cause of death).

PROGNOSIS Relentless progression. Mean survival is about 3 years. Bulbar onset and young onset have worse prognosis.

Multiple sclerosis (MS)

DEFINITION Inflammatory demyelinating disease of the central nervous system.

Relapsing-remitting MS: Commonest form. Characterised by clinical attacks of demyelination with complete recovery in between attacks.

Clinically isolated syndrome: Single clinical attack of demyelination; (does not qualify as MS); 10–50% progress to developing MS.

Primary progressive MS: Steadily accumulation of disability with no clear relapsing-remitting pattern.

Marburg variant[2]: Severe fulminant variant of MS leading to advanced disability of death within a period of weeks. Distinct from acute disseminated encephalomyelitis (ADEM)[2].

AETIOLOGY Unknown. Autoimmune basis with postulated environmental trigger in a genetically susceptible individual. Immune-mediated damage to CNS myelin results in impaired conduction along axons. There is also associated grey matter atrophy.

Risk factors: A role for EBV exposure and prenatal vitamin D levels have been proposed based on epidemiological studies. Strong concordance in monozygotic versus dizygotic twins (25% vs 3%). Geographical variation (temperate>tropical) with individuals carrying the risk of their pre-pubertal (<13 years) country of origin.

EPIDEMIOLOGY Prevalence in UK is one in 1000 (rare in Far East). ♀:♂ 2:1. Usually presents at 20–40 years.

HISTORY Varies depending on site of inflammation.

Optic neuritis (commonest): Unilateral deterioration in visual acuity and colour perception. Pain on eye movement.

Sensory system: Pins and needles, numbness, burning.

Motor: Limb weakness, spasms, stiffness, heaviness.

Autonomic: Urinary urgency, hesitancy, incontinence, impotence.

Psychological: Depression, psychosis.

Uhthoff's phenomenon: Transient increase or recurrence of symptoms due to conduction block precipitated by a rise in body temperature.

EXAMINATION

Optic neuritis[1]: Impaired visual acuity (most common), loss of coloured vision. On fundoscopy, in active disease, there is a swollen optic nerve head, in chronic disease, there may be optic atrophy.

Visual field testing: Central scotoma (optic nerve affected) or field defects (optic radiations affected).

Relative afferent pupillary defect: Tested with a swinging torch test. Both pupils contract when light is shone on the unaffected side, both pupils dilate when light is 'swung' to the diseased (eye).

Internuclear opthalmoplegia: Lateral horizontal gaze produces a failure of adduction of the contralateral eye. This indicates a lesion of the contralateral medial longitudinal fasciculus.

Sensory: Paraesthesia (vibration and joint position sense loss more common than pain and temperature).

Motor: UMN signs (e.g. spastic weakness, brisk reflexes).

Cerebellar: Limb ataxia (intention tremor, past-pointing and dysmetria on finger-nose test and heel-shin test), dysdiadochokinesis, ataxic wide-based gait, scanning speech.

Lhermitte's phenomenon: Electric shock-like sensation in arms and legs precipitated by neck flexion.

---

[1] Neuromyelitis optica (Devic's syndrome): Rare demyelinating condition which is typified by optic neuritis and extensive transverse myelitis. Associated with anti-aquaporin-4 antibodies.

[2] Acute disseminated encephalomyelitis (ADEM): Uncommon acute monophasic CNS demyelinating condition thought to be a post-viral autoimmune phenomenon. Neurological deterioration may be so severe that intubation may be required. Treated with high dose steroids.

INVESTIGATIONS   Diagnosis based on two or more CNS lesions with corresponding symptoms, separated in time and space (McDonald criteria).

Lumbar puncture: Microscopy to exclude other infective or inflammatory causes. CSF electrophoresis shows unmatched oligoclonal bands.

MRI-brain, cervical and thoracic spine (with gadolinium): Plaque detection is highlighted as high-signal lesions. Gadolinium enhancement indicates an active lesion.

Evoked potentials: Visual, auditory or somatosensory evoked potentials (VEP, BEP, SEP) may show delayed conduction velocity. VEPs are delayed in ~90% of patients with MS.

MANAGEMENT

Multidisciplinary management: Combined care involving neurologists, specialist nurses, physiotherapists, psychologists and pain team.

Acute attacks: Corticosteroids (IV methylprednisolone 1 g daily for 5 days) hastens recovery but not degree of recovery. Infection must first be ruled out. If poor response to high-dose corticosteroids: plasma exchange.

Relapsing–remitting MS:
- β-Inteferon or glatarimer SC injections may reduce relapse frequency by ~33% by modulating T-helper cell activity.
- Natalizumab (monoclonal against α4-integrin preventing T-cell movement into the CNS) monthly IV infusions reduces relapses by ~69% and disability progression.
- Mitoxantrone should be reserved for patients with rapidly advancing disease who have failed other therapies.
- Newer oral agents (cladiribine, fingolomid) have been shown to be superior to β-Inteferon, reducing relapse rate by ~50%.

Progressive MS: Clinical trials have shown no or limited effectiveness for the available treatments.

Symptomatic treatment:
- *Bladder disturbances*: Anticholinergics (e.g. oxybutynin), intermittent self-catheterization.
- *Spasticity*: Baclofen, gabapentin or tizanidine if generalised. Botox injections if localised. Consider intrathecal baclofen if immobile.
- *Neuropathic pain*: Consider carbamazepine or gabapentin.
- *Depression*: Psychological support, antidepressants.
- *Fatigue*: Modafinil has been shown to be beneficial.

COMPLICATIONS   Progressive disability, cognitive impairment. The expanded disability status scale (EDSS) is a standardised method of quantifying disability.

Complications of treatment: Treatment with natazulimab carries a 1 in 1000 risk of progressive multifocal leukoencophalopathy (PML)[3].

PROGNOSIS   Relapsing-remitting MS can eventually result in residual disability followed by a secondary progressive phase. 10% have a benign course (one or more initial episodes, then no symptoms for many years).

---

[3] Progressive multifocal leukoencephalopathy (PML): Caused by the reactivation of latent JC virus infection which destroys oligodendrocytes and can mimic an MS relapse. Potentially fatal with no specific treatment.

Myasthenia gravis

DEFINITION   An autoimmune disease affecting the neuromuscular junction producing weakness of skeletal muscles.

AETIOLOGY   Impairment of neuromuscular junction transmission, most commonly due to auto-antibodies against the nicotinic acetylcholine receptor (nAChR). A paraneoplastic subtype (Lambert–Eaton myasthenic syndrome) is caused by auto-antibodies against pre-synaptic calcium ion channels impairing acetylcholine release.
Myasthenia gravis is associated with other autoimmune conditions (e.g. pernicious anaemia) and thymoma development. Breakdown in immune tolerance thought to arise in thymus (75% have thymoma).

EPIDEMIOLOGY   Prevalence is 8–9 in 100 000. More common in females at younger ages, but equal gender distribution in middle age.

HISTORY   Muscle weakness that worsens with repetitive use or towards end of day.
In Lambert–Eaton syndrome, the muscle weakness improves after repeated use.
Ocular symptoms: Drooping eyelids, diplopia.
Bulbar symptoms: Facial weakness ('myasthenic snarl'), disturbed hypernasal speech, difficulty in smiling, chewing or swallowing (nasal regurgitation of fluids).

EXAMINATION   May be generalized (affecting many muscle groups), bulbar (affecting bulbar muscles) or ocular (affecting only the eyes).
Eyes: Bilateral ptosis, may be asymmetrical. Complex opthamoplegia. Test for ocular fatiguability by ask patient to sustain upward gaze for 1 min and watch for progressive ptosis.
'Ice on eyes' test: Placing ice-packs on closed eyelids for 2 min can improve neuromuscular transmission, reducing ptosis. Considered positive when ptosis improves by ≥2 mm from baseline.
Bulbar: Reading aloud may provoke dysarthria or nasal speech after 3 min.
Limbs: Test the power of a muscle before and after repeated use of the muscle (e.g. 20 repetitions).

INVESTIGATIONS   *Blood*:CK (to exclude myopathies). Serum acetylcholine receptor antibody (positive in 80%), TFT (associated hyperthyroidism). Atypical features may warrant testing of anti-MUSK antibody (uncommon variant) and anti-voltage-gated-calcium-channel antibody (Lambert–Eaton syndrome).
Tensilon test: Short-acting anti-cholinesterase (e.g. edrophonium) increases acetylcholine levels by blocking its metabolism and causes rapid and transient improvement in clinical features. Generally avoided due to risk of bradycardia (atropine and cardiac resuscitation equipment must be kept at hand) and subjectivity of most clinical features.
Nerve Conduction Study: Repetitive stimulation demonstrating decrements of the muscle action potential. May differentiate between myasthenic gravis and Lambert–Eaton myasthenic syndrome.
EMG: Single-fibre EMG may demonstrate 'jitter' (variability in latency from stimulus to muscle potential) indicating fluctuation in neuromuscular conduction.
CT-thorax and/or CXR: To visualize thymoma in the mediastinum or malignancies in the lung.

MANAGEMENT   *Symptomatic treatment*:Cholinesterase inhibitors (e.g. pyridostigmine, neostigmine), beware of bradycardia and diarrhoea.
Acute treatment: Bulbar and generalized myasthenia can be life-threatening if the airway or respiratory muscles are affected. Vital capacity monitoring should be performed to assess for this risk. IV immunoglobulin and plasma exchange provides rapid immunosuppression and can be used to for severely affected patients.
Immunosuppresssion: Prednisolone (can worsen symptoms initially), azathioprine and ciclosporin are useful agents for chronic control of disease.

Surgical: Thymectomy is beneficial only in those with a thymoma or early-onset generalized myasthenic gravis. Fifty percent improvement after 2 years.

COMPLICATIONS   Myaesthenic crisis (respiratory failure requiring intubation and mechanical ventilation) may be caused by infections, aspiration, physical and emotional stress, and changes in medication.

Cholinergic crisis caused by excessive cholinesterase inhibitor use presents as agitation, sweating, fever, flush, hypersalivation, pupillary miosis, muscle fasciculations and muscle weakness.

Fetal or neonatal myasthenia (caused by transplacental antibodies transfer from mother with myasthenia gravis).

PROGNOSIS   Disease restricted to ocular muscles only has a good outcome. Maximum extent of involvement in an individual patient usually manifests itself within the first 5–7 years, although the disease may wax and wane in severity.

Myotonic dystrophy

DEFINITION   Autosomal dominant condition characterized by muscle wasting, weakness and myotonia (abnormal sustained contraction of muscle).

AETIOLOGY   Type 1 myotonic dystrophy (DM1) is caused by expansion of CTG nucleotide triplet repeats at the 3' untranslated region (UTR) of the *DMPK* gene (dystrophia myotonica protein kinase gene on chromosome 19). The disease has earlier onset or increased severity in the offspring than in the parents as a result of further triplet repeat expansion in succeeding generations. This phenomenon is called anticipation.
Type 2 myotonic dystrophy (DM2) is caused by the expansion of a CCTG repeat of the *ZNF9* gene (zinc finger protein 9 gene on chromosome 3). In general, DM2 is a less severe disease than DM1.

EPIDEMIOLOGY   Most common form of adult-onset muscular dystrophy. Annual incidence one in 8000. Usual onset age 20–50 years.

HISTORY   Progressive weakness (hands, legs, sternomastoids) and myotonia.
Inability to release the grip.
Mental impairment.
Symptoms of associated conditions, e.g. cataracts, hypogonadism, diabetes mellitus, cardiomyopathy, cardiac conduction defects, cholecystitis.

EXAMINATION   Facial muscle wasting and weakness gives 'myopathic facies' with lack of facial expression. Wasting of frontalis and temporalis. Bilateral ptosis, weakness of sternomastoids. Unable to release the grip. Frontal balding (in men).
Percussion myotonia: Striking the thenar eminence provokes slow flexion of the thumb.
Signs of associated conditions, e.g. cataracts, testicular atrophy.

INVESTIGATIONS   *EMG*: Characteristic abnormal spontaneous electrical discharge during insertion of the electrode into the muscle. The spontaneous discharge ↓ with time.
DNA mutation analysis: Expansion of the CTG triplet repeat in the 3' UTR of the gene.
Blood: Creatine kinase (may be raised).
ECG (annual): To screen for cardiac conduction disturbances.
Echocardiography: If symptoms or signs of myocardial dysfunction are present.
Forced vital capacity (FVC): Periodic measurement.

MANAGEMENT   Management of physical disability is best provided by a multidisciplinary team. Low-intensity exercise training program (after exercise testing with ECG monitoring in patients with cardiac symptoms or an abnormal baseline ECG).
Swallowing assessment. Monitoring of cardiac and respiratory function.
Severe myotonia: phenytoin for adults, oral mexiletine for children. Genetic counselling.

COMPLICATIONS   Neurological, endocrine and cardiac complications as above. ↑ Risk of complications with general anaesthesia. Hypogammaglobulinaemia.

PROGNOSIS   Most patients do not live past 50 years.

Neurofibromatosis

DEFINITION   Neurofibromatosis (NF) is an autosomal dominant genetic disorder affecting cells of neural crest origin, resulting in the development of multiple neurocutaneous tumours.

Type 1 NF (von Recklinghausen's disease): Characterized by peripheral and spinal neurofibromas, multiple *café au lait* spots, freckling (axillary/inguinal), optic nerve glioma, Lisch nodules (on iris), skeletal deformities, phaeochromocytomas and renal artery stenosis.

Type 2 NF: Characterized by schwannomas, e.g. bilateral vestibular schwannomas (acoustic neuromas), peripheral/spinal schwannomas, meningiomas, gliomas, cataracts.

AETIOLOGY   Multiple mutations have been described in tumour suppressor genes NF1 and NF2.

Type 1 NF: Mutations in NF1 gene (chromosome 17) which encodes neurofibromin (a GTPase activating protein). Mutations in neurofibromin result in excessive activity of the proto-oncogene *p21-ras*.

Type 2 NF: Mutations in NF2 (chromosome 22) which encodes merlin (or schwannomin).

EPIDEMIOLOGY   Incidence is one in 3000 births for type 1 NF and one in 40 000 for type 2 NF. No gender or racial predilection.

HISTORY   Positive family history (but 50% are caused by new mutations).

Type 1 NF: Skin lesions, learning difficulties (in 40%), headaches, disturbed vision (optic gliomas, in ~15%), precocious puberty (may indicate lesions of the pituitary from optic glioma involving the chiasm).

Type 2 NF: Hearing loss, tinnitus, balance problems, headache, facial pain or numbness.

EXAMINATION   *Type 1 NF*: >5 *café au lait* macules of >5 mm (pre-pubertal individuals) or >15 mm (post-pubertal individuals), neurofibromas (appear as cutaneous nodules or complex plexiform neuromas), freckling in armpit or groin, Lisch nodules (hamartomas on iris), spinal scoliosis.

Type 2 NF: Few or no skin lesions, sensorineural deafness with facial nerve palsy or cerebellar signs if schwannoma large (*see* Acoustic neuroma).

INVESTIGATIONS

Ophthalmological assessment

Audiometry

MRI brain and spinal cord: For vestibular schwannomas, meningiomas and nerve root neurofibromas.

Skull X-ray: Sphenoid dysplasia in type 1 NF.

Genetic testing: Possible but difficult as the NF1 gene is very long.

MANAGEMENT   Education and genetic counselling. Surveillance for complications.

Type 1 NF: Monitoring growth, neurodevelopmental, puberty and school progress, blood pressure, vision, hearing, skin lesions and scoliosis.

Type 2 NF: Regular hearing assessment and MRI follow-up of CNS lesions.

Surgery: Removal of vestibular schwannomas, removal of painful or disfiguring tumours, treatment of scoliosis or bone deformities.

COMPLICATIONS   *Type 1 NF*: Plexiform neurofibromas can undergo malignant transformation to malignant peripheral nerve sheath tumours (5–8% lifetime risk): present with chronic pain, change in consistency or rapid growth.

Tumours can compress spinal nerve roots or stenose aqueduct of Sylvius causing obstructive hydrocephalus.

PROGNOSIS   Life expectancy appears to be shortened in type 1 NF. Malignant peripheral nerve sheath tumour is an aggressive and potentially fatal malignancy (5-year event-free survival ~20%).

Parkinson's disease

DEFINITION   Neurodegenerative disease of the dopaminergic neurones of the substantia nigra, characterized by bradykinesia, rigidity, tremor and postural instability.

AETIOLOGY   *Sporadic and idiopathic (most common)*: Unknown. Environmental toxins and oxidative stress have been proposed (e.g. pesticides, wood pulp).
Secondary:
- Neuroleptic therapy (e.g. in schizophrenia).
- Vascular insults (e.g. basal ganglia or midbrain strokes).
- MPTP toxin from illicit drug contamination.
- Post-encephalitis (e.g. influenza).
- Repeated head injury (e.g. boxing).

Familial forms: Genes mutations that cause Parkinson's Disease are in LRRK2, PARK2 (Parkin), PARK7, PINK1 and SNCA (α-synuclein) genes.

EXAMINATION   Very common: 1–2% of >60-year-olds. Annual incidence is 20 in 100000. Mean age of onset is ∼57 years.

HISTORY   Insidious onset.
Tremor at rest, usually noticed in hands.
Stiffness and slowness of movements.
Difficulty initiating movements (e.g. getting out of chair, rolling in bed).
Frequent falls.
Smaller hand writing (micrographia).
Insomnia, mental slowness (bradyphenia).

EXAMINATION   *Tremor*: Classically 'pill rolling' rest tremor in the hands of about 4–6 Hz frequency. Decreased on action or flexed posture. Usually asymmetrical.
Rigidity: Lead pipe rigidity of muscle tone, with superimposed tremor (cogwheel rigidity). Rigidity can be enhanced by distraction (asking the patient to keep raising and lowering the other arm).
Gait: Stooped, 'simian', shuffling, small-stepped gait with reduced arm swing. Freezing (difficulty in initiation of walking).
Postural instability: Falls easily with little pressure from the back (propulsion) or the front (retropulsion).
Other features: Frontalis overactivation (furrowing of the brow), expressionless face (hypo-mimia), soft monotonous voice (hypophonia), impaired olfaction on formal testing. There may be mild impairment of up-gaze and tendency to drool (sialorrhoea). Involuntary movements in one part of the face associated with voluntary movement in another part of the face (synkinesis).
Psychiatric: Depression is very common. Cognitive problems and dementia may occur in late disease.

PATHOLOGY/PATHOGENESIS   Degeneration of midbrain dopaminergic neurones projecting from the substantia nigra to the striatum (caudate nucleus and putamen). Surviving neurones often contain eosinophilic cytoplasmic inclusions (Lewy bodies). Patients only symptomatic after >70% neuronal loss. Nigrostriatal dopaminergic deficiency causes abnormalities of plasticity in the basal ganglia and cerebral cortex.

INVESTIGATIONS   Diagnosis is clinical.
Levodopa trial: Timed walking and clinical assessment after levodopa may be informative. Antiemetic (domperidone) may be needed.
Blood: Serum ceruloplasmin (excludes Wilson's disease in young onset).
CT or MRI brain: Useful for excluding other causes of gait decline (e.g. hydrocephalus, vascular disease).

Dopamine transporter scintigraphy (DAT-scan): Reduction in striatum and putamen. May be necessary for distinguishing from essential tremor.

MANAGEMENT Underlying neurodegenerative process is still not treatable.
Medical: Symptomatic therapy by dopamine replacement.
- L-DOPA with peripheral DOPA decarboxylase inhibitor (carbidopa, benserazide); varying formulations. Most effective treatment but long-term therapy has serious complications.
- Dopamine receptor agonists, oral agents (e.g. ropinirole, pramipexole) and parental agents (apomorphine subcutaneous pump, patch).
- Anticholinergics (e.g. benzatropine, amantadine) have a modest effect on tremor.
- COMT inhibitor (e.g. entacapone) may reduce end-of-dose deterioration, especially when combined with levodopa.
- MAO-B inhibitor (e.g. selegiline).
- Rivastigmine (anti-cholinesterase) has been shown to be beneficial for Parkinson's Disease patients with dementia.

Surgery: Stereotactic thalamotomy, pallidotomy and deep brain stimulation (subthalamic nucleus) can substantially reduce levodopa requirements (and thus levodopa-induced dyskinesias).
Other: Physiotherapy, occupational and speech therapy is vital in maintaining a reasonable quality of life.

COMPLICATIONS Depression, dementia, autonomic dysfunction (postural hypotension, constipation, urinary retention or overflow incontinence, erectile dysfunction), death (usually from pneumonia or pulmonary embolism).
Treatment complications (develops over months and years on chronic levodopa therapy):
- 'On–off' motor fluctuations.
- Peak dose dyskinesias (typically choreaform, dance-like).
- 'On–off' dystonia (e.g. typically in feet).
- Impulse control disorders (e.g. pathological gambling, hypersexuality, punding behaviour).

PROGNOSIS Progressive but variable in rate. Optimal treatment can delay impact of disability by 5–10 years.

---

[1]Other akinetic rigid syndromes (poorly responsive to levodopa):
- *Diffuse Lewy body disease*: Cognitive fluctuations and visual hallucinations, dementia.
- *Multiple system atrophy (Shy–Drager syndrome)*: Autonomic failure, cerebellar and extrapyramidal features.
- *Progressive supranuclear palsy*: Impairment of voluntary vertical saccades (upgaze first, then downgaze) dementia.
- *Cortico-basal degeneration*: Dystonia, dyspraxia, 'alien hand syndrome', dementia.

Stroke

DEFINITION Rapid permanent neurological deficit from cerebrovascular insult. Also defined clinically, as focal or global impairment of CNS function developing rapidly and lasting >24 h (see Transient ischaemic attack).
Can be subdivided by location (anterior circulation or posterior circulation) or by pathological process (infarction, haemorrhage).

AETIOLOGY
Infarction (80%):
- Thrombosis: In the elderly, this arises from atherosclerosis within cerebral vessels affecting mainly small vessels (causing lacunar infarcts) and less commonly large vessels (e.g. middle cerebral artery). Can also arise from prothrombotic states (e.g. dehydration or thrombophilia).
- Emboli: From intimal flap of carotid dissection, atheromatous plaques in the carotid arteries or from the heart (e.g. atrial fibrillation). Rarely they can arise from venous circulation and pass through a right–left heart defect (e.g. VSD).
- Hypotension: If below the autoregulatory range maintaining cerebral blood flow, infarction results in the 'watershed' zones between different cerebral artery territories.
- Others: Vasculitis, cocaine.
Haemorrhage (10%): Hypertension, Charcot–Bouchard microaneurysm rupture, amyloid angiopathy, arteriovenous malformations. Less commonly, trauma, tumours, arteriovenous malformations, vasculitis.

EPIDEMIOLOGY Common. Annual incidence is two in 1000. Third most common cause of death in industrialized countries. Most patients are in seventh decade. Young strokes (<50 years merit extensive investigation).

HISTORY Sudden onset (deterioration within seconds).
Weakness, sensory, visual or cognitive impairment, impaired coordination, or consciousness.
Head or neck pain (in carotid or vertebral artery dissection).
Enquire time of onset (critical for emergency management if <4.5 h).
Enquire if history of atrial fibrillation, MI, valvular heart disease, carotid artery stenosis, recent neck trauma or pain.

EXAMINATION Examine for underlying cause (e.g. atrial fibrillation, heart murmurs, carotid bruit, fundoscopy).
Infarction:
- Anterior circulation
  o Anterior cerebral: Lower limb weakness (motor cortex), confusion (frontal lobe).
  o Middle cerebral: Facial weakness, hemiparesis (motor cortex), hemisensory loss (somatosensory cortex), apraxia, hemineglect (parietal lobe), receptive or expressive dysphasia (language centres), quadrantanopia (superior or inferior optic radiations).
- Small vessels (lacunar): Disease in the deep perforating arteries:
  o Internal capsule or pons: Pure sensory or motor deficit (or combination of both).
  o Thalamus: Loss of consciousness, hemisensory deficit.
  o Basal ganglia: Hemichorea, hemiballismus, parkinsonism.
- Posterior circulation
  o Posterior cerebral: Hemianopia.
  o Anterior inferior cerebellar artery: Vertigo, ipsilateral ataxia, ipsilateral deafness (or tinnitus), ipsilateral facial weakness.
  o Posterior inferior cerebellar artery (lateral medullary syndrome of Wallenberg): Vertigo ipsilateral ataxia, ipsilateral Horner's syndrome, ipsilateral hemifacial sensory loss, dysarthria and contralateral spinothalamic sensory loss.
  o Basilar artery: Combination of cranial nerve pathology and impaired consciousness (emergency).

- *Multiple lacunar infarcts*: Vascular dementia, urinary incontinence, gait apraxia ('marche à petits pas', shuffling small-stepped gait, with upright posture and often normal or excessive arm-swing).
Haemorrhage:
- Intracerebral: Headache, meningism, focal neurological signs, nausea and vomiting, signs of raised ICP, seizures.
- Subarachnoid: (*see* Subarachnoid haemorrhage).

PATHOLOGY/PATHOGENESIS Ischaemic brain becomes soft due to vasogenic oedema from breakdown of blood–brain barrier and prone to haemorrhagic transformation. This can cause secondary damage to the CNS.

INVESTIGATIONS *Blood*: FBC, U&E, glucose, clotting profile, lipids (consider thrombophilia screen especially in young patients).
ECG: To identify any arrhythmias which pre-dispose to embolism.
Echocardiogram: Identifies cardiac thrombus, valvular endocarditis or other sources of embolism. Consider bubble contrast study for right-to-left shunt (e.g. VSD).
Carotid Doppler ultrasound: Important to exclude carotid artery disease.
CT-head: For rapid detection of haemorrhages. Often normal especially in lacunar infarcts or very early in the stroke (<6 h).
MRI-brain: Rarely available acutely, but much higher sensitivity for infarction. Diffusion-weighted imaging (DWI) can differentiate between recent strokes (<2 weeks) and old strokes.
CT-cerebral angiogram: To detect artery dissections or intracranial stenosis. Alternatively MRA with T1-fat-saturation can be useful.

MANAGEMENT *Hyperacute stroke*: If <4.5 h from onset and haemorrhage excluded on CT-head, intravenous thrombolysis may be considered. Do not give aspirin in first 24 h. Follow local protocols due to very strict inclusion and exclusion criteria (NINDS and ECASS3 trials, IST3 trial for thrombolysis <6 h is ongoing).
Acute ischaemic stroke:
- Aspirin or clopidogrel to prevent further thrombosis once haemorrhage excluded on CT-head.
- Heparin anti-coagulation may be considered in certain subgroups where there is a high risk of emboli recurrence or stroke progression (e.g. carotid dissection, recurrent cardiac emboli, critical carotid artery stenosis).
- Formal swallow assessment is essential (nasogastric tube may be required).
- Close nursing and GCS monitoring.
- Thromboprophylaxis (but no evidence of net benefit from graded compression stockings in CLOTS trial).
- Hemicraniectomy may be indicated for mass effect from infarcted tissue in the first 48 h (DESTINY and HAMLET trials).
Intracerebral haemorrhage: Control hypertension and seizures. IV mannitol and hyperventilation helps lower intracranial pressure. Evacuation of haematoma or ventricular drainage may be required.
Secondary prevention: Aspirin and dipyridamole, warfarin anticoagulation (if atrial fibrillation), stop smoking, control hypertension and hyperlipidaemia, treatment of carotid artery disease.
Surgical treatment: Carotid endartectomy within 2 weeks of stroke or TIA reduces risk of further stroke in ECST and NASCET trials, although carries a significant peri-operative risk. May be considered in:
- symptomatic stenosis of 70–99% (ECST criteria),
- symptomatic stenosis of 50–99% (NASCET criteria) or
- crescendo TIAs not responding to medical treatment.

Stroke (continued)

The role of surgical treatment in asymptomatic disease is controversial.

Multidisciplinary rehabilitation (best managed by specialist stroke unit): Speech and language therapy, occupational therapy, physiotherapy. And neuropsychology.

COMPLICATIONS Cerebral oedema (↑ ICP and local compression), immobility, infections (e.g. pneumonia, UTI, from pressure sores), DVT, cardiovascular events (arrhythmias, MI, cardiac failure), death.

PROGNOSIS Stroke: 10% mortality in first month. Up to 50% of those who survive remain dependent. Ten percent have a recurrence in 1 year. Generally, poorer for haemorrhages than for infarction.

Subarachnoid haemorrhage

DEFINITION Arterial haemorrhage into the subarachnoid space.

AETIOLOGY Rupture of a saccular aneurysm at the base of the brain (usually at Circle of Willis): 85%.
Perimesencephalic haemorrhage (e.g. parenchymal haemorrhages tracking onto surface of brain): 10%.
Arteriovenous malformations, bleeding diatheses, vertebral or carotid artery dissection with intracranial extension, mycotic aneurysms, drug abuse (e.g. cocaine, amphetamines): 5%.
Associated with hypertension, smoking, excess alcohol intake, saccular aneurysms are associated with polycystic kidney disease, Marfan's syndrome, pseudoxanthoma elasticum and Ehlers–Danlos syndrome.

EPIDEMIOLOGY Annual incidence is 10 in 100 000. Peak age of incidence in the fifth decade.

HISTORY Sudden onset severe headache (classically described 'as if hit at the back of the head').
Nausea, vomiting, neck stiffness, photophobia.
↓ Level of consciousness.

EXAMINATION *Meningism*: Neck stiffness, Kernig's sign (resistance or pain on knee extension when hip is flexed) because of irritation of the meninges by blood. Pyrexia may also occur.
Glasgow Coma Scale (see next page): Assess and regularly monitor for deterioration.
Signs of increased intracranial pressure: Papilloedema, IV or III cranial nerve palsy. Hypertension and bradycardia.
Fundoscopy: Rarely subhyaloid haemorrhage (between retina and vitreous membrane).
Focal neurological signs: Usually develop on second day and are caused by ischaemia from vasospasm and reduced brain perfusion. Aneurysms may cause pressure on cranial nerves causing ophthalmoplegia (classically III nerve or VI nerve palsy).

INVESTIGATIONS *Blood*: FBC, U&E, ESR/CRP, clotting (? bleeding diathesis).
CT scan: Hyperdense areas in the basal regions of the skull (caused by blood in the subarachnoid space). Identifies any intraparenchymal or intraventricular haemorrhages as well.
Angiography (CT or intra-arterial): To detect the source of bleeding if the patient is a candidate for surgery or endovascular treatment.
Lumbar puncture: ↑ Opening pressure, ↑ red cells, few white cells, xanthochromia (straw-coloured CSF) because of breakdown of Hb, confirmed by spectrophotometry of CSF supernatant after centrifugation.

MANAGEMENT *Acute*: Resuscitate, bed-rest, analgesia and obtain neurosurgical review. IV fluids (to maintain a degree of hypertension to keep brain perfused). Nimodipine (calcium-channel antagonist) should be given to reduce vasospasm. Monitor fluid balance and sodium levels as associated with SIADH or cerebral salt-wasting syndrome.
Interventional neuroradiology: Coiling (usually with platinum) of the aneurysm.
Surgical: Clipping or wrapping the aneurysm.
Arteriovenous malformations: May be managed by interventional radiology, radiotherapy and/or surgery.

COMPLICATIONS Obstructive hydrocephalus (CSF flow blocked in the ventricles by blood clot), communicating hydrocephalus (as meninges and arachnoid villi are damaged by the haemorrhage). Major neurological deficits depending on the site of haemorrhage.

Subarachnoid haemorrhage (continued)

PROGNOSIS   High, with >30 % mortality in the first few days. Significant risk of a severe
rebleed in the first 2 months. Worse prognosis with subsequent episodes of rebleeding.
Lower mortality in cases of perimesencephalic subarachnoid haemorrhage and arteriovenous malformations than bleeding from aneurysms.

[1]The Glasgow Coma Scale is a rapid measure of consciousness. Made up of three components, totalling 15.

Score	Eyes	Verbal	Motor
6			Obeys commands
5		Oriented	Localising pain
4	Spontaneously	Confused	Withdrawal to pain
3	To speech	Inappropriate	Abnormal flexion to pain
2	To pain	Incomprehensible	Extending to pain
1	None	None	None

Subdural haemorrhage

DEFINITION A subdural haemorrhage (SDH) is a collection of blood that develops between the surface of the brain and the dura mater.
Acute: Within 72 h. *Subacute*: 3–20 days. *Chronic*: After 3 weeks.

AETIOLOGY Trauma causing rapid acceleration and deceleration of the brain results in shearing forces which tear veins ('bridging veins') that travel from the dura to the cortex. Bleeding occurs between the dura and arachnoid membranes.
In children, non-accidental injury should always be considered.

EPIDEMIOLOGY *Acute*: Tend to occur in younger patients/associated with major trauma (5–25% of cases of severe head injury). More common than extradural haemorrhage.
Chronic: More common in elderly, studies report incidence of 1–5 per 100 000.

HISTORY *Acute*: History of trauma with head injury, patient has ↓ conscious level.
Subacute: Worsening headaches 7–14 days after injury, altered mental status.
Chronic: Can present with headache, confusion, cognitive impairment, psychiatric symptoms, gait deterioration, focal weakness, seizures.
There may not be a history of fall or trauma; hence have low index of suspicion especially in the elderly and alcoholics.

EXAMINATION *Acute*: ↓ GCS. With large haematomas resulting in midline shift, an ipsilateral fixed dilated pupil may be seen (compression of the ipsilateral third nerve parasympathetic fibres), pressure on brainstem: ↓ consciousness, bradycardia.
Chronic: Neurological examination may be normal; there may be focal neurological signs (III or VI nerve dysfunction, papilloedema, hemiparesis or reflex asymmetry).

INVESTIGATIONS *CT head*: Crescent- or sickle-shaped mass, concave over brain surface (an extradural is lentiform in shape), CT appearance changes with time. Acute subdurals are hyperdense, becoming isodense over 1–3 weeks (such that presence may be inferred from signs such as effacement of sulci, midline shift, ventricular compression and obliteration of basal cisterns); and chronic subdurals are hypodense (approaching that of CSF).
MRI-brain: Has higher sensitivity especially for isodense or small SDHs.

MANAGEMENT *Acute*: ALS protocol with priorities of cervical spine control and ABC. With a head injury, there is a significant risk of cervical spine injury. Disability: GCS, pupillary reactivity. If signs of raised ICP, head elevation and consider osmotic diuresis with mannitol and/or hyperventilation. Once stabilised, obtain CT-head.
Conservative: Especially if small and minimal midline shift (SDH < 10 mm thickness, and midline shift <5 mm).
Surgical: Prompt Burr hole or craniotomy and evacuation for symptomatic subdurals >10 mm, with >5 mm midline shift (better outcome if within 4 h). ICP monitoring devices may be placed.
Chronic: If symptomatic or there is mass effect on imaging, surgical treatment with Burr hole or craniotomy and drainage (a drain may be left in for 24–72 h). Asymptomatic SDH without significant mass effect is best managed conservatively with serial imaging to monitor for spontaneous resorption. Haematomas that have not fully liquefied may require craniotomy with membranectomy.
Children: Younger children may be treated by percutaneous aspiration via an open fontanelle or if this fails, placement of a subdural to peritoneal shunt.

COMPLICATIONS Raised ICP, cerebral oedema pre-disposing to secondary ischaemic brain damage, mass effect (transtentorial or uncal herniation).
Post-op: Seizures are relatively common, recurrence (Up to 33% for SDH), intracerebral haemorrhage, subdural empyema, brain abscess or meningitis, tension pneumocephalus.

Subdural haemorrhage (continued)

PROGNOSIS   *Acute*: Underlying brain injury is the most important factor on outcome.
Chronic: Generally have a better outcome than acute SDHs, reflecting lower incidence of underlying brain injury, with good outcomes in 3/4 of those treated by surgery.

Acromegaly

DEFINITION   Constellation of signs and symptoms caused by hypersecretion of GH in adults. (Excess GH before puberty results in gigantism.)

AETIOLOGY   Most cases are a result of GH-secreting pituitary adenoma.
Rarely: Excess GHRH causing somatotroph hyperplasia from hypothalamic ganglioneuroma, bronchial carcinoid or pancreatic tumours.

EPIDEMIOLOGY   Rare. Annual incidence of five in 1 000 000. Age at diagnosis: 40–50 years.

HISTORY   Very gradual progression of symptoms over many years (often only detectable on serial photographs).
May complain of rings and shoes becoming tight.
↑ Sweating, headache, carpal tunnel syndrome.
Symptoms of hypopituitarism (hypogonadism, hypothyroidism, hypoadrenalism). Visual disturbances (caused by optic chiasm compression).
Hyperprolactinaemia (irregular periods, ↓ libido, impotence).

EXAMINATION   *Hands*: Enlarged spade-like hands with thick greasy skin. Signs of carpal tunnel syndrome (*see* Carpal tunnel syndrome). Pre-mature osteoarthritis (arthritis also affects other large joints, temporomandibular joint).
Face: Prominent eyebrow ridge (frontal bossing) and cheeks, broad nose bridge, prominent nasolabial folds, thick lips, ↑ gap between teeth, large tongue, prognathism, husky resonant voice (thickening vocal cords).
Visual field loss: Bitemporal superior quadrantanopia progressing to bitemporal hemianopia (caused by pituitary tumour compressing the optic chiasm).
Neck: Multi-nodular goitre.
Feet: Enlarged.

INVESTIGATIONS   *Serum IGF-1*: Useful screening test. GH stimulates liver IGF-1 secretion (IGF-1 varies with age of patient and ↑ during pregnancy and puberty).
Oral glucose tolerance test: Failure of suppression of GH after 75 g oral glucose load (false-positive results are seen in anorexia nervosa, Wilson's disease, opiate addiction).
Pituitary function tests: 9 a.m. cortisol, free T4 and TSH, LH, FSH, testosterone (in men) and prolactin (to test for hypopituitarism).
MRI of the brain: To image the pituitary tumour and effect on the optic chiasm.

MANAGEMENT   *Surgical*: Trans-sphenoidal hypophysectomy is the only curative treatment.
Radiotherapy: Adjunctive treatment to surgery.
Medical: If surgery is contra-indicated or refused.
SC somatostatin analogues (octreotide, lanreotide). Side-effects: abdominal pain, steatorrhoea glucose intolerance, gallstones, irritation at the injection site.
Oral dopamine agonists (bromocriptine, cabergoline). Side-effects: nausea, vomiting, constipation, postural hypotension (↑ dose gradually and take it during meals), psychosis (rare).
GH antagonist (pegvisomant)
Monitor: GH and IGF1 levels can be used to monitor disease control. Pituitary function tests, echocardiography, regular colonoscopy and blood glucose.

COMPLICATIONS   *CVS*: Cardiomyopathy, hypertension.
Respiratory: Obstructive sleep apnoea.
GI: Colonic polyps.
Reproductive: Hyperprolactinaemia (30%).
Metabolic: Hypercalcaemia, hyperphosphataemia, renal stones, diabetes mellitus, hypertriglyceridaemia.

Acromegaly (continued)

Psychological: Depression, psychosis (resulting from dopamine agonist therapy).

Complications of surgery: Nasoseptal perforation, hypopituitarism, adenoma recurrence, CSF leak, infection (meninges, sphenoid sinus).

PROGNOSIS   Good with early diagnosis and treatment, although physical changes are irreversible.

Adrenal insufficiency

DEFINITION   Deficiency of adrenal cortical hormones (e.g. mineralocorticoids, glucocorticoids and androgens).

AETIOLOGY   *Primary (Addison's disease)*: Autoimmune (>70%).
Infections: Tuberculosis, meningococcal septicaemia (Waterhouse–Friderichsen syndrome), CMV (HIV patients), histoplasmosis.
Infiltration: Metastasis (e.g. lung, breast, melanoma), lymphomas, amyloidosis.
Infarction: Secondary to thrombophilia
Inherited: Adrenoleukodystrophy[1], ACTH receptor mutation.
Surgical: After bilateral adrenalectomy.
Secondary: Pituitary or hypothalamic disease.
Iatrogenic: Sudden cessation of long-term steroid therapy.

EPIDEMIOLOGY   Most common cause is iatrogenic. Primary causes are rare (annual incidence of Addison's is eight in 1 000 000).

HISTORY   *Chronic presentation*: Non-specific vague symptoms such as dizziness, anorexia, weight loss, diarrhoea, vomiting, abdominal pain, lethargy, weakness, depression.
Acute presentation (Addisonian crisis): Acute adrenal insufficiency with major haemodynamic collapse often precipitated by stress (e.g. infection or surgery).

EXAMINATION   Postural hypotension.
Increased pigmentation: Generalized but more noticeable on buccal mucosa, scars, skin creases, nails, pressure points (resulting from melanocytes being stimulated by ↑ ACTH levels).
Loss of body hair in women (androgen deficiency).
Associated autoimmune conditions: e.g. vitiligo.
Addisonian crisis: Hypotensive shock, tachycardia, pale, cold, clammy, oliguria.

INVESTIGATIONS   *Confirm the diagnosis*: 9 a.m. serum cortisol < 100 nmol/L is diagnostic of adrenal insufficiency. If 9 a.m. cortisol > 550 nmol/L: adrenal insufficiency is unlikely. Patients with 9 a.m. cortisol of between 100 and 550 nmol/L should have a *short ACTH stimulation test (short Synacthen test)*: IM 250 µg tetracosactrin (synthetic ACTH) is given. Serum cortisol <550 nmol/L at 30 min indicates adrenal failure.
Identify the level of defect ACTH: ↑ in primary disease and ↓ in secondary disease. *Long Synacthen test*: One milligram tetracosactrin is given and cortisol is measured at 0, 30, 60, 90 and 120 min then at 4, 6, 8, 12 and 24 h. Patients with primary adrenal insufficiency show no increase after 6.
Identify the cause: Autoantibodies (against 21-hydroxylase). Abdominal CT or MRI. Other tests e.g. adrenal biopsy for microscopy, culture, PCR depending on the suspected causes.
Check TFTs
Investigations in 'Addisonian crisis': FBC (neutrophilia), U&E (↑ urea, ↓ Na +, ↑ K +), ESR or CRP (↑ in acute infection), Ca^{2+} (may be ↑), glucose (↓), blood cultures, urinalysis, culture and sensitivity (UTI may have triggered the crisis). CXR: May identify cause (e.g. tuberculosis, carcinoma) or precipitant of crisis (e.g. infection).

MANAGEMENT   *Addisonian crisis*: Rapid IV fluid rehydration (0.9% saline, 1 L over 30–60 min, 2–4 L in 12–24 h). 50ml of 50 % dextrose to correct hypoglycaemia. IV 200 mg hydrocortisone bolus followed by 100 mg 6 hourly (until BP is stable). Treat the precipitating cause (e.g. antibiotics for infection). Monitor temperature, pulse, respiratory rate, BP, sat O_2 and urine output.

---

[1]Adrenoleukodystrophy is an X-linked inherited disease characterized by adrenal atrophy and demyelination.

Adrenal insufficiency (continued)

Chronic: Replacement of glucocorticoids with hydrocortisone (three times/day) and mineralocorticoids with fludrocortisone. Hydrocortisone dosage needs to be increased during acute illness or stress. If associated with hypothyroidism, give hydrocortisone *before* thyroxine (to avoid precipitating an Addisonian crisis).

Advice: Steroid warning card, Medic-alert bracelet, emergency hydrocortisone ampoule, patient education.

COMPLICATIONS   Hyperkalaemia. Death during an Addisonian crisis.

PROGNOSIS   Adrenal function rarely recovers, but normal life expectancy can be expected if treated.

Type I (autosomal recessive disorder caused by mutations in the *AIRE* gene which encodes a nuclear transcription factor.): Addison's disease, chronic mucocutaneous candidiasis, hypoparathyroidism.

Type II (Schmidt's syndrome): Addison's disease, diabetes mellitus Type 1, hypothyroidism, hypogonadism.

†Polyglandular syndromes:
Type I (autosomal recessive disorder caused by mutations in the AIRE gene which encodes a nuclear transcription factor): α Addison's disease, chronic mucocutaneous candidiasis, hypoparathyroidism.
Type II (Schmidt's syndrome): α Addison's disease, type 1 diabetes mellitus, hypothyroidism, hypogonadism.

Carcinoid syndrome

DEFINITION   Constellation of symptoms caused by systemic release of humoral factors (biogenic amines, polypeptides, prostaglandins) from carcinoid tumours.

AETIOLOGY   Carcinoid tumours are slow-growing neuroendocrine tumours mostly derived from serotonin-producing enterochromaffin cells. They produce secretory products such as serotonin, histamine, tachykinins, kallikrein and prostaglandin. May be classified into fore-, mid- or hindgut tumours. 75–80% of patients with the carcinoid syndrome have small bowel carcinoids. Common sites for carcinoid tumours include appendix and rectum, where they are often benign and non-secretory. Also found in other parts of large intestine, stomach, thymus, bronchus and other organs. Hormones released into the portal circulation are metabolized in the liver. Thus symptoms typically do not appear until there are hepatic metastases (resulting in the secretion of tumour products into the hepatic veins), or release into the systemic circulation from bronchial or extensive retroperitoneal tumours.

EPIDEMIOLOGY   Rare, annual UK incidence is one in 1 000 000. Asymptomatic carcinoid tumours are more common and may be an incidental finding after rectal biopsy or appendectomy. Ten percent of patients with multiple endocrine neoplasia (MEN) type 1 have carcinoid tumours.

HISTORY   Paroxysmal flushing, diarrhoea, crampy abdominal pain, wheeze, sweating, palpitations.

EXAMINATION   Facial flushing, telangiectasia, wheeze.
Right-sided heart murmurs: Tricuspid stenosis, regurgitation or pulmonary stenosis.
Nodular hepatomegaly in cases of metastatic disease.
Carcinoid crisis: Profound flushing, bronchospasm, tachycardia and fluctuating blood pressure.

INVESTIGATIONS   *24-h urine collection*: 5-HIAA levels (a metabolite of serotonin, false positive with high intake of certain fruit/drugs e.g. bananas and avocados, caffeine, paracetamol).
Blood: Plasma chromogranin A and B, fasting gut hormones.
CT or MRI scan: To localizes the tumour.
Radioisotope scan: Radiolabelled somatostatin analogue (e.g. indium-111 octreotide) helps localize tumour.
Investigations for MEN-1: (*see* footnote to Hyperparathyroidism).

MANAGEMENT   *Carcinoid crisis*: Octreotide infusion, also IV antihistamine and hydrocortisone.
Multidisciplinary approach (endocrinologists/gastroenterologists, oncologists, radiologists and surgeons).
Advice: Avoid precipitating factors e.g. alcohol, strenuous exercise.
Somatostatin analogues (e.g. *octreotide*) inhibit hormone release and tumour growth. Radiolabelled octreotide may be beneficial (receptor-targeted therapy).
Interferon-α: May be given on its own or added to long-acting somatostatin analogues if the patient is not responding to the maximum dosage of somatostatin analogues.
Supportive: Ondansetron and cyproheptadine (5-HT antagonists) can alleviate symptoms, rehydration (for diarrhoea), antiemetics and anti-diarrhoeal treatment (codeine, loperamide).
Surgery: Should be considered for resectable nodal or hepatic metastasis, extraintestinal (bronchial and ovarian) carcinoids. Small intestinal carcinoids may be resected even in the presence of metastases, to prevent fibrosing mesenteritis. Valve surgery for symptomatic carcinoid heart disease. A potential peri-operative carcinoid crisis should be prevented by prophylactic treatment with octreotide.

Carcinoid syndrome (continued)

Hepatic artery embolization: For patients with non-resectable multiple and hormone secreting tumours. Two types: particle and chemoembolization.

COMPLICATIONS Electrolyte imbalance (secondary to diarrhoea), metastases, bowel obstruction (due to fibrosis near a gut primary), tricuspid and pulmonary valve stenosis with consequent right heart failure, pellagra: dermatitis, glossitis, diarrhoea, dementia (due to niacin deficiency caused by diversion of dietary tryptophan for the synthesis of large amounts of serotonin).

PROGNOSIS Median survival is usually 5–10 years but can range up to 20 years. Earlier detection and treatment should improve quality of life and survival.

Congenital adrenal hyperplasia

DEFINITION Inherited disorders of adrenal steroid synthesis.

AETIOLOGY Autosomal recessive genetic defects in the steroid synthesis pathway result in ↓ cortisol (and, in some cases, ↓ aldosterone) synthesis. This produces a secondary rise in pituitary ACTH secretion causing hyperplasia of the adrenal glands and build-up of precursor steroids and in most cases androgenic steroids. Common defective enzymes include 21-hydroxylase (most common), 11β-hydroxylase and 17α-hydroxylase.

EPIDEMIOLOGY Annual incidence of 21-hydroxylase deficiency and 11β -hydroxylase deficiency are one in 10 000 and one in 100 000, respectively. The rest are less common.

HISTORY AND EXAMINATION *21-Hydroxylase deficiency* (↓ aldosterone, ↑ androgens):
Classic: Salt-losing crisis in infants (hypotension, hyponatraemia, hyperkalaemia). *Females*: Ambiguous genitalia (cliteromegaly, fused labia). *Males*: Precocious puberty.
Non-classic or late-onset CAH: Hirsutism, acne and menstrual irregularity in young women, early pubarche or sexual precocity in school age children, or there may be no symptoms.
11 β-Hydroxylase deficiency (↑11-deoxycorticosterone: a mineralocorticoid, ↑ androgens): Hypertension, hypokalaemia.
Females: Ambiguous genitalia. *Males*: Precocious puberty.
17α-Hydroxylase deficiency (↑ aldosterone, ↓ androgens): Hypertension, hypokalaemia. *Females*: Failure to develop secondary sexual characteristics at puberty. *Males*: Ambiguous genitalia.

INVESTIGATIONS *Blood*: 9 a.m. follicular phase 17OH-progesterone (↑ in 21-hydroxylase deficiency and 11β-hydroxylase deficiency), testosterone, LH, FSH, U&Es. *ACTH stimulation test*: Inappropriately elevated 17OH-progesterone levels after IM synthetic ACTH. *Karyotyping*: Confirms gender of infant with ambiguous genitalia. *Genetic analysis* may be performed to identify specific *CYP21* mutations. *Men who desire future fertility*: Serum testosterone level, semen analysis and testicular ultrasound.

MANAGEMENT *Acute salt-losing crisis*: IV saline, dextrose and hydrocortisone.
Glucocorticoid replacement with dexamethasone or hydrocortisone. Fludrocortisone in salt-losers.
Monitor growth in children, serum 17OH-progesterone, DHEAS, androstenedione and testosterone (goal: slightly above the normal range). Monitor plasma renin activity and U&Es in patients on mineralocorticoids.
Children with ambiguous genitalia: Careful evaluation by an experienced team of paediatric endocrinologists, geneticists and paediatric surgeons (reconstructive surgery at age 2–6 months). Psychosocial support.
Non-classic CAH: If not pursuing fertility, oral contraceptives or cyproterone acetate (anti-androgen). Those who desire fertility should receive glucocorticoids; if do not ovulate add clomiphene citrate. Males do not usually require treatment unless they have testicular masses (*see* Complications) or oligospermia (in a man desiring fertility).
CAH and pregnancy: The male partner must be screened for CAH. If 17OH-progesterone levels are elevated, genotyping must be done. If the male partner is heterozygote, then the foetus is at risk of inheriting CAH and developing virilization. Thus pre-natal dexamethasone is given to the mother as soon as the pregnancy is recognized.

COMPLICATIONS Reduced fertility (caused by hyperandrogenaemia due to inadequate glucocorticoid therapy or structural abnormalities due to androgen excess in utero or suboptimal surgical reconstruction). Short final adult height (because of pre-mature epiphyseal closure). Testicular adrenal rests (ectopic adrenal tissue which is stimulated by the increased ACTH).

PROGNOSIS Undiagnosed infants may die from salt-losing crisis. Otherwise, quality of life is usually good.

Cushing's syndrome

DEFINITION   Syndrome associated with chronic inappropriate elevation of free circulating cortisol.

AETIOLOGY   *ACTH-dependent (80%)*
- Excess ACTH secreted from a pituitary adenoma: Cushing's disease (80%).
- ACTH secreted from an ectopic source, e.g. small-cell lung carcinomas, pulmonary carcinoid tumours (20%).

ACTH-independent (20%)
- Excess cortisol secreted from a benign adrenal adenoma (60%).
- Excess cortisol secreted from an adrenal carcinoma (40%).

Rare: ACTH-independent micro- or macronodular adrenal hyperplasia[1].

EPIDEMIOLOGY   Incidence reported as 2–4/1000000 per year, but may be more common. Endogenous Cushing's syndrome is more common in females. Peak incidence is 20–40 years.

HISTORY   Increasing weight and fatigue. Muscle weakness, myalgia, thin skin, easy bruising, poor wound healing, fractures (resulting from osteoporosis).
Hirsutism, acne, frontal balding. Oligo- or amenorrhoea, depression or psychosis.

EXAMINATION
Facial fullness, *facial plethora*, interscapular fat pad.
Proximal muscle weakness, thin skin, *bruises*.
Central obesity, pink/purple striae on abdomen, breast, thighs.
Kyphosis (due to vertebral fracture). Poorly healing wounds.
Hirsutism, acne, frontal balding.
Hypertension. Ankle oedema (salt and water retention as a result of mineralocorticoid effect of excess cortisol).
Pigmentation in ACTH-dependent cases.
(Signs in *italic* are more discriminatory)

INVESTIGATIONS   Must only be performed in patients with a high pre-test probability.
Blood: Non-specific changes include hypokalaemia (particularly in ectopic Cushing's), ↑ glucose.
Initial high-sensitivity tests:
Urinary free cortisol (two or three 24 h urine collections). *Late-night salivary cortisol. Overnight dexamethasone suppression test. Low dose dexamethasone suppression test* (LDDST). LDDST involves giving 0.5 mg dexamethasone orally every 6 h for 48 h. In Cushing's syndrome, serum cortisol measured 48 h after the first dose of dexamethasone fails to suppress below 50 nmol/L.
Tests to determine the underlying cause:
ACTH-independent (adrenal adenoma/carcinoma): ↓ Plasma ACTH. CT or MRI of adrenals.
ACTH-dependent (pituitary adenoma): ↑ Plasma ACTH. Pituitary MRI. High-dose dexamethasone suppression test (largely abandoned in centres where inferior petrosal sinus sampling is available). Inferior petrosal sinus sampling: Central: peripheral ratio of venous ACTH > 2:1 (or >3:1 after CRH administration) in Cushing's disease.

ACTH-dependent (ectopic):
If lung cancer is suspected: CXR, sputum cytology, bronchoscopy, CT scan. Radiolabelled octreotide scans to detect carcinoid tumours as they express somatostatin receptors.

MANAGEMENT   In iatrogenic cases, discontinue administration, lower steroid dose or use an alternative steroid-sparing agent if possible.
Medical: Pre-operative or if unfit for surgery. Inhibition of cortisol synthesis with metyrapone or ketoconazole. Treat osteoporosis and provide physiotherapy for muscle weakness.
Surgical:
Pituitary adenomas: Trans-sphenoidal adenoma resection (hydrocortisone replaced until pituitary function recovers).
Adrenal adenoma/carcinoma: Surgical removal of tumour (plus adjuvant therapy with mitotane for adrenal carcinoma).
Ectopic ACTH production: Treatment is directed at the tumour.
Radiotherapy: In those who are not cured and have persistent hypercortisolaemia after transsphenoidal resection of the tumour. Stereotactic radiotherapy provides less irradiation to surrounding tissues.
In refractory cases of Cushing's disease, bilateral adrenalectomy may be performed.

COMPLICATIONS   Diabetes, osteoporosis, hypertension. Pre-disposition to infections.
Complications of surgery: CSF leakage, meningitis, sphenoid sinusitis, hypopituitarism. Complications of radiotherapy: Hypopituitarism, radionecrosis, small ↑ risk of second intracranial tumours and stroke.
Bilateral adrenalectomy may rarely be complicated by development of Nelson's syndrome (locally aggressive pituitary tumour causing skin pigmentation due to excessive ACTH secretion).

PROGNOSIS   In the untreated, 5-year survival rate is 50%. Depression usually persists for many years following successful treatment.

---

[1] *Micronodular adrenal hyperplasia* may be isolated or occur as part of Carney's complex (autosomal dominant syndrome characterized by spotty skin pigmentation, endocrine tumours and myxomas of the skin, heart, breast). Three responsible genes have so far been identified: *PRKAR1A*, *PDE11A*, and *MYH8*. *Macronodular adrenal hyperplasia:* Ectopic adrenal expression of G protein coupled receptors or ↑ expression/activity of some eutopic receptors. McCune–Albright syndrome is a rare variant caused by activating mutations of the α-subunit of stimulatory G protein. It is characterized by café au lait spots, polyostotic fibrous dysplasia, precocious puberty and other endocrine disorders. Surgical bilateral adrenalectomy is used in patients with micronodular adrenal hyperplasia and most patients with macronodular adrenal hyperplasia.

Diabetes insipidus

DEFINITION   A disorder of inadequate secretion of or insensitivity to vasopressin (ADH) leading to hypotonic polyuria.

AETIOLOGY   Failure of ADH secretion by the posterior pituitary (central/cranial) or insensitivity of the collecting duct to ADH (nephrogenic). Water channels (aquaporins) fail to activate and the luminal membrane of the collecting duct remains impermeable to water. This results in large volume hypotonic urine and polydipsia.

Central (Cranial)	Nephrogenic
Idiopathic	Idiopathic
Tumours (e.g. pituitary tumours)	Drugs (e.g. lithium)
Infilitrative (e.g. sarcoidosis)	Post-obstructive uropathy
Infection (e.g. meningitis)	Pyelonephritis
Vascular (e.g. aneurysms, Sheehan syndrome)	Pregnancy
Trauma (e.g. head injury, neurosurgery) DIDMOAD[1]	Osmotic diuresis (e.g. diabetes mellitus)

EPIDEMIOLOGY   Depends on aetiology, but median age of onset is 24 years.

HISTORY   Polyuria, nocturia and polydipsia (excessive thirst). Enuresis and sleep disturbances in children.
Other symptoms depend on the aetiology.

EXAMINATION   Cranial diabetes insipidus has few signs if patients drink adequate fluids. Urine output is often >3 L/24 h.
If fluid intake < fluid output, signs of dehydration may be present (e.g. tachycardia, reduced tissue turgor, postural hypotension, dry mucous membranes).
Signs of the cause (e.g. visual field defect).

INVESTIGATIONS
Blood: U&E and Ca^{2+} (Na^+ may be rise secondary to dehydration). ↑ Plasma osmolality. ↓ Urine osmolality.
Water deprivation test: Water is restricted for 8 h. Plasma and urine osmolality are measured every hour over the 8 h. Weigh the patient (hourly) to monitor the level of dehydration; stop the test if the fall in body weight is >3%. Desmopressin (2 μg IM) is given after 8 h and urine osmolality is measured.

Normal	Water restriction causes a rise in plasma osmolality and ↑ ADH secretion. This leads to ↑ water reabsorption in the collecting ducts. Urine is concentrated. (Urine osmolality > 600 mosmol/kg)	
Diabetes insipidus	Lack of ADH activity means that urine is unable to be concentrated by the collecting ducts. (Urine osmolality < 400 mosmol/kg)	
	Cranial	Urine osmolality rises by >50%, following administration of desmopressin.
	Nephrogenic	Urine osmolality rises by <45%, following administration of desmopressin.

[1] DIDMOAD (Wolfram's syndrome) is characterized by diabetes insipidus, diabetes mellitus, optic atrophy and deafness. It is inherited as an autosomal recessive trait with incomplete penetrance. It is caused by at least two different genes: *WFS1* and *ZCD2*. Wolframin, the product of *WFS1* a transmembrane protein expressed in pancreatic β cells and neurons.

MANAGEMENT   Treat the identified cause if possible.

Cranial diabetes insipidus: Desmopressin (DDAVP), a vasopressin analogue, can be given 10 μg/day, intranasally. In mild disease, chlorpropamide or carbamazepine can be used to potentiate effects of residual vasopressin.

Nephrogenic diabetes insipidus: Sodium and/or protein restriction may help polyuria. Thiazide diuretics.

COMPLICATIONS   Hypernatraemic dehydration. Excess desmopressin therapy may cause hyponatraemia.

PROGNOSIS   Variable depending on cause. Cranial diabetes insipidus may be transient following head trauma. Cure of cranial or nephrogenic diabetes insipidus may be possible on removal of cause, e.g. tumour resection, drug discontinuation.

Diabetes mellitus, Type 1

DEFINITION Metabolic hyperglycaemic condition caused by absolute insufficiency of pancreatic insulin production.

AETIOLOGY Caused by destruction of the pancreatic insulin-producing β-cells, resulting in absolute insulin deficiency. The β -cell destruction is caused by an autoimmune process in 90% of patients.

Likely to occur in genetically susceptible subjects and is probably triggered by environmental agents. Polymorphisms of a number of genes may influence the risk of type 1 diabetes. These include the gene encoding preproinsulin and a number of genes related to immune system function such as HLA-DQβ and HLA-DR, PTPN22 and CTLA-4.

Pancreatic β-cell autoantigens may play a role in the initiation or progression of autoimmune islet injury. These include glutamic acid decarboxylase (GAD), insulin, insulinoma-associated protein 2 (IA-2) and cation efflux zinc transporter (ZnT8).

EPIDEMIOLOGY One of the most common chronic diseases in childhood with a prevalence of 0.25% in the UK. Considerable geographic variation in the incidence. The US and Northern Europe have an incidence of ~8–17/100 000 per year.

HISTORY AND EXAMINATION Often of juvenile onset (<30 years). Polyuria/nocturia (osmotic diuresis caused by glycosuria), polydipsia (thirst), tiredness, weight loss. Symptoms of complications (*see below*) *Diabetic ketoacidosis*: Nausea, vomiting, abdominal pain, polyuria, polydipsia, drowsiness, confusion, coma, Kussmaul breathing (deep and rapid), ketotic breath, signs of dehydration (e.g. dry mucous membranes, ↓ tissue turgor).

Signs of complications: Fundoscopy (to look for diabetic retinopathy). Examination of feet (test for neuropathy: 10 g monofilament testing and vibration sensation; palpate dorsalis pedis and posterior tibial pulses). Measure BP.

Signs of associated autoimmune conditions e.g. vitiligo, Addison's disease, autoimmune thyroid disease.

INVESTIGATIONS *Blood glucose*: Fasting blood glucose >7 mmol/L or random blood glucose >11 mmol/L. Two positive results are needed before diagnosis.

HbA1C: Estimates overall blood glucose levels in past 2–3 months.

FBC: MCV, reticulocytes (↑ erythrocyte turnover causes misleading HbA1c levels).

U&E: Monitor for nephropathy and hyperkalaemia caused by ACE inhibitors.

Lipid profile.

Urine albumin creatinine ratio (to detect microalbuminuria).

Patients presenting with suspected DKA *Blood*: FBC (↑ WCC even without infection), U&E (↑ urea and creatinine from dehydration), LFT, CRP, glucose, amylase (may ↑), blood cultures, ABG (metabolic acidosis with high anion gap), blood/urinary ketones.

Urine: Glycosuria, ↑ ketones, MSU (microscopy, culture).

CXR: To exclude any infection.

ECG: To look for acute ischaemic changes.

MANAGEMENT Diabetic ketoacidosis Consider HDU/ICU input, central line, arterial line and urinary catheter if severe acidosis, hypotensive or oliguric.

Insulin: 50 U of soluble insulin in 50 mL 0.9% saline—start at 0.1 U/kg/h (~6–7 U/h) until capillary ketones <0.3, venous pH >7.30, and venous bicarbonate >18 mmol/L. At this point, if the patient is able to eat and drink, change to SC insulin regimen. If not, change to IV insulin sliding scale. Do not stop insulin infusion until 1–2 h after regular SC insulin is restarted.

Fluids: 500 mL 0.9% saline over 15–30 min until systolic BP >100 mmHg. Then 1 L 2-hourly × 3 and 1 L 3-hourly × 3. IV dextrose is started in conjunction with 0.9% saline when blood glucose reaches 15 mmol/L: 1 L 5% dextrose over 8 h when blood glucose is 7–15 mmol/L and 500 mL 10% dextrose over 4 h when blood glucose is <7 mmol/L.

Potassium replacement (start in the second bag of fluid, if passing urine). Adjust amount of potassium added to fluids according to plasma potassium (If >5.50 mmol/L: Nil. If 2.5–5.5 mmol/L: 40 mmol/L, If <2.5 mmol/L 60–80 mmol/L).

Monitor blood glucose, capillary ketones and urine output hourly, U&Es 4-hourly, and venous blood gas at 0, 2, 4, 8, 12 h and before stopping fixed rate insulin regimen. Monitor phosphate and magnesium daily.

Broad spectrum antibiotics if infection suspected.

Thromboprophylaxis.

NBM for at least 6 h (gastroparesis is common).

NG tube: If GCS is reduced (to prevent vomiting and aspiration).

There is no strong evidence for the use of IV bicarbonate.

Refer to diabetes team for patient education.

Glycaemic control

Advice and patient education: Diabetes nurse specialists and dietitians. *SC insulin*: Short-acting insulin (e.g. Lispro, aspart, glulisine) three times daily before each meal and one long-acting insulin (isophane, glargine, detemir) injection once daily. Injection sites should be rotated.

Insulin pumps may give slightly better glycaemic control. However, they are costly and cumbersome for some patients and ketoacidosis may occur if the pump malfunctions.

Motivated patients can attend DAFNE (dose adjustment for normal eating) courses to learn how to calculate their carbohydrate intake and adjust their insulin doses accordingly.

Monitor: Control of symptoms (e.g. thirst, tiredness), regular finger prick tests by the patient, monitoring HbA1c levels (target <7%) every 3–6 months.[1]

Screening and management of complications. See Diabetes mellitus, Type 2.

Treatment of hypoglycaemia: If ↓ consciousness: 50 ml of 50% glucose IV or 1 mg glucagon IM. If conscious and cooperative: 50 g oral glucose (e.g. in the form of Lucozade®, milk, sugar or 3 dextrose tablets), followed with a starchy snack. Should not drive for 45 min.

Screening and management cardiovascular risk factors See Diabetes mellitus, Type 2.

COMPLICATIONS   *Diabetic ketoacidosis*: ↓ Insulin and ↑ counter-regulatory hormones result in ↑ hepatic gluconeogenesis and ↓ peripheral glucose utilization. Renal reabsorptive capacity of glucose is exceeded causing glycosuria, osmotic diuresis and dehydration. ↑ Lipolysis leads to ketogenesis and metabolic acidosis. Diabetic ketoacidosis may be precipitated by infection (30%), errors in management (15%), newly diagnosed diabetes (10%), other medical disease (5%), no cause identified (40%).

Microvascular: Retinopathy, nephropathy, neuropathy (*see* Diabetes mellitus, Type 2). *Macrovascular*: Peripheral vascular disease, ischaemic heart disease, stroke/TIA. *Susceptible to infections (especially on feet). Complications of insulin treatment*: Weight gain. Fat hypertrophy at insulin injection sites. Hypoglycaemia caused my missing a meal or overdosage of insulin (Patients present with neuroglycopenic and adrenergic signs: personality change, fits, confusion, coma, pallor, sweating, tremor, tachycardia, palpitations, dizziness, hunger and focal neurological symptoms). Hypoglycaemic symptoms may be masked by autonomic neuropathy, β-blockers and brain adapting to recurrent episodes.

PROGNOSIS   Depends on early diagnosis, good glycaemic control and compliance with screening and treatment. Vascular disease and renal failure are major causes of increased morbidity and mortality.

---

[1] Diabetes control and complications trial (DCCT) showed that strict glycaemic control in type 1 diabetes mellitus ↓ the risk of development and progression of diabetic microvascular complications.

Diabetes mellitus, Type 2

DEFINITION   Characterized by ↑ peripheral resistance to insulin action, impaired insulin secretion and ↑ hepatic glucose output.

AETIOLOGY   Multi-factorial (genetic and environmental). *Genetic*: Monozygotic twins have a 90% concordance rate. The lifetime risk for a first-degree relative of a patient with type 2 diabetes is 5–10 times higher than that those without a family history of diabetes. Monogenic causes of type 2 diabetes represent a very small fraction of cases[1]. Several inherited polymorphisms (e.g. in the gene for the transcription factor 7-like 2) may contribute to the risk for diabetes.

Obesity, ↑ plasma *free fatty acid* levels and '*adipokines*' secreted by adipocytes (e.g. leptin, adiponectin, TNF-α, resistin) contribute to peripheral insulin resistance. Chronic hyperglycaemia can have a toxic effect on β-cells (*glucotoxicity*). ↑ Free fatty acid levels may also worsen pancreatic β-cell function (*lipotoxicity*).

Secondary diabetes: *Pancreatic diseases* (chronic pancreatitis, hereditary haemochromatosis, pancreatic cancer, surgical removal of pancreas), *Endocrinopathies* (Cushing's syndrome, acromegaly, phaeochromocytoma, glucagonoma), *Drugs* (e.g. corticosteroids, atypical antipsychotics, protease inhibitors).

EPIDEMIOLOGY   Prevalence in the UK: 5–10%. People of Asian, African and Hispanic descent are at greater risk. The incidence has ↑ over the last 20 years, in parallel with ↑ prevalence of obesity worldwide.

HISTORY   May be incidental finding.

Polyuria, polydypsia, tiredness. Patients may present with hyperosmolar hyperglycaemic state (also known as hyperosmolar non-ketotic state; *See* Complication below). Infections (infected foot ulcers, candidiasis, balanitis or pruritus vulvae).

Assess for other cardiovascular risk factors: hypertension, hyperlipidaemia and smoking.

EXAMINATION   Measure weight and height (calculate body mass index: weight(kg)/height(m)²), waist circumference, blood pressure. Look for signs of complications (*see* Complication). *Diabetic foot*: Both ischaemic and neuropathic signs. Dry skin, reduced subcutaneous tissue, corns and calluses, ulceration, gangrene. Charcot's arthropathy and signs of peripheral neuropathy, foot pulses are ↓ in ischaemic foot. *Skin changes (rare)*: Necrobiosis lipoidica diabeticorum (well-demarcated plaques on the shins or arms with shiny atrophic surface and red–brown edges), granuloma annulare (flesh-coloured papules coalescing in rings on the back of hands and fingers), diabetic dermopathy (depressed pigmented scars on shins).

INVESTIGATIONS   Diabetes mellitus is diagnosed if one or more of the following are present:

- Symptoms of diabetes and a random plasma glucose ≥11.1 mmol/L.
- Fasting plasma glucose ≥7.0 mmol/L (after an overnight fast of at least 8 h).
- Two-hour plasma glucose ≥11.1 mmol/L after a 75 g oral glucose tolerance test.

In the absence of unequivocal hyperglycaemia and acute metabolic decompensation, these criteria should be confirmed by repeat testing on another day.

---

[1] **MODY** (mature onset diabetes of the young) is a rare cause of type 2 diabetes due to mutations transmitted in an autosomal dominant manner. MODY1, MODY3 and MODY5 are due to mutations in the genes encoding hepatocyte nuclear transcription factors 4-α, 1-α and 1-β, respectively. MODY2 is caused by mutations in the glucokinase gene. MODY4 is caused by mutations in the insulin promoter factor-1, a transcription factor that regulates pancreatic development and insulin gene transcription. MODY 6 is caused by mutations of the gene for neurogenic differentiation 1 (NeuroD1).

Monitor: HbA1C, U&Es, lipid profile, estimated glomerular filtration rate (GFR) using the MDRD calculator. Spot urine albumin: Creatinine ratio (to detect microalbuminuria).

MANAGEMENT   *Glycaemic control*: Pharmacologic therapy for glycaemic control in type 2 diabetes is summarized in figure 3. Monitor control of symptoms (e.g. thirst, tiredness), capillary blood glucose (finger prick tests done by the patient) and HbA1C (every 3 months)

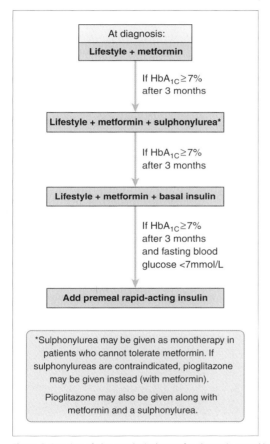

Figure 3 Overview of pharmacologic therapy for glycaemic control in type 2 diabetes

Sulphonylureas (e.g. gliclazide) block ATP-sensitive K^+ channels in β cells, stimulating insulin release (side effects: hypoglycaemia, weight gain). Metformin inhibits hepatic gluconeogenesis (side effects: GI disturbance, rarely lactic acidosis; hence stop in unwell/septic patients). Pioglitazone, a thiazolidinedione, activates PPAR γ and $\downarrow$ peripheral insulin resistance. (Note: rosiglitazone, another thiazolidinedione, is not recommended as associated with $\uparrow$ risk of myocardial infarction and incidence of fractures.)

Diabetes mellitus, Type 2 (continued)

Other less well-validated therapies When hypoglycaemia is particularly undesirable (hazardous jobs): Add pioglitazone or exenatide to metformin instead of sulphonylureas. If weight loss is a major consideration & HbA1C <8% use SC exenatide. Exenatide is a glucagon-like peptide-1 (GLP-1) agonist. GLP-1 is produced by the L-cells in the gut. It ↑ glucose-stimulated insulin secretion, ↓ glucagon release, gastric emptying and appetite. An inhibitor of dipeptidyl peptidase IV, the enzyme that degrades GLP-1 (e.g. sitagliptin), may be considered in patients who have contraindications or intolerance to metformin, sulfonylureas or pioglitazone (e.g. those with chronic kidney disease). Acarbose (inhibits intestinal glucosidases and ↓ carbohydrate digestion); less used because of side-effects (bloating, flatulence).

Screening for and management of complications:

Retinopathy: Regular digital retinal photography, ophthalmology referral and laser photocoagulation if necessary.

Nephropathy: Monitor U&Es and estimated GFR using the MDRD calculator, spot urine analysis (albumin: creatinine ratio), BP control, ACE inhibitors/angiotensin receptor blockers, monitor K^+.

Neuropathy: Regular examination and inspection of the feet for ulcers, 10 g monofilament testing, joint vibration, foot hygiene, amitriptyline, duloxetine, gabapentin or capsaicin cream for painful neuropathy.

Vascular disease: Regular examination of foot pulses.

Diabetic foot: Educate to examine feet regularly. Diabetic footwear. Podiatry assessment. For infections: clean and dress regularly, swab for culture and sensitivity, IV antibiotics (e.g. flucloxacillin, co-amoxiclav, cephalosporin and metronidazole). Look for osteomyelitis on X-ray. Surgical debridement or amputation if necessary.

Screen for and treat cardiovascular risk factors: Lose weight, exercise, stop smoking, BP control, all diabetic patients should be started on a statin (CARDS trial). Aspirin in patients with diabetes and an additional cardiovascular risk factor.

Advice and patient education: (INFORM PT)

Information: Diabetic nurses, leaflets, websites, etc. explaining diabetes control, complications.

Nutrition: Optimizing meal plans, diet (complex carbohydrates as opposed to simple sugars, ↓ fat intake).

Foot care: Regular inspection, appropriate footwear, role of chiropodist.

Organizations: Local and national support groups.

Recognition and treatment of hypoglycaemia.

Monitoring capillary blood glucose and charting it. Monitoring for ketones during intercurrent illness.

Pregnancy: Strict glycaemic control and planning of conception.

Treatment: Action, duration and administration technique for insulin, change the site of injection (to avoid lipohypertrophy), explain the need to plan exercise.

Hyperosmolar hyperglycaemic state: Management similar to diabetic ketoacidosis (*see* Diabetes, type 1), except use 0.45 % saline if serum Na^+ > 170 mmol/L, and a lower rate of insulin infusion (1–3 U/h). DVT prophylaxis with SC heparin.

COMPLICATIONS *Hyperosmolar hyperglycaemic state*: Due to insulin deficiency, as diabetic ketoacidosis, but patient is usually old and may be presenting for the first time; history is longer (e.g. 1 week); there is marked dehydration, ↑ Na^+, ↑ glucose (>35 mmol/L), ↑ osmolality (>340 mosmol/kg), no acidosis. *Neuropathy*: Distal symmetrical sensory neuropathy, painful neuropathy, carpal tunnel syndrome, diabetic amyotrophy (asymmetrical wasting of proximal muscle), mononeuritis (e.g. III nerve palsy with preservation of pupillary response, VI nerve), autonomic neuropathy (e.g. postural hypotension), gastroparesis (abdominal pain, nausea, vomiting), impotence, urinary retention. *Nephropathy*: Microalbuminuria, proteinuria and, eventually, renal failure. Prone to urinary tract infections and renal papillary necrosis. *Retinopathy*: *Background*: Dot and blot haemorrhages, hard exudates. *Pre-proliferative*: Cotton wool spots, venous beading. *Proliferative*: New vessels on the disc and elsewhere. *Maculopathy*: Macular oedema, exudates within 1 disc diameter of the centre of fovea, haemorrhage within 1 disc diameter of centre of the fovea associated with ↓ visual acuity. Also prone to glaucoma, cataracts, transient visual loss (sudden osmotic changes). *Macrovascular complications*: Ischaemic heart disease, stroke, peripheral vascular disease.

PROGNOSIS The United Kingdom Prospective Diabetes Study (UKPDS) showed that intensive therapy to achieve lower levels of glycaemia ↓ the risk of development and progression of diabetic microvascular complications. The 10-year post-trial monitoring data from the UKPDS show that early intensive glucose control, ↓ the risk for myocardial infarction and all-cause mortality.

Pre-diabetes can be diagnosed based upon a fasting blood glucose test or an oral glucose tolerance test:

- *Impaired fasting glucose* (IFG) is defined as a fasting plasma glucose between 5.6–6.9 mmol/L.
- *Impaired glucose tolerance* (IGT) is defined as a plasma glucose level of 7.8–11.0 mmol/L measured 2 h after a 75 g oral glucose tolerance test.

Individuals with IFG or IGT are at considerable risk for developing type 2 diabetes (40% risk over the next 5 years).

Hyperaldosteronism (primary)

DEFINITION Characterized by autonomous aldosterone overproduction from the adrenal gland with subsequent suppression of plasma renin activity.

AETIOLOGY Excess aldosterone may be secondary to an adrenal adenoma (Conn's syndrome; 70%) or hyperplasia of the adrenal cortex (30%). Rare: Glucocorticoid-suppressible hyperaldosteronism (1–3%) or an aldosterone producing adrenal carcinoma.
Pathophysiology: Excess aldosterone results in: ↑ Na and water retention causing hypertension; ↑ renal K loss and hypokalaemia and suppression of renin because of NaCl retention.

EPIDEMIOLOGY The prevalence in hypertensive patients is 1–2%. Aldosterone producing adenoma occurs more commonly in women and in younger patients (<50 years). Bilateral adrenal hyperplasia occurs more commonly in men and usually presents at an older age.

HISTORY Usually asymptomatic and picked up on routine blood tests.
Symptoms of hypokalaemia: Muscle weakness, polyuria and polydipsia (nephrogenic diabetes insipidus secondary to hypokalaemia), paraesthesia, tetany.

EXAMINATION Hypertension. Complications of hypertension (e.g. retinopathy).

INVESTIGATIONS
Screening tests
↓ *Serum K⁺* (<4 mmol/L), serum Na⁺ usually normal (due to parallel ↑ in the water content of the blood).
↑ *(Inappropriate) urine potassium.*
↑ *Plasma aldosterone concentration: Plasma renin activity ratio*: after stopping anti-hypertensives (6 weeks for spironolactone and 2 weeks for most other anti-hypertensives). If anti-hypertensive therapy is required an α-blocker (e.g. doxazosin) may be used. Hypokalaemia should be corrected prior to the test.
Confirmatory tests
Salt loading: Failure of aldosterone suppression following a sodium load (oral or IV 0.9% sodium chloride) confirms primary hyperaldosteronism. Determining the cause
Postural test: Plasma aldosterone, renin activity and cortisol are measured with patient recumbent at 8 a.m. The tests are repeated after 4 h of being upright (at 12 noon). In adenomas which are mostly ACTH-sensitive, aldosterone secretion ↓ from 8 a.m. until 12 noon. In bilateral adrenal hyperplasia, adrenals respond to standing posture by ↑ renin and thus ↑ aldosterone secretion. This test has a 20% false negative rate.
CT or MRI (abdomen): To visualize the adrenals.
Bilateral adrenal vein catheterization: Allows distinction between Conn's syndrome and bilateral adrenal hyperplasia by measuring adrenal vein aldosterone levels.
Radio-labelled cholesterol scanning: Unilateral uptake in adrenal adenomas; bilateral uptake in bilateral adrenal hyperplasia.

MANAGEMENT *Bilateral adrenal hyperplasia*: Spironolactone (an aldosterone receptor antagonist). Change to eplerenone if spironolactone side effects are intolerable (gynaecomastia, impotence, menstrual irregularities, muscle cramps and gastrointestinal upset). Amiloride (a potassium-sparing diuretic) is alternative. Monitor serum potassium and creatinine, and BP. ACE inhibitors and calcium channel blockers may need to be added. It can take 4–8 weeks for the hypertension to respond to the treatments.
Aldosterone producing adenomas: Adrenalectomy by an experienced endocrine surgeon. Laparoscopic surgery is associated with ↓ post-operative morbidity, hospital stay and expense compared with open laparotomy.
Adrenal carcinoma: Surgery and post-operative mitotane. *GSH* is treated with dexamethasone (0.25 mg in the morning, 0.5 mg at night).

COMPLICATIONS   Complications of hypertension (*see* Hypertension).

PROGNOSIS   Surgery may either cure hypertension (in about 50%) or make it more amenable to anti-hypertensive therapy in those who are not cured (usually the elderly or those with long-standing hypertension).

Hyperparathyroidism

DEFINITION *Primary*: ↑ Secretion of parathyroid hormone (PTH) unrelated to the plasma calcium concentration.
Secondary: ↑ Secretion of PTH secondary to hypocalcaemia.
Tertiary: Autonomous PTH secretion following chronic secondary hyperparathyroidism.

AETIOLOGY *Primary*: Parathyroid gland adenoma(s) or hyperplasia (80% single adenoma, 18% hyperplasia/multiple adenomas). Rarely, parathyroid carcinoma (2%). May be associated with multiple endocrine neoplasia (MEN)[1].
Secondary: Chronic renal failure, vitamin D deficiency.

EPIDEMIOLOGY *Primary*: Annual incidence is five in 100 000. Twice as common in females. Peak incidence 40–60 years.

HISTORY AND EXAMINATION *Primary*: Many patients have mild hypercalcaemia and are asymptomatic.
Hypercalcaemia may present with: polyuria, polydipsia, renal calculi, bone pain, abdominal pain, nausea, constipation, psychological depression and lethargy.
Secondary: May present with symptoms and signs of hypocalcaemia (*See* Osteomalacia) and/ or the underlying cause (chronic renal failure, vitamin D deficiency).

INVESTIGATIONS U&Es, serum calcium (↑ in primary and tertiary, ↓/normal in secondary), phosphate (↓ in primary and tertiary, ↑ in secondary), albumin (to calculate 'corrected' calcium), ↑ alkaline phosphatase, vitamin D (↓ in secondary hyperparathyroidism), PTH levels[2]. Patients with parathyroid carcinomas are more likely to have a marked hypercalcaemia with very high serum PTH levels.
Primary: Hyperchloraemic acidosis (normal anion gap) caused by PTH inhibition of renal tubular reabsorption of bicarbonate.
Urine: The differential diagnosis of primary hyperparathyroidism includes familial hypocalciuric hypercalcaemia (FHH)[3]. Thus in patients with ↑ or inappropriately normal PTH levels, calcium: creatinine clearance ratio should be measured to differentiate between primary hyperparathyroidism (ratio >0.01) and FHH (ratio <0.01). Calcium: creatinine clearance ratio:
Urine calcium (mmol/L) × [Plasma creatinine (μmol/L)/1000]
Plasma calcium (mmol) × Urine creatinine (mmol/L)
Twenty four hour urine collection should be sent for creatinine clearance and calcium measurement.
Renal ultrasound at baseline to look for renal calculi.
*Radiographs (*no longer routinely performed): Subperiostial erosions of phalanges, brown tumours (osteolucent bone defects), diffuse porotic mottling of skull caused by demineralization ('pepper pot' skull), sclerosis of superior and inferior vertebral margins with central demineralization ('rugger jersey' spine), renal calculi/nephrocalcinosis.
Preoperative localization: Ultrasound of neck and technetium sestamibi scan.

---

[1] **MEN type 1** (mutation in menin gene on chromosome 11): Parathyroid adenoma or hyperplasia, pancreatic endocrine tumours, pituitary adenomas. **MEN type 2** (mutation in *RET* gene on chromosome 10): Medullary thyroid carcinoma, phaeochromocytoma and either parathyroid hyperplasia (MEN-2A) or mucosal neuromas on the lips or tongue (MEN-2B).

[2] Patients with hypercalcaemia secondary to malignancy, myeloma and granulomatous conditions (e.g. TB, sarcoidosis and lymphoma, causing excess production of 1,25 dihydroxyvitamin D) have *suppressed* PTH. Patients with hypercalcaemia secondary to malignancy are treated with rehydration and IV pamidronate (a bisphosphonate).

[3] Autosomal dominant disorder caused by inactivating mutations in the gene encoding the calcium-sensing receptor on the parathyroid cells and in the kidneys.

MANAGEMENT
Primary
Acute hypercalcaemia: IV fluids (often 4–6 in the first 24 h). *Conservative management*: In patients who do not meet surgical criteria (*see* below), avoid factors that can exacerbate hypercalcaemia including thiazide diuretics. Maintain adequate hydration (at least 6–8 glasses of water per day), moderate calcium and vitamin D intake.

Surgical: Subtotal parathyroidectomy, total parathyroidectomy (in MEN1). Indications: Symptomatic patients or asymptomatic patients with:

Age <50 years, **B**one mineral density: T-score <2.5, **C**alculi (renal stones), **Cr**eatinine clearance ↓ by 30%, **D**ifficult to do follow up periodically, **El**evated serum calcium >0.25 mmol/L above upper limit of normal or 24-h urinary calcium >10 mmol.

Secondary Treat the underlying renal failure. Calcium and vitamin D supplements.

COMPLICATIONS *Primary*: ↑ PTH results in ↑ bone resorption, ↑ renal tubular calcium reabsorption, 1α- hydroxylation of vitamin D and intestinal calcium absorption, leading to hypercalcaemia.

Secondary: ↑ stimulation of osteoclasts and bone turnover leading to 'osteitis fibrosa cystica'.

Complications of surgery: Hypocalcaemia, recurrent laryngeal nerve palsy (<1%).

PROGNOSIS *Primary*: Surgery is curative for benign disease in most cases.

Secondary or tertiary: As for chronic renal failure.

Hypogonadism, (female)

DEFINITION Characterized by impairment of ovarian function.

AETIOLOGY Primary hypogonadism (hypergonadotrophic)
Gonadal dysgensis: Chromosomal abnormalities (e.g. Turner's syndrome), *FMR1* gene pre-mutation carriers (CGG repeats of between 55 and 200).
Gonadal damage: Autoimmune, iatrogenic (chemotherapy, radiation, surgery).
Secondary hypogonadism (hypogonadotrophic)
Functional: Stress, weight loss, excessive exercise, eating disorders (anorexia nervosa, bulimia).
Pituitary/hypothalamic tumours and infiltrative lesions: Pituitary adenomas, craniopharyn-giomas, haemochromatosis.
Hyperprolactinaemia: Prolactinomas or tumours causing pituitary stalk compression.
Congenital GnRH deficiency: Kallmann's syndrome, idiopathic.

EPIDEMIOLOGY Secondary hypogonadism is a more common cause of an ovulation and amenorrhoea than primary hypogonadism. Turner's syndrome occurs in up to 1.5% of conceptions, 10% of spontaneous abortions and 1 in 2000–2500 live births.

HISTORY *Symptoms of oestrogen deficiency*: Night sweats, hot flush, vaginal dryness and dyspareunia. ↓ Libido, infertility. *Symptoms of the underlying cause.*

EXAMINATION *Pre-pubertal hypogonadism*
Delayed puberty (primary amenorrhoea, absent breast development, no secondary sexual characteristics).
Eunuchoid proportions (e.g. long legs, ↑ arm span for height).
Post-pubertal hypogonadism:
Regression of secondary sexual characteristics (loss of secondary sexual hair, breast atrophy). Perioral and periorbital fine facial wrinkles.
Signs of the underlying cause/associated conditions
Hypothalamic/pituitary disease: Visual field defects.
Kallmann's syndrome: Anosmia.
Turner's syndrome: Short stature, low posterior hairline, high arched palate, widely spaced nipples, wide carrying angle, short fourth and fifth metacarpals, congenital lymphoedema.
Patients with autoimmune primary ovarian failure: Signs of other autoimmune diseases e.g. hyperpigmentation in Addison's disease or vitiligo.

INVESTIGATIONS ↓ Serum oestradiol. Serum FSH and LH: ↑ in primary hypogonadism (due to ↓ feedback inhibition by ovarian oestradiol and inhibin). ↓ or inappropriately normal FSH/LH in secondary hypogonadism.
Investigations to determine the aetiology
Primary: Karyotype (to look for chromosomal abnormalities: complete or partial deletion of the X chromosome in Turner's syndrome, or the presence of a Y chromosome). Pelvic imaging (ultrasound and/or MRI): in patients with primary amenorrhoea, to demonstrate the presence or absence of the uterus and vagina and vaginal or cervical outlet obstruction (Müllerian agenesis, androgen insensitivity[1], transverse vaginal septum, imperforate hymen).

---

[1] *Androgen insensitivity syndrome* is caused by mutations in the androgen receptor gene on the X chromosome. Patients are phenotypically female but have XY karyotype and a male range serum testosterone. Removal of the gonads is deferred until immediately after pubertal maturation.

In unexplained pre-mature ovarian failure: screening for pre-mutation in the *FMR1* gene after appropriate genetic counselling and informed consent[2].

Secondary: Pituitary function tests (9 a.m. cortisol, TFTs, prolactin), visual field testing, hypothalamic-pituitary MRI, smell tests for anosmia. Serum transferrin saturation if hereditary haemochromatosis is suspected.

Investigation of the associated conditions

Turner's syndrome: Periodic echocardiography and cardiology follow-up, Renal ultrasound.

Autoimmune oophoritis: Evaluate for autoimmune adrenal insufficiency (by measuring 21-hydroxylase antibodies and if positive, an ACTH stimulation test).

MANAGEMENT   *Secondary hypogonadism in females*: Treat the underlying cause.

Induce puberty: Low-dose ethinyloestradiol, gradually increasing dose over puberty. Cyclical oral progesterone is added (first 2 weeks of each month) with the onset of breakthrough bleeding.

In adults: Oestrogen/progesterone replacement (oral contraceptive pill).

Induce ovulation in secondary hypogonadism: Pulsatile GnRH or gonadotrophin replacement therapy (with pelvic ultrasound monitoring to avoid ovarian hyperstimulation).

Surgery: Gonadectomy in patients with XY or XO/XY genotype (The presence of a Y chromosome ↑ the risk of gonadoblastomas).

Treatment of short stature in Turner's syndrome: Recombinant GH. Oxandrolone (anabolic steroid) may be added when 9–12 years.

COMPLICATIONS   Infertility. Osteoporosis. ischaemic heart disease. *Turner's syndrome*: Cardiac (aortic dissection, bicuspid aortic valve, coarctation of aorta, hypertension), gastro-intestinal (angiodysplasia, coeliac disease, abnormal liver function tests), renal anomalies (horseshoe kidneys, abnormal vascular supply), endocrine (↑ risk of hypothyroidism and diabetes mellitus).

PROGNOSIS   Prognosis varies with the underlying cause.

---

[2] Women with the *FMR1* pre-mutation are at risk of having a child with mental retardation as pre-mutations are unstable when transmitted by females and can expand to a full mutation causing fragile X syndrome. Male carriers of the FMR1 pre-mutations also at risk of developing ataxia and tremor (fragile X-associated tremor/ataxia syndrome).

Hypogonadism, (male)

DEFINITION A syndrome of ↓ testosterone production, sperm production or both.

AETIOLOGY *Primary (hypergonadotrophic) hypogonadism:*
Gonadal dysgensis: Klinefelter's syndrome (XXY), undescended testes (cryptorchidism).
Gonadal damage: Infection (e.g. mumps), torsion, trauma, autoimmune, iatrogenic (chemotherapy, surgery, radiation).
Rare causes: Defects in enzymes involved in testosterone synthesis, myotonic dystrophy.
Secondary (hypogonadotrophic) hypogonadism:
Pituitary/hypothalamic lesions: (see Hypopituitarism).
GnRH deficiency: Kallmann's syndrome (associated with anosmia), idiopathic
Hyperprolactinaemia
Systemic/chronic diseases
Rare causes: Genetic mutations[1]. Secondary hypogonadism may be seen in a number of rare syndromes:
Prader–Willi syndrome: Loss of a critical region on chromosome 15 causing obesity and short stature, small hands, almond-shaped eyes, learning difficulty/postnatal hypotonia.
Laurence–Moon–Biedl syndrome: Obesity, polydactyly, retinitis pigmentosa, learning difficulty.

EPIDEMIOLOGY Primary hypogonadism accounts for 30–40% of cases of male infertility; secondary hypogonadism accounts for 1–2% (10–20% of cases of male infertility are secondary to disorders of sperm transport and 40–50% are non-classifiable). The most common cause of primary hypogonadism is Klinefelter's syndrome (one in 500–1000 live births).

HISTORY Delayed puberty (if the onset is before puberty). ↓ Libido, impotence, infertility. Symptoms of the underlying cause e.g. Klinefelter's syndrome: intellectual dysfunction and behavioural abnormalities which cause difficulty in social interactions.

EXAMINATION Measure testicular volume using Prader's orchidometer (ellipsoids of different sizes). Normal adult testicular volume is 15–25 ml.
Prepubertal hypogonadism:
Signs of delayed puberty (high-pitched voice, ↓ pubic/axillary/facial hair, small or undescended testes, small phallus), gynaecomastia, eunuchoid proportions: arm span > height, lower segment > upper segment (due to delayed fusion of the epiphyses and continued growth of long bones).
Features of the underlying cause e.g. cryptorchidism, anosmia in Kallmann's syndrome.
Postpubertal hypogonadism:
↓ Pubic/axillary/facial hair, soft and small testes, gynaecomastia, fine perioral wrinkles.
Features of the underlying cause e.g. visual field defects due to a pituitary tumour, signs of systemic/chronic illness.

INVESTIGATIONS Serum total testosterone, SHBG and albumin (to calculate serum free testosterone), LH and FSH
Primary: ↓ Testosterone, ↑ LH and FSH (due to ↓ negative feedback).
Secondary: ↓ Testosterone, ↓ or inappropriately normal LH and FSH levels.
Determine the level of defect:
Primary: Karyotype (to exclude Klinefelter's syndrome).

Secondary: Pituitary function tests (9 a.m. cortisol, TFTs, prolactin), MRI of the hypothalamic-pituitary area, visual field testing, smell tests for anosmia. Iron studies (ferritin and transferrin saturation) if hereditary haemochromatosis is suspected.

---

[1] Mutations in the genes encoding GPR54 (the kisspeptin receptor), GnRH receptor, LH, FSH, leptin, leptin receptor, DAX1 (associated with congenital adrenal hypoplasia), LHX3, LHX4, HESX1 and PROP-1 (transcription factors necessary for early differentiation of the pituitary).

Bone age: In boys with delayed puberty; determined by the comparison of the radiograph of the patient's bones in the left hand and wrist with the bones of a standard atlas (allows assessment of skeletal maturation and the potential for future skeletal growth).

MANAGEMENT Treat the underlying cause if possible (e.g. dopamine agonists for prolactinoma).

Prepubertal: Testosterone replacement, gradually ↑ dose over puberty, monitor growth velocity and bone age.

Postpubertal: Testosterone replacement therapy (testosterone gel, intramuscular, subcutaneous implants or patches)

Side effects: Acne, prostate enlargement (obstructive symptoms), polycythaemia, fluid retention, sleep apnoea, mood fluctuations, side effects of the particular route of administration.

Follow-up and monitoring: Symptoms, digital rectal examination (to look for prostate enlargement), PSA, haemoglobin/haematocrit, testosterone levels. Sleep study if obstructive sleep apnoea is clinically suspected.

Secondary hypogonadism: Gonadotrophin (hCG and FSH) replacement therapy or pulsatile gonadotrophin-releasing hormone (GnRH) therapy.

Men who desire fertility: In vitro fertilization for moderate oligospermia, intracytoplasmic sperm injection for severe oligospermia.

COMPLICATIONS Infertility. Osteoporosis.

Klinefelter's syndrome: Predisposition to develop chronic bronchitis, bronchiectasis, emphysema; germ cell tumours, breast cancer, possibly non-Hodgkin lymphoma, varicose veins, leg ulcers and diabetes mellitus.

PROGNOSIS Normal life expectancy.

Hypopituitarism

DEFINITION   Deficiency of one or more of the hormones secreted by the anterior pituitary. Panhypopituitarism is deficiency of all pituitary hormones.

AETIOLOGY   *Pituitary masses:* Most commonly adenomas. Other parapituitary tumours (e.g. craniopharyngioma, meningioma, glioma, metastases), cysts (arachnoid cyst, Rathke's cleft cyst).
Pituitary trauma: Radiation, surgery or skull base fracture.
Hypothalamus (functional): Anorexia, starvation, over-exercise.
Infiltration: Tuberculosis, sarcoidosis, haemochromatosis, histiocytosis X.
Vascular: Pituitary apoplexy,[1] Sheehan's syndrome.[2]
Infection: Meningitis, encephalitis, syphilis (rare), fungal abscess.
Genetic mutations: Pit-1 and Prop-1 genes.

EPIDEMIOLOGY   Annual incidence and prevalence of pituitary adenomas: ~1 in 100 000 and nine in 100 000, respectively.

HISTORY AND EXAMINATION   Symptoms or signs depending on aetiology (e.g. bitemporal hemianopia caused by a pituitary mass).
Symptoms and signs according to type of hormone deficiency.

Hormone	Features
GH	*Children:* Short stature (<third centile/not in keeping with parental height)
	Adults: Low mood, fatigue, ↓ exercise capacity/muscle strength, ↑ abdominal fat mass
LH or FSH	Delayed puberty
	Females: Loss of secondary sexual hair, breast atrophy, menstrual irregularities, dyspareunia, ↓ libido, infertility
	Males: Loss of secondary sexual hair, gynaecomastia, ↓ small or soft testes, ↓ libido, impotence
ACTH	(*see* Adrenal insufficiency)
TSH	(*see* Hypothyroidism)
Prolactin	Absence of lactation (in Sheehan's syndrome[2])

Pituitary apoplexy: Life-threatening hypopituitarism with headache, visual loss and cranial nerve palsies.

INVESTIGATIONS   *Pituitary function tests:*
- *Basal tests:* 9 a.m. cortisol, LH, FSH, testosterone, oestradiol, IGF-1, prolactin, free T4 and TSH.
- *Dynamic tests (rarely performed):* Insulin-induced hypoglycaemia (contraindicated in patients with epilepsy, IHD, hypoadrenalism). Give 0.15 U/kg IV insulin. In hypopituitarism, peak GH and cortisol response to insulin-induced hypoglycaemia are <20 mU/L and <550 nmol/L, respectively.

Short Synacthen test: (*see* Adrenal insufficiency).
MRI or CT of brain.
Visual field testing.

---

[1] Pituitary apoplexy is the haemorrhage or infarction of a pituitary tumour.

[2] Sheehan's syndrome is pituitary infarction, haemorrhage and necrosis following post-partum haemorrhage.

MANAGEMENT
Hormone replacement:
Hydrocortisone: 20 mg in morning, 10 mg in evening (double oral dose for febrile illnesses, IM hydrocortisone at times of surgery). Should be provided with Medicalert bracelet and steroid card.
L-thyroxine: ~100 μg daily (always taken after hydrocortisone to avoid Addisonian crisis).
Sex hormones: Testosterone in males. Oestrogen ± progestogerone in females.
Growth hormone: SC 1.2 unit/day in adults. Children require specialist supervision.
Posterior pituitary deficiency (damaged to pituitary stalk): Desmopressin (vasopressin analogue) 10–20 μg/dayintranasally.

COMPLICATIONS   Adrenal crisis, hypoglycaemia, myxoedema coma, infertility. Osteoporosis; dwarfism (children).
Complications of the pituitary mass: Optic chiasm compression, hydrocephalus (third ventricular compression), temporal lobe epilepsy.

PROGNOSIS   Good with lifelong hormone replacement.

Hypothyroidism

DEFINITION The clinical syndrome resulting from insufficient secretion of thyroid hormones.

AETIOLOGY *Primary* ($\downarrow$ thyroid hormone production):
Acquired:
Autoimmune (Hashimoto's) thyroiditis (cellular and antibody-mediated).
Iatrogenic (post-surgery, radioiodine, medication for hyperthyroidism).
Severe iodine deficiency or iodine excess (Wolff–Chaikoff effect).
Thyroiditis
Congenital: Thyroid dysgenesis
Inherited defects in thyroid hormone biosynthesis
Secondary (<5% of cases):
Pituitary or hypothalamic disease (e.g. tumours) resulting in $\downarrow$ TSH or TRH and $\downarrow$ stimulation of thyroid hormone production.

EPIDEMIOLOGY The frequency of hypothyroidism varies from 0.1 to 2% of adults. $\female$: $\male$ ~ 6:1. Age of onset commonly >40 years, but can occur at any age. Iodine deficiency is seen in mountainous areas (e.g. Alps, Himalayas).

HISTORY Onset is usually insidious.
Cold intolerance, lethargy, weight gain, constipation, dry skin, hair loss, hoarse voice.
Mental slowness, depression, dementia, cramps, ataxia, paraesthesia.
Menstrual disturbances (irregular cycles, menorrhagia) in females.
History of surgery or radioiodine therapy for hyperthyroidism.
Personal or family history of other autoimmune conditions e.g. Addison's disease, type 1 diabetes mellitus, pernicious anaemia and pre-mature ovarian failure.
Myxoedema coma (severe hypothyroidism usually seen in the elderly): Hypothermia, hypoventilation, hyponatraemia, heart failure, confusion and coma.

EXAMINATION *Hands:* Bradycardia, cold hands.
Head/Neck/Skin: Pale puffy face, goitre, oedema, hair loss, dry skin, vitiligo.
Chest: Pericardial or pleural effusions.
Abdomen: Ascites.
Neurological: Slow relaxation of reflexes, signs of carpal tunnel syndrome.

INVESTIGATIONS
Blood: TFT: Primary: $\downarrow$ T_4/T_3 and $\uparrow$ TSH (due to reduced negative feedback). Secondary: $\downarrow$ T_3/T_4 and $\downarrow$ or inappropriately normal TSH.
(Subclinical hypothyroidism is characterized by normal serum free T_4 and T_3 and $\uparrow$ TSH.)
FBC: Normocytic anaemia
U&Es: May show $\downarrow$ Na^+.
Cholesterol: May be $\uparrow$.
In suspected secondary cases: Pituitary function tests, pituitary MRI and visual field testing

MANAGEMENT
Chronic: Levothyroxine (25–200 µg/day). Rule out underlying adrenal insufficiency and treat before starting thyroid hormone replacement to avoid Addisonian crisis. Adjust dosage depending on TFT and clinical picture (monitor at 6 weeks). In patients with ischaemic heart disease, start at low dose (25 µg/day) and gradually increase at 6 week intervals if ischaemic symptoms do not deteriorate.
Myxoedema coma: Oxygen, rewarming, rehydration, IV T_4/T_3, IV hydrocortisone (in case hypothyroidism is secondary to hypopituitarism), treat the underlying disorder e.g. infection.

COMPLICATIONS Myxoedema coma, myxoedema madness (psychosis with delusions and hallucinations or dementia) in severe hypothyroidism (may be seen in the elderly after starting levothyroxine treatment).

PROGNOSIS Lifelong levothyroxine replacement therapy required. Myxoedema coma has a mortality of up to 80%.

Osteomalacia and rickets

DEFINITION Osteomalacia is a disorder of mineralization of bone matrix ('osteoid'). Rickets is a disorder of defective mineralization of cartilage in the epiphyseal growth plates of children.

AETIOLOGY
Vitamin D[1] deficiency:
Lack of sunlight exposure. Dietary deficiency or malabsorption (small bowel disease e.g. coeliac disease/inflammatory bowel disease, extensive bowel surgery, gastrectomy, pancreatic insufficiency). $\downarrow$ 25-hydroxylation of vitamin D (liver disease, anticonvulsants). $\downarrow$ 1α-hydroxylation (chronic kidney disease, hypoparathyroidism, mutations in the gene encoding 1α-hydroxylase). Vitamin D resistance (mutations in the vitamin D receptor gene).
Renal phosphate wasting:
Fanconi's syndrome (phosphaturia, glycosuria, amino aciduria). Renal tubular acidosis (type 2). Hereditary hypophosphataemic rickets (X-linked or autosomal dominant). Tumour-induced osteomalacia[2].

EPIDEMIOLOGY Now uncommon in industrialized countries. More common in females.

HISTORY *Osteomalacia*: Bone pain (especially axial skeleton), weakness, malaise.
Rickets: Hypotonia, growth retardation, and skeletal deformities.

EXAMINATION *Osteomalacia*: Bone tenderness, proximal muscle weakness, waddling gait. Signs of hypocalcaemia may be present:
Trousseau's sign: Inflation of the sphygmomanometer cuff to above the systolic pressure for >3 min causes tetanic spasm of wrist and fingers.
Chvostek's sign: Tapping over the facial nerve causes twitching of the ipsilateral facial muscles.
Rickets: Bossing of frontal and parietal bones. Swelling of costochondral junctions (rickety rosary). Bow legs in early childhood, 'knock knees' in later childhood. Short stature.

INVESTIGATIONS *Blood*: $\downarrow$ or normal Ca^{2+}, $\downarrow$ phosphate, $\uparrow$ Alk Phos, $\downarrow$ 25 (OH) vitamin D. $\uparrow$ PTH (secondary hyperparathyroidism). Check U&Es, ABG (Patients with renal tubular acidosis have normal anion gap hyperchloraemic metabolic acidosis.)
$\uparrow$ Phosphate excretion (If renal phosphate wasting is not the cause of the hypophosphataemia, the fractional excretion of phosphate should be well below 5%).
Radiographs: May appear normal or show osteopenia. Looser's zones or pseudofractures (radiolucent bands) in ribs, scapula, pubic rami or upper femur.
Bone biopsy after double tetracycline labelling: Tetracycline is deposited at the mineralization front as a band. After two courses of tetracycline (separated by a period of days), the distance between the bands of deposited tetracycline is reduced in osteomalacia. Not usually performed as osteomalacia can be diagnosed from the history, examination, laboratory and radiologic studies.

MANAGEMENT Vitamin D and calcium replacement. Monitor 24 h urinary calcium, serum calcium, phosphate, Alk Phos, PTH and vitamin D.
Treat the underlying cause (e.g. advice on diet and sunlight exposure).
X-linked hypophosphataemia: Oral phosphate and 1,25 (OH)$_2$ vitamin D.

---

[1] Vitamin D is obtained from diet (e.g. fish and eggs) or synthesized in the skin from 7-dehydrocholesterol. Vitamin D is activated by hydroxylation into 1,25-(OH)$_2$ vitamin D in the liver and kidney.

[2] Caused by $\uparrow$ fibroblast growth factor-23 (FGF-23) which causes $\uparrow$ renal phosphate loss ('phosphate diabetes').

COMPLICATIONS   Bone deformities, hypocalcaemia may cause epileptic seizures, cardiac arrhythmias, hypocalcaemic tetany, depression.

PROGNOSIS   Symptoms and radiological appearances improve with vitamin D treatment. Bone deformities in children tend to be permanent.

Osteoporosis

DEFINITION   Reduced bone density (defined as <2.5 standard deviations below peak bone mass achieved by healthy adults, i.e. T-score <−2.5) resulting in bone fragility and increased fracture risk.
Osteopenia is defined as a T-score between −1.0 and −2.5.

AETIOLOGY   *Primary*: Idiopathic (<50 years), post-menopausal.
Secondary:
* *Malignancy*: Myeloma, metastatic carcinoma.
* *Endocrine*: Cushing's disease, thyrotoxicosis, primary hyperparathyroidism, hypogonadism.
* *Drugs*: Corticosteroids, heparin.
* *Rheumatological*: Rheumatoid arthritis, ankylosing spondylitis.
* *Gastrointestinal*: Malabsorption syndromes (e.g. coeliac disease, partial gastrectomy), liver disease (primary biliary cirrhosis), anorexia.

ASSOCIATIONS/RISK FACTORS   Age, family history, low BMI, low calcium intake, smoking, lack of physical exercise, low exposure to sunlight, alcohol abuse, late menarche, early menopause, hypogonadism.

EPIDEMIOLOGY   Common. In >50-year-olds, one-third of women, one-twelfth of men. Causes >200 000 fractures annually in UK (especially hip fractures). More common in caucasians than in afro-carribeans.

HISTORY   Often asymptomatic until characteristic fractures occur.
Femoral neck fractures (commonly after minimal trauma). Vertebral factures (loss of height or stooped posture or acute back pain after lifting).
Colles' fracture of the distal radius after fall onto outstretched hand.

EXAMINATION   Often no signs until complications develop:
* tenderness on percussion (over vertebral fractures);
* thoracic kyphosis (if multiple vertebral fractures); and
* severe pain with leg shortened and externally rotated (in a femoral neck fracture).

INVESTIGATIONS
Blood: Ca^{2+}, PO_4^{3-} and AlkPhos are normal in primary osteoporosis (unless a result of secondary causes).
X-ray radiography: Usually to diagnose fractures when symptomatic. Often normal (>30% loss in density before showing radiolucency, abnormal trabeculae or cortical thinning evident), biconcave vertebrae, crush fractures.
Isotope bone scans: Can highlight stress or microfractures, but not commonly used.
Bone densitometry (dual-energy X-ray absorptiometry): For obtaining T and Z scores of bone density:
* *T-score*: The number of standard deviations the bone mineral density measurement is above or below the young normal mean bone mineral density. T-score is used to define osteoporosis.
* *Z-score*: The number of standard deviations the measurement is above or below the age-matched mean bone mineral density. Z-score may be helpful in identifying patients who may need a work-up for secondary causes of osteoporosis.

MANAGEMENT   *Primary prevention*: Regular weight-bearing exercise, calcium-rich diet, avoidance of smoking and excess alcohol, hormone replacement therapy (if not contraindicated). In patients who are on corticosteroids, consider use of bisphosphonates as prophylaxis.
Osteopenia: Calcium supplements (>1 g/day) and vitamin D supplements.

Osteoporosis: Treat the underlying cause e.g. Testosterone replacement in hypogonadal men.

The WHO *FRAX*® calculator[1] is used to calculate the 10-year probability of hip/major osteoporotic fracture. For patients at high risk: consider pharmacologic treatment.

- *Bisphosphonates* (e.g. alendronate): Pyrophosphate analogues that adsorb onto bone surfaces and exert an inhibitory effect on osteoclasts and ↓ bone turnover. May cause oesophagitis.
- *Strontium ranelate*: In patients who do not tolerate bisphosphonates.
- *Nasal Calcitonin*: If pain is a prominent problem, frequent side effects: nausea/flushing.
- *Raloxifene*: An alternative in post-menopausal women with osteoporosis.
- *Hormone replacement therapy* is no longer a first-line treatment for osteoporosis.
- *Synthetic PTH (Teriparatide)* is indicated in patients with severe osteoporosis (T score <−2.5 and at least one fragility fracture) who do not tolerate bisphosphonates or do not respond to them (i.e. continue to fracture after 1 year of therapy).

COMPLICATIONS   Pain, disability, loss of independence with fractures; 20% of those sustaining hip fractures will need long-term residential care.

PROGNOSIS   Further loss of bone density can be stopped or slowed with treatment.

[1] http://www.sheffield.ac.uk/FRAX/index.htm

Paget's disease of bone

DEFINITION Characterized by excessive bone remodelling at one (monostotic) or more (polyostotic) sites resulting in bone that is structurally disorganized.

AETIOLOGY Unknown. Genetic factors and viral infection may play a role as suggested by familial and pathologic studies.

Excessive bone resorption by abnormally large osteoclasts is followed by increased bone formation by osteoblasts in a disorganized fashion. This results in an abnormal ('mosaic') pattern of lamellar bone. The marrow spaces are filled by an excess of fibrous tissue with a marked increase in blood vessels.

EPIDEMIOLOGY Common in older age, 3% of all >50-year-olds, 10% of all >80-year-olds. Men and women are equally affected.

HISTORY May be asymptomatic. May present with insidious onset pain, aggravated by weight bearing and movement (may be caused by Pagetic process, associated degenerative joint disease or stress fractures), headaches, deafness, increasing skull size.

EXAMINATION Bitemporal skull enlargement with frontal bossing. Spinal kyphosis.
Anterolateral bowing of femur, tibia or forearm.
Skin over involved bone may be warm (as a result of ↑ vascularity).
Sensorineural deafness (compression of vestibulocochlear nerve).

INVESTIGATIONS *Bloods*: ↑ Alk Phos, but Ca^{2+} and PO_4^{3-} normal (except if immobilized).
Bone radiographs: Enlarged, deformed bones with mixed lytic/sclerotic appearance, lack of distinction between cortex and medulla, skull: osteoporosis circumscripta, enlargement of frontal and occipital areas, associated with a 'cotton wool' appearance.
Bone scan (^{99m}TC MDP): To asses the extent of skeletal involvement, but is not specific for diagnosis. Pagetic bone lesions are seen as focal areas of markedly ↑ uptake ('hot spots').
Resorption markers (for monitoring of disease activity): Urinary hydroxyproline.

MANAGEMENT The primary indication for treatment is the presence of symptoms.
Bisphosphonates (three courses of IV pamidronate fortnightly):
Treatment usually suppresses disease activity for 12–18 months.
Recurrent disease usually responds to retreatment. Side effects: low grade fever, flu-like symptoms, ocular complications and osteonecrosis of the jaw are rare. Oral risedronate (30 mg/day for 2 months) is an effective alternative to IV pamidronate, but may cause oesophagitis.
Calcitonin (subcutaneous injections) may be used.
Stress fractures are treated by bed rest, analgesia.
Surgical decompression: For spinal cord compression, spinal stenosis or basilar invagination complicated by neural compromise. Fracture fixation, joint replacement for associated degenerative joint disease.

COMPLICATIONS Stress fractures, accelerated osteoarthritis.
Skull enlargement, which can cause sensorineural deafness, platybasia (upward bulging of the floor of the posterior cranial fossa in the region of foramen magnum) and hydrocephalus. Neurological deficits from impingement of spinal cord and foramina.
High-output cardiac failure.
Osteosarcoma develops in ∼1% of patients (suggested by increasingly severe bone pain).

PROGNOSIS Bisphosphonate treatment can result in prolonged remission. Sarcoma development is associated with very poor prognosis.

Phaeochromocytoma

DEFINITION Catecholamine-producing tumours that usually arise from chromaffin cells of the adrenal medulla but are extra-adrenal in about 10% of cases. Ten percent are bilateral and 10% are malignant. Extra-adrenal phaeochromocytomas are referred to as 'paragangliomas'.

AETIOLOGY Cause of sporadic cases unknown. May be familial in up to 30% of patients.
Familial cases may be seen in patients with: multiple endocrine neoplasia type 2a (MEN2a), von Hippel-Lindau (VHL) syndrome, neurofibromatosis type 1 (NF1) and mutations in the genes encoding subunits of the mitochondrial enzyme succinate dehydrogenase: *SDHB, SDHD, SDHC.*
Mutations in *VHL, SDHB* and *SDHD* may contribute to the pathogenesis of tumours via dysregulation of the HIF-1 (hypoxia-inducible factor 1) and HIF-2 transcription factors.

EPIDEMIOLOGY Rare. <0.2% of hypertensive patients.

HISTORY Paroxysmal episodes of headache, sweating:
Cardio/respiratory: Palpitations, chest pain, dyspnoea. *GI:* Epigastric pain, nausea, constipation.
Neuro/psychiatric: Weakness, tremor, anxiety.

EXAMINATION Hypertension (50–70%): Two-thirds sustained, one-third paroxysmal. Postural hypotension: Secondary to ↓ plasma volume. Pallor, tachycardia, fever, weight loss.

INVESTIGATIONS *24-h urine collections* (in acid-containing bottle) for measurement of catecholamines (adrenaline, noradrenaline, dopamine) and if available fractionated metanephrines. Urinary creatinine should be measured to verify an adequate collection. Certain drugs may ↑ measured catecholamines e.g. tricyclic antidepressants, levodopa. Blood glucose, Ca^{2+} (may be ↑), K^+ (may be ↓).
Plasma free metanephrines: In patients at high risk (sensitivity of 99%).
Tumour localization: CT or MRI scan.
[123]*I-MIBG scintigraphy:* For large (>10 cm) phaeochromocytomas (↑ risk of malignancy) or paraganglioma (↑ risk of multiple tumours and malignancy), or if CT or MRI is negative, but diagnosis considered likely due to clinical and biochemical evidence.
Screen for associated conditions: MEN 2a: Serum calcium and calcitonin.
VHL: Ophthlamoscopy, MRI posterior fossa and renal USS.
NF 1: Clinical examination for neurofibromas, café-au-lait spots and axillary freckling.
Genetic testing and counselling: For mutations in *VHL, SDHB, SDHD* and *RET* genes in patients with onset at a young age (<20 years), family history, evidence of one of the familial disorders mentioned above or bilateral tumours.

MANAGEMENT
α-*blockade:* Phenoxybenzamine. Rehydrated (1L 0.9% saline) before alpha-blockade to prevent sudden hypotension.
β-*blockade:* Propranolol 2–3 days after starting phenoxybenzamine. Never start β-blockers before α-blockers as hypertension may be worsened.
Surgery: Laparoscopic adrenalectomy by an experienced endocrine surgeon. 24-hour urine catecholamines should be measured about 2 weeks after surgery to assess cure.
Metastatic disease: Should be resected if possible. Long term α- and β-blockade. Chemotherapy (with dacarbazine, cyclophosphamide and vincristine) may control the symptoms. Radiotherapy for bony metastases.
Follow-up: Life-long to detect recurrence. Malignant phaeochromocytomas appear histologically similar to benign.

Phaeochromocytoma (continued)

COMPLICATIONS   Atrial or ventricular fibrillation, myocardial infarction, dilated cardio-myopathy, stroke, hypertensive encephalopathy, diabetes mellitus.

PROGNOSIS   Surgical resection may result in resolution of hypertension in 75% of patients. Recurrence rate <10%. 5 year survival for benign tumours is about 96%. 5-year survival in metastatic disease is 35%.

Polycystic ovary syndrome (PCOS)

DEFINITION Characterized by oligomenorrhoea/amenorrhoea and hyperandrogenism (clinical or biochemical). Frequently associated with obesity, insulin resistance, type 2 diabetes and dyslipidaemia.

AETIOLOGY Environmental factors (e.g. related to diet and the development of obesity) and genetic variants (possibly in genes regulating gonadotrophin, insulin and androgen synthesis, secretion and action, weight and energy regulation) may influence development of PCOS. Hyperinsulinaemia results in increased ovarian androgen synthesis and reduced hepatic SHBG synthesis (resulting in ↑ free androgens).

EPIDEMIOLOGY PCOS is the most common cause of infertility in women. Affects 6–8% of women.

HISTORY Menstrual irregularities (oligomenorrhoea or amenorrhoea), dysfunctional uterine bleeding, infertility.
Symptoms of hyperandrogenism: hirsutism, male-pattern hair loss, acne.

EXAMINATION Hirsutism, male pattern hair loss and acne.
Acanthosis nigricans (sign of severe insulin resistance): velvety thickening and hyperpigmentation of the skin of axillae or neck.

INVESTIGATIONS *Blood*: ↑ LH, ↑ LH: FSH ration (>3). ↑ Testosterone, androstenedione and DHEA-S. ↓ SHBG.
Tests to exclude hyperprolactinaemia (serum prolactin), hypo/hyperthyroidism (thyroid function tests), congenital adrenal hyperplasia (17OH-progesterone), and Cushing's syndrome (if clinically suspected).
Look for impaired glucose tolerance/type 2 diabetes: fasting glucose, HbA1c (oral glucose tolerance test if either abnormal).
Fasting lipid profile.
Transvaginal USS: Twelve or more follicles in each ovary, measuring 2–9 mm and/or ↑ ovarian volume >10 mL.

MANAGEMENT Reduce weight, exercise and stop smoking.
Oligomenorrhoea: Oral contraceptive pill, or intermittent progestin therapy.
Hirsutism: Oral contraceptive pill, (ethinyl oestradiol plus a progestin with minimal androgenic effect or anti-androgenic effect e.g. cyproterone acetate or drospirenone). Oestrogen component ↑ serum SHBG and ↓ serum free androgen levels. Inhibition of gonadotrophin secretion by oral contraceptive therapy, results in ↓ ovarian androgen secretion. If not satisfied with the clinical response after 4–6 months, anti-androgens e.g. spironolactone or flutamide may be added. Anti-androgens should not be prescribed without reliable contraception.
Eflornithine hydrochloride (*Vaniqa*) cream is a topical treatment used to inhibit hair growth.
Cosmetic measures (e.g. electrolysis).
Metformin is a reasonable adjunct to diet and exercise for patients with PCOS who are obese.
Clomifene citrate to initiate ovulation induction if modest weight loss does not restore ovulatory cycles (induces gonadotrophin release by occupying hypothalamic oestrogen receptors and interfering with feedback mechanisms).

COMPLICATIONS Infertility, recurrent miscarriage, endometrial carcinoma (due to chronic unopposed oestrogen), diabetes mellitus, cardiovascular complications, obstructive sleep apnoea

PROGNOSIS Wide spectrum of severity; lifestyle and medical interventions are generally successful.

Syndrome of inappropriate ADH (SIADH)

DEFINITION   Characterized by continued secretion of ADH, despite the absence of normal stimuli for secretion (i.e. ↑ serum osmolality or ↓ blood volume).

AETIOLOGY
Brain: Haemorrhage/thrombosis, meningitis, abscess, trauma, tumour, Guillain–Barré syndrome.
Lung: Pneumonia, TB, abscess, aspergillosis, small cell carcinoma.
Tumours: Small cell lung cancer, lymphoma, leukaemia, pancreas, prostate, mesothelioma, sarcoma, thymoma. It may be caused by ectopic ADH secretion.
Drugs: Vincristine, opiates, carbamazepine, chlorpropamide.
Metabolic: Porphyria, alcohol withdrawal.

EPIDEMIOLOGY   Hyponatraemia is the most common electrolyte imbalance seen in hospitals. <50% of all severe hyponatraemia are due to SIADH.

HISTORY
Mild hyponatraemia (Na$^+$: 125–135 mmol/L) may be asymptomatic.
Headache, nausea/vomiting, muscle cramp/weakness, irritability, confusion, drowsiness, convulsions and coma.
Symptoms of the underlying cause.

EXAMINATION
Mild hyponatraemia: No signs.
Severe hyponatraemia: ↓ Reflexes, extensor plantar reflexes.
Signs of the underlying cause.
The hyponatraemia in SIADH is dilutional from ↑ body water and not ↓ total body Na$^+$.

INVESTIGATIONS
↓ Na$^+$, creatinine (renal function), glucose, serum protein and lipids (to exclude pseudohyponatraemia seen with ↑ protein or lipids).
Free T4 and TSH (exclude hypothyroidism), short ACTH stimulation test (to exclude adrenal insufficiency).
SIADH diagnosis: ↓ Plasma osmolality and [Na$^+$] and ↑ urine osmolality (>100 mosmol/kg) and ↑ Na$^+$ (>20 mmol/L). The presence of the above and absence of hypovolaemia/hypotension, oedema, renal failure, adrenal insufficiency and hypothyroidism are required for a diagnosis of SIADH.
Investigations for identifying the cause: CXR, CT chest/abdomen/pelvis, MRI/CT head.

MANAGEMENT   Treat the underlying cause.
Water restriction (0.5–1 L/day). If ineffective, give demeclocycline (↓ responsiveness of the collecting tubule cells to ADH).
Vasopressin (V$_2$) receptor antagonists e.g. tolvaptan are likely to be useful in moderate chronic hyponatraemia if water restriction is insufficient.
In severe cases (seizures and ↓ consciousness), give slow IV hypertonic 3% saline (and furosemide) with close monitoring. The change in [Na$^+$] must not exceed 10 mmol/L in the first 24 h and 18 mmol/L in the first 48 h. Rapid correction can result in central pontine myelinolysis.

COMPLICATIONS   Convulsions, coma, death. Central pontine myelinolysis (quadreparesis, respiratory arrest, fits) occurs with rapid correction of hyponatraemia.

PROGNOSIS   Depends on the underlying cause. High morbidity and mortality with [Na$^+$] <110 mmol/L. Up to 50% mortality with central pontine myelinolysis.

Thyrotoxicosis

DEFINITION   Syndrome resulting from an excess of circulating free thyroxine (T4) and/or free tri-iodothyronine (T3). Thyrotoxicosis may be either due to ↑ thyroid hormone synthesis (hyperthyroidism) or ↑ release of stored thyroid hormone from an inflamed thyroid gland (thyroiditis).
Patients with '*subclinical hyperthyroidism*' have normal T_3 and T_4 levels and ↓ TSH.

AETIOLOGY   Graves' disease. Toxic multinodular goitre. Toxic adenoma.
Thyroiditis (post-partum or de Quervain's thyroiditis, presumed to be post-viral).
Rare: TSH-secreting pituitary tumours (secondary hyperthyroidism).
Drugs (amiodarone, self-administration of T_4).
Choriocarcinoma (↑ hCG which is structurally similar to TSH).*Graves' disease*: Plasma IgG to thyroid TSH receptor stimulates thyroid hyperplasia and thyroid hormone hypersecretion, causing exaggerated thyroid hormone action and autonomic overactivity.

EPIDEMIOLOGY   Thyrotoxicosis affects 1% of ♀ and 0.1% of ♂. Graves' disease accounts for 70–80% of all cases of hyperthyroidism. Toxic multinodular goitre is the commonest cause of hyperthyroidism in the elderly.

HISTORY   Heat intolerance, sweating, palpitations, anxiety and irritability.
Weight loss (despite good appetite), diarrhoea, pruritus.
Exertional dyspnoea.
Menstrual irregularities in females, ↓ libido, impotence in males.
Graves' ophthalmopathy: Blurred vision, double vision, eye grittiness, eye protrusion.
de Quervain's thyroiditis: Flu-like illness, tender goitre.

EXAMINATION   *General*: Underweight, restless, irritable, sweating. There may be signs of associated autoimmune conditions e.g. vitiligo.
Hands: Tremor, warm, moist, rapid or irregular pulse, onycholysis, acropachy, palmar erythema.
BP: Wide pulse pressure.
Eyes: Lid retraction and lid lag (caused by ↑ catecholamine sensitivity of levator palpebrae superioris), signs of Graves' ophthalmopathy: periorbital oedema, proptosis (secondary to ↑ glycosaminoglycans secreted by fibroblasts stimulated by activated T cell cytokines and TSH receptor antibodies), chemosis (conjunctival oedema), ↑ tears, opthalmoplegia, optic nerve atrophy (caused by compression).
Thyroid: Goitre or bruit.
Neurological: Proximal muscle weakness, hyper-reflexia.
Signs specific to Graves' disease: Thyroid acropachy (clubbing), Graves' ophthalmopathy (*see* above), pretibial myxoedema (raised pigmented orange-peel textured nodules or plaques on the shins).
Thyroid crisis: Hyperpyrexia, signs of dehydration, tachycardia, restlessness, coma.

INVESTIGATIONS
Thyroid function tests: *Primary hyperthyroidism*: ↑ T_4, ↑ T_3, ↓ TSH. *Secondary hyperthyroidism*: ↑ T_4, ↑ T_3, ↑ or inappropriately normal TSH.
Radioisotope uptake scan ([99]Technetium pertechnetate).
Graves' disease: Diffuse ↑ uptake, *Toxic multinodular goitre*: multiple areas of ↑ radio-isotope uptake ('hot' nodules) with suppression of uptake in the rest of the gland. *Solitary toxic adenoma*: single area of ↑ radio-isotope uptake ('hot nodule) with suppression of uptake in the rest of the gland. *de Quervain's thyroiditis*: absent uptake.
TSH receptor-stimulating antibodies are positive in Graves' disease. This test is expensive and the aetiology of thyrotoxicosis can often be determined with a combination of thyroid function tests and a radioisotope uptake scan.

Thyrotoxicosis (continued)

CT or MRI of orbits (STIR sequence): Assessment and follow-up of patients with Graves' ophthalmopathy.

MANAGEMENT *Acute thyroid crisis*: Propylthiouracil, propranolol, IV hydrocortisone (inhibits peripheral conversion of $T_4 \rightarrow T_3$), potassium iodide or Lugol's iodine. Rehydrate and control temperature. Treat the underlying cause.

All patients with primary hyperthyroidism should be told about the three options available for treatment:

1. *Medical*: Antithyroid drugs (ATD): carbimazole or propylthiouracil (both inhibit thyroid peroxidase and hormone synthesis), β-blockers. ATD may rarely cause agranulocytosis. Patients must be told to stop ATD, tell their doctor and have their FBC checked if they develop fever, sore throat, mouth ulcers or any signs of infection.
2. *Radioactive iodine*: Must avoid pregnancy for 4 months and close contact with pregnant women and young children for 2 weeks after radioactive iodine therapy.
3. *Surgery*: Reserved for patients with large goitres causing upper airway obstruction or dysphagia, and those who cannot take ATD (e.g. due to allergy/agranulocytosis) and are either pregnant or have moderate/severe Graves' ophthalmopathy (which may be exacerbated by radioiodine). *Preoperative preparation*: Control hyperthyroidism with ATD. Give oral potassium iodide and propranolol. Examination of vocal cords by ENT specialists.

Ophthalmopathy: Corneal protection (artificial tears, lateral tarsorrhaphy), surgery for realignment.

COMPLICATIONS Thyrotoxic crisis. Heart failure. Osteoporosis. Infertility. Complications of surgery (recurrent laryngeal nerve palsy, hypothyroidism, hypoparathyroidism) or radioiodine (exacerbation of ophthalmopathy, hypothyroidism, recurrence).

Patients with subclinical hyperthyroidism have ↑ long-term risk of atrial fibrillation and ↓ bone density.

PROGNOSIS Many patients eventually become hypothyroid.

Cellulitis

DEFINITION   Acute non-purulent spreading infection of the subcutaneous tissue, causing overlying skin inflammation.

AETIOLOGY   Often results from penetrating injury (e.g. intravenous cannulation), local lesions (e.g. insect bites, sebaceous cysts, surgery) or fissuring (e.g. in anal fissures, toe web spaces), which allows pathogenic bacteria to enter the skin. In rare cases of septicaemia, it can arise spontaneously from blood-borne sources.
Most common organisms: *Streptococcus pyogenes* and *Staphylococcus aureus*. Methicillin-resistant *Staphylococcus aureus* (MRSA) is not uncommon.
If occurring in the orbit, *Haemophilus influenzae* is the most common cause. The infection often arises from adjacent sinuses.

EPIDEMIOLOGY   Very common. Main risk factors are skin break, poor hygiene and poor vascularization of tissue (e.g. diabetes mellitus).

HISTORY   There may be history of a cut, scratch or injury.
Periorbital: Painful swollen red skin around eye.
Orbital cellulitis: Painful or limited eye movements, visual impairment.

EXAMINATION
Lesion: erythema, oedema, warm tender indistinct margins. Pyrexia may signify systemic spread.
Exclude abscess: Test for fluid thrill or fluctuation. Aspirate if pus suspected.
Periorbital: Swollen eyelids. Conjunctival injection.
Orbital cellulitis: Proptosis, impaired acuity and eye movement. Test for relative afferent pupillary defect, visual acuity and colour vision (to monitor optic nerve function).

INVESTIGATIONS
Blood: WCC, blood culture.
Discharge: Culture and sensitivity.
Aspiration: As it is often non-purulent, it is not usually necessary.
CT/MRI scan: When orbital cellulitis is suspected (to assess the posterior spread of infection).

MANAGEMENT
Medical: Oral penicillins (e.g. flucloxacillin, benzylpenicillin, coamoxiclav) or tetracyclines are effective in most community-acquired cases. In the hospital, treat empirically using local microbiological guidelines but change depending on sensitivity of any cultured organisms. Intravenous use may be necessary.
Surgical: Orbital decompression may be necessary in orbital cellulitis. This is an emergency.
Abscess: Abscesses can be aspirated, incised and drained or excised completely.

COMPLICATIONS   Sloughing of overlying skin. Localized tissue damage. In orbital cellulitis, there may be permanent vision loss and spread to brain, abscess formation, meningitis, cavernous sinus thrombosis.

PROGNOSIS   Good with treatment.

Herpes simplex

DEFINITION   Disease resulting from HSV1 or HSV2 infection.

AETIOLOGY   HSV is an α-herpes virus with double-stranded deoxyribonucleic acid (dsDNA). Transmitted via close contact with an individual shedding the virus (e.g. kissing, sexual intercourse).

Pathology/Pathogenesis: Following primary viral infection the virus becomes dormant (classically in trigeminal or sacral root ganglia). Reactivation may occur in response to physical or emotional stresses or immunosuppression. The virus causes cytolysis of infected epithelial cells and vesicle formation.

EPIDEMIOLOGY   90% adults seropositive for HSV1 by 30 years.
35% adults >60 years seropositive for HSV2.
>One-third world population has recurrent HSV infections.

HISTORY   HSV1: Primary infection often asymptomatic; usual symptoms:

• pharyngitis;
• gingivostomatis, may make eating very painful; and
• herpetic whitlow, inoculation of virus into a finger.

Recurrent infection/reactivation (herpes labialis/'cold sore'): prodrome (6 h) peri-oral tingling and burning. Vesicles appear (48 h duration), ulcerate and crust over. Complete healing 8–10 days.
HSV2: Very painful blisters and rash in genital, perigenital and anal area. Dysuria. Fever and malaise.
HSV encephalitis: Usually HSV1 (*see* Encephalitis).
HSV keratoconjunctivitis: Epiphoria (watering eyes), photophobia

EXAMINATION
HSV1 primary infection: Tender cervical lymphadenopathy. Erythematous, oedematous pharynx. Oral ulcers filled with yellow slough (gingivostomatitis). Digital blisters/pustules (herpetic whitlow).
Herpes labialis: Perioral vesicles/ulcers/crusting.
HSV2: Maculopapular rash, vesicles and ulcers (external genitalia, anal margin, upper thighs), inguinal lymphadenopathy, pyrexia.
HSV encephalitis: (*see* Encephalitis).
HSV keratoconjunctivitis: Characterisitic lesion is a dendritic ulcer. May be visualized following staining with 1% fluorescein.

INVESTIGATIONS   Usually a clinical diagnosis and investigations are not warranted.
Vesicle fluid: Electron microscopy, PCR, direct immunofluorescence, growth of virus in tissue culture.
Diagnosis of HSV encephalitis: (*see* Encephalitis).

MANAGEMENT   Topical, oral or IV aciclovir (a nucleoside analogue phosphorylated by viral thymidine kinase to a monophosphate that, when converted to a triphosphate, causes chain termination of viral DNA synthesis). Valaciclovir is a prodrug of aciclovir with better bioavailability.

COMPLICATIONS   **Neonatal HSV:** Acquired during delivery. Skin vesicles, scarring eye disease, encephalitis. May be fatal.
Treatment: caesarian section for mothers with active HSV infection. IV aciclovir to neonate.

HSV in the immunocompromised: Severe local disease may disseminate involving the respiratory and GI tracts.

↑ Transmission of HIV in the presence of HSV2 genital lesions.

Erythema multiforme.

PROGNOSIS   Infection is lifelong. Inter-individual variation in frequency of reactivation.

Human immunodeficiency virus (HIV) infection

DEFINITION   Infection with the human immunodeficiency virus (HIV).

AETIOLOGY   HIV is transmitted by:
1. *Sexual intercourse*: Heterosexual is most common worldwide, but ↑ risk in homosexuals in the West.
2. *Blood (and other body fluids)*: Mother to child (intrauterine, childbirth or breastfeeding), needles (injecting drug users, health care workers), blood product transfusion, organ transplantation.

HIV enters the CD4 lymphocytes following binding of its envelope glycoprotein (gp120) to CD4 and a chemokine receptor. Reverse transcriptase (in viral core) reads RNA to manufacture DNA, which is incorporated into the host genome. Dissemination of virions leads to cell death and eventually to T-cell depletion.

EPIDEMIOLOGY   On the rise in Africa and Asia. >40,000,000 adults affected worldwide.

HISTORY AND EXAMINATION
Three phases:
1. *Seroconversion*: (4–8 weeks post-infection), self-limiting – fever, night sweats, generalized lymphadenopathy, sore throat, oral ulcers, rash, myalgia, headache, encephalitis, diarrhoea.
2. Early/asymptomatic: (18 months to 15 + years), apparently well – some patients may have persistent lymphadenopathy (>1 cm nodes, at 2 + extrainguinal sites for >3 months). Progressive minor symptoms, e.g. rash, oral thrush, weight loss, malaise.
3. *AIDS*: Syndrome of secondary diseases reflecting severe immunodeficiency or direct effect of HIV infection (CD4 cell count <200/mm^3).

Direct effects of HIV infection:
Neurological: Polyneuropathy, myelopathy, dementia.
Lung: Lymphocytic interstitial pneumonitis.
Heart: Cardiomyopathy, myocarditis.
Haematological: Anaemia, thrombocytopenia.
GI: Anorexia, HIV enteropathy (malabsorption and diarrhoea), severe wasting.
Eyes: Cotton wool spots.
Some secondary infections arising from immunodeficiency:
Bacterial: Mycobacteria (lungs, GI, skin), e.g. *Mycobacterium tuberculosis, Mycobacterium avium intracellulare* (late), staphylococci (skin), *Salmonella*, capsulated organisms (*Streptococcus pneumoniae, Haemophilus influenzae*).
Viral: CMV (retinitis, oesophagitis, colitis, pneumonitis, adrenalitis, encephalitis), HSV (encephalitis), varicella zoster virus (VZV) (recurrent shingles), human papillomavirus (HPV) (warts), papovavirus (progressive multifocal leucoencephalopathy with motor, intellectual and speech impairment), Epstein–Barr virus (EBV) (oral hairy leukoplakia on the side of the tongue)
Fungal: Pneumocystis pneumonia (PCP), *Cryptococcus* (meningitis), *Candida* (oral, airway, genital, oesophageal), invasive aspergillosis.
Protozoal: Toxoplasmosis (cerebral abscess, chorioretinitis, encephalitis), cryptosporidia and microsporidia (diarrhoea).
Tumours: Kaposi's sarcoma (cutaneous or conjunctival vascular tumour caused by human herpesvirus [HHV8]), squamous cell carcinoma (particularly cervical or anal), non-Hodgkin's B-cell lymphoma (brain, GI), Hodgkin's lymphoma.

INVESTIGATIONS
HIV testing (after discussion and consent): HIV antibodies (usually positive by 12 weeks after exposure), PCR for viral RNA or incorporated proviral DNA. Monitor CD4 count and viral load.

Other investigations (as appropriate):

PCP: CXR bilateral perihilar/'ground glass' shadowing, bronchoalveolar lavage
Cryptococcal meningitis: Brain CT or MRI, lumbar puncture – cerebrospinal fluid (CSF) microscopy (India ink staining), culture, ELISA for antigen.
CMV (colitis): Colonoscopy and biopsy (cytomegalic cells with inclusions)
Toxoplasmosis: Brain CT or MRI shows ring-enhancing lesions.
Cryptosporidia/microsporidia: Stool microscopy.

MANAGEMENT Best delivered by providers with specific training and considerable expertise.

Goals: Viral load <50 copies/mL, ↑ CD4 counts and prevention of HIV-related complications.

Highly Active Antiretroviral Treatment (HAART):[1]

Two nucleoside reverse transcriptase inhibitors (tenofovir/emtricitabine or abacavir/lamivudine and zidovudine/lamivudine), plus either
- one non-nucleoside reverse transcriptase inhibitor (e.g. efavirenz, nevirapine); or
- one protease inhibitor (e.g. ritonavir).

Abacavir should only be administered if HLA-B*5701 screening is negative (associated with an ↑ risk of abacavir hypersensitivity).
Test for resistance by genotyping.
HAART may be delayed while treating a known opportunistic infection to ↓ likelihood of immune reconstitution inflammatory syndrome (IRIS) (*see* Complications).

Treatment of Infections:

PCP: IV co-trimoxazole, steroids (severe cases)
Cryptococcus: IV amphotericin B or fluconazole and long-term oral fluconazole
Aspergillus fumigatus: IV amphotericin B
CMV: Ganciclovir.
Toxoplasmosis: Pyrimethamine and sulfadiazine, folinic acid.

Treatment of Tumours:

Kaposi's sarcoma: Radiotherapy for localized and chemotherapy for systemic disease

Social and Psychological Help:

Postexposure prophylaxis: 0.3% risk without treatment. Triple therapy (4 weeks).
Prevention: Condoms and safe sex education, screening blood products, avoid sharing needles.

COMPLICATIONS Complications of secondary infections, drug side effects (e.g. myelosuppression with zidovudine, renal failure with amphotericin B, lipodystrophy with protease inhibitors), drug interactions (e.g. with TB treatments).

IRIS: Inflammatory response associated with worsening of pre-existing infections within 7 days to a few months after initiation of HAART. IRIS is a diagnosis of exclusion. Drug reaction or resistance, non-compliance and persistently active infection should be excluded first. For example, abacavir hypersensitivity may be confused with IRIS.

PROGNOSIS Viral load (plasma [HIV RNA]) and CD4 count are good predictors of disease progression, response to treatment and long-term prognosis.

[1] Indicated for CD4 count <350/mm³, rapidly falling CD4 count, rapidly rising viral load or serious symptomatic HIV-related illness. Treatment and pregnancy guidelines are available at the British HIV Association website, http://www.bhiva.org/cms1191540.asp.

Infectious mononucleosis

DEFINITION   Clinical syndrome caused by primary EBV infection. Also known as glandular fever.

AETIOLOGY   EBV is a γ-herpes virus (dsDNA), present in pharyngeal secretions of infected individuals and is transmitted by close contact, e.g. kissing or sharing eating utensils.
EBV infection of the oropharyngeal epithelial cells leads to B cell infection with incorporation of the viral DNA into host DNA. Infected B cells disseminate and proliferate in lymphoid tissue throughout the body. There is humoral (heterophile antibodies, *see* Investigations) and cellular (T cells-mediated) immune response and production of interleukin (IL)-2 and interferon-γ cytokines. The atypical lymphocytes, in the peripheral blood are primarily activated CD8+ T cells. Despite these immune responses, which control the initial lytic infection, EBV remains latent in lymphocytes. Reactivation may occur following stress or immunosuppression.

EPIDEMIOLOGY   Common (UK annual incidence 1 in 1000).
2 age peaks: 1–6 years (usually asymptomatic) and 14–20 years; >90% of adult population are EBV immunoglobulin (Ig) G positive.

HISTORY
Incubation period: 4–8 weeks May have abrupt onset: sore throat, fever, fatigue, headache, malaise, anorexia, sweating, abdominal pain

EXAMINATION   Pyrexia.
Oedema and erythema of pharynx, fauces and soft palate, with white/creamy exudate on the tonsils which becomes confluent within 1–2 days, palatal petechiae. Cervical/generalized lymphadenopathy, splenomegaly (50–60%), hepatomegaly (10–20%). Jaundice (5–10%), widespread maculopapular rash in patients who have received ampicillin.

INVESTIGATIONS
Blood: FBC (leukocytosis), LFT (↑ aminotransferases).
Blood film: Lymphocytosis (>20% atypical lymphocytes).
Paul–Bunnell/Monospot test: Detects the presence of heterophile antibodies that are produced in response to EBV infection but are not actually against EBV antigens (10–15% are heterophile Ab negative especially if <14 years).
Throat swabs (culture and antigen testing) to exclude streptococcal tonsillitis.
IgM or IgG to EBV viral capsid antigen (VCA): Usually present at the onset of clinical illness. Only needed in patients with compatible syndrome and negative Monospot test.
IgG against EBNA (Epstein–Barr nuclear antigen): Appear 6-12 weeks after the onset of symptoms. The presence of IgG EBNA, or the absence of IgG and IgM VCA, excludes acute primary EBV infection and should prompt consideration of CMV, HIV infection and toxoplasmosis.

MANAGEMENT   Bed rest, paracetamol or non-steroidal anti-inflammatory drugs (NSAIDs) for fever, throat discomfort and malaise.
Corticosteroids may be indicated for severe cases (e.g. haemolytic anaemia, severe tonsilar swelling, obstructive pharyngitis).
Caution: Nearly 100% of patients with infectious mononucleosis develop a widespread maculopapular rash when given amoxicillin or ampicillin.
Advice: Advise against contact sports for 2 weeks, as increased risk of splenic rupture (*see* Complications).

COMPLICATIONS   Lethargy for several months following the acute infection.
Respiratory: Airway obstruction by oedematous pharynx, secondary bacterial throat infections, pneumonitis.
Haematological: Haemolytic or aplastic anaemia, thrombocytopenia.

GI/renal: Splenic rupture (caused by persistent splenomegaly), fulminant hepatitis, pancreatitis, mesenteric adenitis, renal failure.

CNS: Guillain–Barré syndrome, encephalitis, viral meningitis, brachial plexitis.

EBV-associated malignancy: Burkitt's lymphoma (sub-Saharan Africa), nasopharyngeal carcinoma (China), post-transplant lymphoma, Hodgkin's lymphoma (usually mixed cellularity type).

PROGNOSIS Most make an uncomplicated recovery in 3–21 days. Immunodeficiency and death can occur very rarely.[1]

[1] Duncan's syndrome or X-linked lymphoproliferative (XLP) syndrome is the aberrant immune response to EBV leading to acute liver necrosis and immunodeficiency. Among infected children, >50% die.

Infective arthritis

DEFINITION   Joint inflammation resulting from intra-articular infection. Also known as septic arthritis.

AETIOLOGY   May be idiopathic, although in most cases, there is systemic infection allowing for haematogenous spread, recent orthopaedic procedures, osteomyelitis, diabetes, immunosuppression, alcoholism. Common organisms are:

Bacteria:
All ages: Staphylococcus aureus, Mycobacterium tuberculosis.
<4 years: Strepotococcus pneumoniae, Strepotococcus pyogenes, Neisseria meningitidis, Gram-negative rods.
16–40 years: Mainly *Neisseria gonorrhoea*
Viruses: Rubella, mumps, HBV, parvovirus B19.
Fungi: Candida.

EPIDEMIOLOGY   Most common in children and the elderly.

HISTORY   Fever.
Excruciating joint pain, redness, swelling and loss of joint function.
Usually affecting single large joint (polyarthritis in the immunosuppressed).
Tuberculous arthritis is much more insidious and chronic.

EXAMINATION   Painful, hot, swollen and immobile joint with overlying erythema.
Severe pain prevents passive movement.
Pyrexia.
Look for signs of aetiology (e.g. small pustules near joint in N. gonorrhoea).

INVESTIGATIONS
Joint aspiration (very important): Aspirate is usually grossly purulent. Send synovial fluid for cytology, polarizing microscopy (for gout or pseudogout crystals), culture and sensitivity. Polymerase chain reaction (PCR) if suspected viral aetiology.
Blood: FBC (↑ WCC, ↑ neutrophils); ↑ CRP and ESR. Blood cultures for microscopy, culture and sensitivity. Viral serology may also be useful.
Plain joint radiographs: Affected joint may initially be normal. Useful when assessing joint damage in later films.
MRI scan: Useful in detecting associated osteomyelitis.

MANAGEMENT[1]
Emergency: Temporary joint immobilization with a splint, analgesia. Immediate joint aspiration followed by antibiotic therapy. (Note that joint aspiration only provides symptomatic relief.)
High-dose IV antibiotics for 2 weeks, then switch to oral for up to 4 weeks. Follow local antibiotic guidelines, but common regimens are:
• Flucloxacillin/Clindamycin and cefuroxime/gentamicin
• Cefuroxime and vancomycin

Change depending on culture and sensitivity.
Viral arthritis is typically a self-limiting condition, and no antiviral therapy required.
Surgery: Joint aspiration via arthroscopy or open debridement may be necessary (especially in hip joints).
Physiotherapy: Best carried out as early as possible.

---

[1] Coakley G. Mathews C. Field M. et al. BSR & BHPR, BOA, RCGP and BSAC guidelines for management of the hot swollen joint in adults. *Rheumatology.* 2006 **45** (8): 1039–41

COMPLICATIONS   Septicaemia. Dislocation. Epiphyseal destruction in children. Ankylosis. Juxta-articular osteoporosis. Spinal cord compression in spinal tuberculosis (Pott's disease). Chronic osteomyelitis.

PROGNOSIS   Complete recovery in 70% of patients, especially with early appropriate antibiotic treatment. Full recovery may take several months. Risk of permanent joint damage in severe cases or if treatment is delayed.

Infective endocarditis

DEFINITION Infection of intracardiac endocardial structures (mainly heart valves).

AETIOLOGY The endocardium can be colonized by virtually any organism, but the most common are:

1. *Streptococci* (40%): Mainly α-haemolytic *Streptococcus viridans* or *Streptococcus bovis*.
2. *Staphylococci* (35%): *Staphylococcus aureus* and occasionally *Staphylococcus epidermidis* (in IV drug users)
3. *Enterococci* (20%): Usually *Enterococcus faecalis*.
4. *Other organisms:* HACEK (*Haemophilus, Actinobacillus, Cardiobacterium, Eikenella, Kingella*), *Coxiella burnetii*, histoplasma.

Vegetations form as a result of lodging of the organisms on the heart valves during a period of bacteraemia. These vegetations are made up of platelets, fibrin and infective organisms and are poorly penetrated by the cellular or humoral immune system. Vegetations proceed to destroy the valve leaflets, invade the myocardium or aortic wall leading to abscess cavities. Activation of the immune system also causes formation of immune complexes leading to cutaneous vasculitis, glomerulonephritis or arthritis.

Associations/Risk Factors: Abnormal valves (e.g. congenital, post-rheumatic, calcification/ degeneration), prosthetic heart valves, turbulent flow (e.g. patent ductus arteriosus or VSD), recent dental work and bacteraemia. *S. bovis* may be associated with GI malignancy.

EPIDEMIOLOGY Incidence 16–22 per million per year (United Kingdom).

HISTORY Fever with sweats/chills/rigors (may be relapsing and remitting).
Malaise, arthralgia, myalgia, confusion (particularly in elderly).
Skin lesions.
Inquire about recent dental surgery or IV drug abuse.

EXAMINATION Pyrexia, tachycardia, signs of anaemia.
Clubbing (if long-standing).
New regurgitant murmur or muffled heart sounds (right-sided lesions may imply IV drug use).
Frequency: Mitral > aortic > tricuspid > pulmonary.
Splenomegaly.
Vasculitic lesions: Petechiae particularly on retinae (Roth's spots), pharyngeal and con-junctival mucosa; Janeway lesions (painless palmar macules, which blanch on pressure); Osler's nodes (tender nodules on finger/toe pads); splinter haemorrhages (nail-bed haemorrhages).

INVESTIGATIONS
Blood: FBC ($\uparrow$ neutrophils, normocytic anaemia), $\uparrow$ ESR and CRP, U&Es, rheumatoid factor positive
Urinalysis: Microscopic haematuria, proteinuria
Blood culture: At least three sets 1 h apart (ensure aseptic technique). Culture and sensitivity is vital, but empirical treatment should be started first. Cultures remain negative in 2–5%.
Echocardiography: Transthoracic. Transoesophageal echocardiography is much more sensitive for the detection of endocarditis; especially useful for the detection of vegeta-tions and valve abscess, diagnosis of prosthetic valve endocarditis and assessment of embolic risk.
Other investigations: ECG (abscesses can cause conduction changes), CXR (septic pul-monary emboli: focal lung infiltrates $\pm$ central cavitation; particularly in tricuspid valve endocarditis).
Dukes' classification for diagnosis of endocarditis: (2 major, 1 major + 3 minor or all minor).

Major criteria: Positive blood culture in two separate samples. Positive echocardiogram (vegetation, abscess, prosthetic valve dehiscence, new valve regurgitation).

Minor criteria: High-grade pyrexia (temperature >38°C). Risk factors (abnormal valves, IV drug use, dental surgery). Positive blood culture, but not major criteria. Positive echocardiogram, but not major criteria. Vascular signs.

MANAGEMENT Antibiotics for 4–6 weeks (at least 6 weeks for prosthetic valve endocarditis).

On clinical suspicion: Benzylpenicillin + gentamicin (empirical treatment); gentamicin dosage adjusted for peak serum level of 3–4 μg/ml, trough <1 μg/ml

Streptococci: Continue as above (alternatives – ceftriaxone, vancomycin).

Staphylococci: Flucloxacillin/vancomycin + gentamicin (for prosthetic valves: vancomycin + gentamicin + rifampin)

Enterococci: Ampicillin + gentamicin

HACEK: Ampicillin or ceftriaxone + gentamicin

Culture negative: Vancomycin + gentamicin

Surgery: If poor response or deterioration, urgent valve replacement is indicated. Surgical replacement of the prostheses. In 'kissing' mitral valve vegetations, the mitral valve may be salvageable.

Antibiotic prophylaxis for patients with a history of infective endocarditis undergoing high risk procedures: Dental, incision or biopsy of respiratory mucosa, procedures in patients with GI/GU tract infection, procedures on infected skin or musculoskeletal tissue, prosthetic heart valve placement. For patients undergoing a dental procedure: 2 g oral amoxicillin 30–60 min before the procedure.

COMPLICATIONS Valve incompetence, intracardiac fistulae or abscesses, aneurysm formation, heart failure. Renal failure, glomerulonephritis. Arterial emboli from the vegetations (brain, kidneys, lungs, spleen).

PROGNOSIS Fatal if untreated. Even when treated, 15–30% mortality.

Malaria

DEFINITION   Infection with protozoan *Plasmodium* (*Plasmodium falciparum*, *Plasmodium vivax*, *Plasmodium ovale* and *Plasmodium malariae*). The most serious is *Plasmodium falciparum*, which is potentially fatal.

AETIOLOGY
The *Plasmodium* spp. are transmitted by the bite of the female *Anopheles* mosquito. The protozoa infect red blood cells (RBCs) and grow intracellularly.
1. Injection of sporozoites into the bloodstream by the bite of the female *Anopheles* mosquito.
2. Invasion and replication in hepatocytes (exoerythrocytic schizogeny). *P. vivax* and *P. ovale* may develop into dormant hypnozoites and cause relapse within months or even years.
3. Parasites may reinvade the blood (at this point they are called merozoites). Inside RBCs, parasites develop from ring forms (trophozoites) to multinucleated schizonts (erythrocytic schizogeny).
4. The RBCs rupture and release merozoites, which may reinfect new RBCs. Some differentiate into male and female gametocytes.
5. Gametocytes are taken up by the *Anopheles* mosquitoes, develop into sporozoites in their gut and migrate to the salivary gland of the mosquito to be transmitted in their bite.

Certain populations have some innate immunity (e.g. sickle cell trait, G6PD deficiency, pyruvate kinase deficiency, thalassaemias).

EPIDEMIOLOGY   Endemic in tropics. Affects 250 million people worldwide yearly. There are about 2000 reported cases and 10 deaths caused by malaria (mainly *P. falciparum*) annually in the United Kingdom.

HISTORY   High degree of clinical suspicion in any feverish traveller (incubation up to 1 year, but usually 1–2 weeks). Cyclical symptoms of high fever, flulike symptoms, severe sweating and shivering cold/rigors.
Peak temperature may coincide with rupture of the intra-erythrocytic schizonts:
• every 48 h for *P. falciprum* (malignant tertian);
• every 72 h for *P. malariae* (benign quartan); and
• every 48 h for *P. vivax* and *P. ovale* (benign tertian).

Cerebral malaria: Headache, disorientation, coma.

EXAMINATION   Pyrexia/rigors, anaemia, hepatosplenomegaly.

INVESTIGATIONS
Thick/thin blood film (using Field's or Giemsa's stain): Measure daily for detection and quantitative count of level of intracellular ring forms. Has to be negative for 3 days to exclude malaria. >2% in *P. falciparum* malaria is severe.
Blood: FBC (Hb, platelets), U&E, LFT, ABG (pH).
Urinalysis: Test for blood or protein.
Quantitative buffy coat (QBC) test: Acridine orange stains parasite nucleus. Lower sensitivity than blood films.
Immunochromatographic (ICT) test: Detects histidine-rich protein 2 found only in *P. falciparum*. Lower sensitivity than blood films.

MANAGEMENT[1]
Uncomplicated malaria:
For *P. malariae, P. vivax, P. ovale:*
1. Oral chloroquine
2. Add Primaquine in *P. vivax* and *P. ovale* (to destroy hypnozoites)

---

[1]Lalloo DG, Shingadia D, Pasvol G, et al. UK malaria treatment guidelines. *J. Infect.* 2007; **54**:111–21.

For *P. falciparum:*
1. Oral quinine + doxycycline, or
2. Co-artem (combination if artemether + lumefantrin), or
3. Malarone (combination of atovaquone + proguanil).

Severe malaria (Impaired consciousness, renal impairment, acidosis, hypotension, hypoglycaemia, DIC, haemoglobinuria):
1. IV quinine + oral doxycycline, or
2. Artesunate + oral doxycyline

Prophylaxis: From day before travel to 28 days from day of return.

	Drug	Dose
Areas of chloroquine resistanc	Mefloquine	250 mg/week
	Doxycycline	100 mg/day
	Atovaquone-proguanil (Malorone®)	250/100 mg/day
Areas of low chloroquine resistance	Proguanil and chloroquine	200 mg/day 300 mg/week

Public health: Personal awareness and protection (netting, long sleeves, time of day, insect repellants). Malaria is a notifiable disease.

COMPLICATIONS   *P. falciparum* can cause cerebral malaria, Blackwater fever (intravascular haemolysis → haemoglobinuria → renal failure), DIC and shock, metabolic acidosis, hypoglycaemia, splenic rupture.
Pregnancy: abortion, stillbirth and low birth weight.

PROGNOSIS   *P. falciparum* malaria is life threatening. The others are more benign.

Sepsis and systemic inflammatory response syndrome (SIRS)

DEFINITION

SIRS: When two or more of the following are present:

- Heart rate >90/min
- Temperature <36°C or >38°C,
- Tachypnea >20/min or $PaCO_2$ <4.3 kPa (32 mmHg),
- WCC <4000 or >12,000 cells/mm^3 or >10% immature neutrophils

Sepsis: SIRS + infection.
Severe sepsis: Sepsis + organ dysfunction, hypotension or hypoperfusion.
Septic shock: Sepsis-induced hypotension despite adequate fluid resuscitation.

AETIOLOGY   SIRS is a common inflammatory response to a wide variety of physiological insults, can be caused by infection, ischaemia, inflammation e.g. pancreatitis, trauma, burns. Can progress to multiple organ dysfunction syndrome (MODS) – altered organ function in an acutely ill patient so that haemostasis cannot be maintained without intervention.

Pathology/Pathogenesis: Following an insult, local cytokines incite an inflammatory response to fight infection and promote healing. Cytokines are released into circulation to improve the local response. This acute-phase response is usually controlled by a decrease in the proinflammatory mediators and by the release of endogenous antagonists. If homeostasis is not restored, a cycle of uncontrolled pro-inflammatory amplification arises with inflammation and coagulation dominant resulting in microcirculatory thrombosis, hypoperfusion, ischaemia, loss of circulatory integrity and tissue injury.

EPIDEMIOLOGY   Extremes of age and concomitant comorbidities negatively affect the outcome.

HISTORY   Depends on the aetiology whether infectious, traumatic, ischaemic or inflammatory.

EXAMINATION   Thorough systematic examination for diagnosis with attention to vital signs, urine output, mental status. Respiratory rate is a sensitive sign of severity of illness.

INVESTIGATIONS

Blood: FBC, U&E, LFT, amylase, cardiac enzymes. Inflammatory markers include CRP and ESR, with newer IL6, IL8 pro-calcitonin and LPS binding protein.
ABG: Provides important information on severity of acidosis, lactate.
Cultures: Blood, sputum, urine, lines, other potentially infected sites CSF, joint fluid, ascites or pleural effusions.
Imaging studies: To locate/sample source of infection.

MANAGEMENT

Immediate stabilization of the patient: Resuscitation according to ABC. In sepsis, prompt institution of empirical antibiotics and support organ function. Targeted and protocol-driven early 'goal-directed therapy' of fluid and inotropic support has been shown to improve the outcome from sepsis with a standardized approach formulated into 'The Surviving Sepsis Campaign' goals include:

- central venous pressure 8–12 mmHg,
- mean arterial pressure ≥65 mm Hg,
- urine output ≥0.5 ml/kg/h, and
- central venous oxygen saturation ≥70%

Supportive measures: Critical care support, glycemic control, nutrition, DVT and stress ulcer prophylaxis. Acute renal failure often develops during the sepsis and may require renal replacement therapy. Even if renal function is normal in a septic patient, early high-volume continuous veno-venous haemofiltration may still be advocated. It is thought that this process may remove some of the pro-inflammatory or pro-coagulant cytokines that drive the septic cascade.

Activated Protein C: The PROWESS (Recombinant Human Activated Protein C Worldwide Evaluation in Severe Sepsis) study showed that recombinant activated protein C (drotrecogin-α) reduces mortality in severe sepsis (Avoid in patients with increased risk of bleeding).

Surgical: Acute surgical problems should be managed appropriately e.g. drainage of abscesses, removal/debridement of infected tissue.

COMPLICATIONS   Multiorgan dysfunction; renal failure, coagulopathy, liver failure, ARDS, death.

PROGNOSIS

Mortality rates: SIRS ~7%, severe sepsis 30% and septic shock (>50%). These increase by 15–20% for each additional organ failure.

Tuberculosis (TB)

DEFINITION   Granulomatous disease caused by *Mycobacterium tuberculosis*.
Primary: Initial infection may be pulmonary (acquired by inhalation from the cough of an infected patient) or, occasionally, gastrointestinal.
Miliary TB: Results when there is haematogenous dissemination.
Post-primary: Caused by reinfection or reactivation.

AETIOLOGY   *M. tuberculosis* is an intracellular organism (also known as acid-fast bacilli, AFB) which survives after being phagocytosed by macrophages.

EPIDEMIOLOGY   Annual mortality 3 million (95% in developing countries); annual UK incidence 6000. Incidence in Asian immigrants >30 times native UK white population.

HISTORY AND EXAMINATION   TB is a multi-system disease.
Primary TB: Mostly asymptomatic, may have fever, malaise, cough, wheeze, erythema nodosum and phlyctenular conjunctivitis (allergic manifestations).
Miliary TB: Fever, weight loss, meningitis, yellow caseous tubercles spread to other organs (e.g. in bone and kidney may remain dormant for years).
Post-primary TB: Fever/night sweats, malaise, weight loss, breathlessness, cough, sputum, haemoptysis, pleuritic pain, signs of pleural effusion, collapse, consolidation, fibrosis.
Non-pulmonary TB: Particularly in immunocompromised.
Lymph nodes: Suppuration of cervical lymph nodes leading to abscesses or sinuses, which discharge pus and spread to skin (scrofuloderma).
CNS: Meningitis, tuberculoma.
Skin: Lupus vulgaris (jellylike reddish-brown glistening plaques).
Heart: Pericardial effusion, constrictive pericarditis.
Gastrointestinal: Subacute obstruction, change in bowel habit, weight loss, peritonitis, ascites.
Genitourinary: Urinary tract infection symptoms, renal failure, epididymitis, endometrial or tubal involvement, infertility.
Adrenal: Insufficiency.
Bone/joints: Osteomyelitis, arthritis, paravertebral abscesses and vertebral collapse (Pott's disease), spinal cord compresson from abscesses.

INVESTIGATIONS
Sputum/pleural fluid/bronchial washings: Microscopy (Ziehl–Neelsen stain), culture (takes up to 6 weeks). Low sensitivity.
Tuberculin tests: Positive in previous exposure to *M. tuberculosis* or BCG. Strongly positive results may indicate infection.
Mantoux test: Intradermal injection of PPD, induration and erythema after 72 h.
Heaf test: Place drop of PPD on forearm, fire spring-loaded needled gun, read after 3–7 days. Graded according to papule size and vesiculation.
Interferon-γ tests: In latent TB, exposure of host T cells to TB antigens causes release of interferon. Specificity is high (negative with BCG vaccination) so can be used to diagnose latent TB if tuberculin test is positive.
CXR: *Primary infection:* Peripheral consolidation, hilar lymphadenopathy.
Miliary: Fine shadowing.
Post-primary: Upper lobe shadowing, streaky fibrosis and cavitation, calcification, pleural effusion, hilar lymphadenopathy.
HIV testing: Recommended to coincident disease (2% may be HIV positive).
CT, lymph nodes, pleural biopsy, sampling of other affected systems: (e.g. CSF).

MANAGEMENT   Needs to be treated by specialist physician.

Antimicrobial therapy: Combined therapy necessary to prevent resistance. Rising incidence of multiresistant TB. Directly observed therapy may be necessary. Treat for 6 months in pulmonary, 12 months for bone or brain.

1. *Rifampicin: Side effects – orange body fluids, enzyme inducing*
2. *Isoniazid: Side effects – pyridoxine deficiency, peripheral neuropathy.*
3. *Ethambutol: Side effects – optic neuropathy*
4. *Pyrazinamide: Side effects – ↑ urate/arthralgia, hepato-toxicity*
5. *Streptomycin: Only for highly resistant organisms*

Advice: Explain side effects and importance of compliance to treatment. Consider *steroids* for pericardial, cerebral or bone involvement.

Public health: Notifiable disease. Isolate if respiratory until 2 weeks on treatment. Contact tracing using a combination of CXR, tuberculin test, check BCG status and/or interferon-γ testing. Consider chemoprophylaxis (e.g. isoniazid).

Prevention: BCG vaccination, a live attenuated strain derived from *Mycobacterium bovis*, provides 60–80% efficacy. It should be considered as protection against extrapulmonary TB only.

COMPLICATIONS

Primary TB: Lobar collapse (especially middle lobe) and bronchiectasis (Brock's syndrome), pleural effusion, pneumonic spread, miliary disease disseminated in lung or throughout body.

Post-primary TB: Pleural effusion, empyema, aspergilloma, adenocarcinoma, laryngeal disease, swelling of bronchial lymphatics and airflow obstruction, haemoptysis, distant spread.

PROGNOSIS   Excellent if pulmonary TB and treated. Overall mortality 8% if extrapulmonary TB, relapse because of non-adherence, resistance, cavitation, empyema, latency.

Urinary tract infections

DEFINITION   Characterized by presence of >100,000 of colony-forming units per millilitre of urine. Urinary tract infections (UTI) may affect bladder (cystitis), kidney (pyelonephritis) or prostate (prostatitis).

AETIOLOGY   Usually transurethral ascent of normal colonic organisms. The most common organism is *Escherichia coli*, others include *Proteus mirabilis*, *Klebsiella* and *Enterococci* (more common in hospitals).

EPIDEMIOLOGY
Common in females: 30% of women experience UTI at some point in their lives.
UTI may be seen in 5% of pregnant women, 2% of young non-pregnant women, 20% of elderly living at home and 50% of institutionalized elderly.
UTI is rare in children and young men (if present, suspect an underlying cause).

HISTORY   May be clinically silent (asymptomatic bacteruria).
Cystitis: Frequency, urgency, dysuria (pain on micturition), haematuria, suprapubic pain, smelly urine.
Pyelonephritis (acute): Fever, malaise, rigors, loin/flank pain.
Prostatitis: Fever, low back/perineal pain, irritative and obstructive symptoms (e.g. hesitancy, urgency, intermittency, poor stream, dribbling).
Elderly: Malaise, nocturia, incontinence, confusion.
Up to 30% of women with UTI symptoms may not have bacteruria.

EXAMINATION   May be asymptomatic.
Cystitis: Fever, abdominal/suprapubic/loin tenderness, bladder distension.
Pyelonephritis: Fever, loin/flank tenderness.
Prostatitis: Tender, swollen prostate.

INVESTIGATIONS
Mid-stream urine for:
Dipstick test: For blood, protein, leucocytes, nitrites (urinary bacteria reduce nitrates to nitrites).
Microscopy, culture and sensitivity: $\geq 10^5$ colonies/mL indicates a significant bacteriuria, but in the presence of UTI symptoms, the threshold is lower, in women ($>10^2$/mL) and in men ($>10^5$/mL).
If there is sterile pyuria (pus cells with no organisms), consider if this may be partially treated UTI, tuberculosis stones, tumour, interstitial nephritis or renal papillary necrosis.
Imaging: Renal ultrasound or intravenous urogram may be considered in:
* women with frequent UTIs; and
* in children and men.

This is to exclude predisposing structural/functional abnormalities.

MANAGEMENT
Cystitis: If symptomatic, consider local microbiological policies, commonly used agents are oral co-trimoxazole, trimethoprim, nitrofurantoin or amoxicillin (in females) and ciprofloxacin (males).
Pyelonephritis: IV gentamicin, cefuroxime or ciprofloxacin.
Catheterized patients: Obtain a culture and consider changing the catheter. Do not treat unless the patient is symptomatic as catheters invariably become colonized.
Prophylaxis: High fluid intake. Regular micturation to keep bladder empty. Cranberry-based products reduce the frequency of recurrence. In some cases, low-dose long-term (6–12 months) antibiotics for women with frequent UTIs.
Surgical: Rarely necessary. May be necessary for relief of any obstruction and removal of any renal calculi.

COMPLICATIONS   Renal papillary necrosis (in those with underlying renal disease, e.g. diabetes mellitus or stones).
Renal/perinephric abscess (seen on renal ultrasound).
Pyonephrosis (pus in palvicalyceal system).
Gram-negative septicaemia.

PROGNOSIS   Mostly resolve with treatment. Among pregnant women, 20% develop acute pyelonephritis if not treated; however, there is a high relapse rate.

Varicella zoster

DEFINITION Primary infection is called varicella (chickenpox). Reactivation of the dormant virus in the dorsal root ganglia, causes zoster (shingles). Confusingly also known as herpes zoster in some texts.

AETIOLOGY VZV is an herpes ds-DNA virus. Highly contagious, transmission is by aerosol inhalation or direct contact with the vesicular secretions.

EPIDEMIOLOGY Chickenpox peak incidence occurs at 4–10 years. Shingles peak incidence occurs at >50 years. About 90% of adults are VZV IgG positive (previously infected).

HISTORY Incubation period 14–21 days.
Chickenpox: Prodromal malaise, mild pyrexia, sudden appearance of intensely itchy spreading rash affecting the face and trunk more than the extremities, the oropharynx, conjunctivae and genitourinary tract. As vesicles weep and crust over, new vesicles appear. Contagious from 48 h before the rash and until all the vesicles have crusted over (within 7–10 days).
Shingles: May occur after a period of stress. Tingling/hyperaesthesia in a dermatomal distribution, followed by painful skin lesions. Recovery in 10–14 days.

EXAMINATION
Chickenpox (disseminated varicella): Macular papular rash evolving into crops of vesicles with areas of weeping (exudate) and crusting (vesicles, macules, papules and crusts may all be present at one time), skin excoriation (from scratching), mild pyrexia.
Shingles: Vesicular macular papular rash, in a dermatomal distribution, skin excoriation.

PATHOLOGY/PATHOGENESIS Viral inhalation and infection of upper respiratory tract. Viral replication in regional lymph nodes, liver and spleen. By week 2–3 infection spreads to skin producing rash then leading to clinical resolution. Virus remains latent in dorsal root ganglia (lifelong). Reactivation causes virus to travel down sensory axon to produce dermatomal shingles rash.

INVESTIGATIONS Both chickenpox and shingles are usually clinical diagnoses.
Vesicle fluid: Electron microscopy, direct immunofluorescence, cell culture, viral PCR (all rarely necessary).
Chickenpox: Consider HIV testing especially in adults with prior history of varicella infection.

MANAGEMENT
Chickenpox (primary infection):
Children: Treat symptoms (calamine lotion, analgesia, antihistamines).
Adults: Consider aciclovir, valaciclovir or famciclovir if within 24 h of rash onset especially if elderly, smoker, immunocompromised or pregnant (especially second or third trimester).
Shingles (reactivation): Aciclovir, valaciclovir or famciclovir if within 72 h of appearance of the rash if elderly, immunocompromised or ophthalmic involvement. Low-dose amitriptyline may benefit those with moderate/severe discomfort. Simple analgesia (paracetamol).
Prevention: VZIG may be indicated in the immunosuppressed and in pregnant women exposed to varicella zoster. Chickenpox vaccine is licensed in the United Kingdom, but no guidelines available for appropriate use.

COMPLICATIONS
Chickenpox: Secondary infection, scarring, pneumonia, encephalitis, cerebellar syndrome, congenital varicella syndrome.[1]

---

[1] Congenital varicella syndrome is characterized by scarring, ophthalmic defects, limb dysplasia and CNS abnormalities. Occurs in 1–2% of offspring of mothers who developed chickenpox ≤20 weeks' gestation.

Shingles: Postherpetic neuralgia, zoster opthalmicus (rash involves opthalmic division of trigeminal nerve), Ramsay Hunt's syndrome,[2] sacral zoster may lead to urinary retention, motor zoster (muscle weakness of myotome at similar level as involved dermatome).

PROGNOSIS Depends on the complications. Worse in pregnancy, the elderly and immunocompromised.

---

[2] Ramsay Hunt's syndrome is the reactivation of virus in geniculate ganglion causing zoster of the ear and facial nerve palsy. Vesicles may be seen behind the pinna of the ear or in the ear canal.

Anaemia, aplastic

DEFINITION   Characterized by diminished haematopoietic precursors in the bone marrow and deficiency of all blood cell elements (pancytopaenia).

AETIOLOGY
Idiopathic (>40%): May be due to destruction or suppression of the stem cell by autoimmune mechanisms.

Acquired: Drugs (chloramphenicol, gold, alkylating agents, antiepileptics, sulphonamides, methotrexate, nifedipine), chemicals (DDT, benzene), radiation, viral infection (B19 parvovirus, HIV, EBV), paroxysmal nocturnal haemoglobinuria (see Anaemia, haemolytic).

Inherited: Fanconi's anaemia,[1] dyskeratosis congenita (associated with reticulated hyperpigmented rash, nail dystrophy and mucosa leukoplakia).

EPIDEMIOLOGY
Annual incidence: 2–4 in 1,000,000. Can occur at any age. Slightly more common in males.

HISTORY   Slow (months) or rapid (days) onset.
Anaemia: Tiredness, lethargy, dyspnoea.
Thrombocytopaenia: Easy bruising, bleeding gums, epistaxis.
Leukopenia: ↑ Frequency and severity of infections.

EXAMINATION
Anaemia: Pale.
Thrombocytopaenia: Petechiae, bruises.
Leukopaenia: Multiple bacterial or fungal infections. No hepatomegaly, splenomegaly or lymphadenopathy.

INVESTIGATIONS
Blood: FBC (↓ Hb, ↓ platelets, ↓ WCC, normal MCV, low or absent reticulocytes).
Blood film: To exclude leukaemia (absence of abnormal circulating white blood cells).
Bone marrow trephine biopsy: For diagnosis (hypocellular marrow with a decrease in all elements; the marrow space is composed mostly of fat cells and marrow stroma) and exclusion of other causes (lymphoma, leukaemia, malignancies, myeloma, myelofibrosis).
Criteria for severe aplastic anaemia (AA):
Marrow showing <25 % of normal cellularity, OR Marrow showing <50 % of normal cellularity, <30% of the cells are haematopoietic plus 2 of the following:
- neutrophils $< 0.5 \times 10^9$/L
- platelets $< 20 \times 10^9$/L
- reticulocytes $< 40 \times 10^9$/L

Fanconi's anaemia: Presence of increased chromosomal breakage in lymphocytes cultured in the presence of DNA cross-linking agents e.g. mitomycin C.

MANAGEMENT
Treat the underlying cause: E.g. withdrawal of potentially causative drugs
Supportive: Blood and platelet transfusions, antibiotics for infections, consider antibiotic prophylaxis.
For patients with severe AA: *Allogeneic haematopoietic cell transplantation:* For patients <20 years with an HLA-matched sibling or those 20–45 years in otherwise excellent health with a fully HLA-matched sibling donor. Curative. *Immunosuppressive therapy (combined use of anti-thymocyte globulin, cyclosporine, and corticosteroids, with or*

---

[1]Fanconi anaemia: Rare autosomal recessive or X-linked disorder caused by an error of DNA repair. Characterized by familial aplastic anaemia, short stature, abnormality of thumbs, café au lait spots, microcephaly, hypogonadism and renal tract defects.

Anaemia, aplastic (continued)

without granulocyte-colony stimulating factor): For patients who do not have a matched sibling donor OR those >45 years (because of the high risk of graft versus host disease). Patients relapsing after successful treatment can be re-treated with this regimen.

COMPLICATIONS Bleeding, infections. Complications of bone marrow transplantation (e.g. infection, graft vs host disease). Patients with Fanconi anaemia are at high risk for developing a myelodysplastic syndrome, acute myeloid leukaemia, and squamous cell carcinoma of the head and neck.

PROGNOSIS Depends on patient age (worse outcome in older patients) and the severity of pancytopaenia. >70 % of patients with severe AA will be dead within 1 year if not successfully treated.

Anaemia, haemolytic

DEFINITION   Premature erythrocyte breakdown causing shortened erythrocyte life span
($<$120 days) and anaemia.

AETIOLOGY

Hereditary	
Membrane defects	Hereditary spherocytosis,[1] elliptocytosis (elliptical erythrocytes).
Metabolic defects	G6PD deficiency.[2] Pyruvate kinase deficiencies (autosomal recessive).
Haemoglobinopathies	Sickle cell disease, thalassaemia (see Sickle cell anaemia and Thalassaemias).
Acquired	
Autoimmune	Warm or cold antibodies[3] attach to erythrocytes causing intravascular haemolysis and extravasular haemolysis.
Isoimmune	Transfusion reaction, haemolytic disease of the newborn.
Drugs	Penicillin, quinine (through formation of drug–antibody–erythrocyte complex).
Trauma	Microangiopathic haemolytic anaemia caused by red cell fragmentation in abnormal microcirculation (e.g. haemolytic uraemic syndrome, DIC, malignant hypertension, pre-eclampsia), artificial heart valves.
Infection	Malaria, sepsis.
Paroxysmal nocturnal haemoglobinuria	↑ Complement-mediated lysis caused by ↓ synthesis of protein cellular anchor of complement-degrading proteins.

EPIDEMIOLOGY   Common. Genetic causes are prevalent in African, Mediterranean,
Middle Eastern populations. Hereditary spherocytosis is the most common inherited haemolytic anaemia in northern Europe.

HISTORY   Jaundice, haematuria, anaemia. Ask about systemic illness, family, drug and
travel history.

EXAMINATION   Pallor (anaemia), jaundice, hepatosplenomegaly.

INVESTIGATIONS
Blood: FBC (↓ Hb, ↑ reticulocytes, ↑ MCV, also ↑ unconjugated bilirubin, ↓ haptoglobin), U&E,
folate.
Blood film: Leucoerythroblastic picture, macrocytosis, nucleated erythrocytes or reticulocytes, polychromasia. Identifies specific abnormal cells, such as spherocytes, elliptocytes,
sickle cells, fragmented erythrocytes, malarial parasites, erythrocyte Heinz bodies
(denatured Hb, stained with methyl violet seen in G6PD deficiency).

---

[1]Hereditary spherocytosis is an autosomal dominant condition where ↓ spectrin (a structural membrane
protein) causes ↓ deformability of erythrocytes.

[2]G6PD deficiency (X-linked): G6PD is important in maintaining glutathione in reduced state. Deficiency
results in susceptibility to oxidative stress (e.g. precipitated by sulphonamides, nitrofurantoin, dapsone,
fava beans).

[3]'Warm' antibodies (IgG) agglutinate erythrocytes at 37°C. Associated with SLE, lymphomas or methyldopa.
'Cold' antibodies (IgM) agglutinate erythrocytes in at room temperature or colder. Associated with
infections (e.g. Mycoplasma, EBV) or lymphomas.

Anaemia, haemolytic (continued)

Urine: ↑ Urobilirubinogen. If intravascular haemolysis, there is haemoglobinuria and haemosiderinuria.

Direct Coombs' test: Identifies erythrocytes coated with antibodies (agglutinins) using antihuman globulin. Warm agglutinin and cold agglutinin.

Osmotic fragility test or Spectrin mutation analysis: To identify membrane abnormalities.

Ham's test: Lysis of erythrocytes in acidified serum in paraxosymal nocturnal haemoglobinuria. More recently – red cells are analyzed, using monoclonal antibodies to the GPI-anchored proteins (CD55 and CD59) and flow cytometry.

Hb electrophoresis or enzyme assays: When other causes excluded.

Bone marrow biopsy (rarely required): Erythroid hyperplasia.

MANAGEMENT Treat underlying cause and avoid the contributing factor (e.g. cold exposure for cold agglutinins).

Spherocytosis: Folate supplement, splenectomy (postponed until >5 years old), lifetime penicillin, vaccination against encapsulated organisms (e.g. pneumococcus, *Haemophilus influenzae* and meningococcus).

Autoimmune (warm agglutinins): Prednisolone, splenectomy, azathioprine or cyclophosphamide.

Paroxysmal nocturnal haemoglobinuria: Blood transfusions (leucocyte-depleted). Anticoagulants (e.g. warfarin) for thrombotic episodes. Bone marrow transplantation has been successful in some patients.

COMPLICATIONS Depends on cause. All can cause acute renal failure.

Spherocytosis can predispose to gallstones, aplastic, megaloblastic and haemolytic crises and leg ulcers. Paroxysmal nocturnal haemoglobinuria can transform to aplastic anaemia or leukaemia.

PROGNOSIS Mostly normal life expectancy, may be reduced in sickle cell anaemia, β-thalassaemia major and paroxysmal nocturnal haemoglobinuria.

Anaemia, macrocytic

DEFINITION   Anaemia associated with a high MCV of erythrocytes (>100 fl in adults).

AETIOLOGY
Megaloblastic: Deficiency of B_{12} or folate required for conversion of deoxyuridate to thymidylate, DNA synthesis and nuclear maturation.

Vitamin B_{12}: $\downarrow$ Absorption (post-gastrectomy, pernicious anaemia,[1] terminal ileal resection or disease e.g. Crohn's disease, bacterial overgrowth, pancreatic insufficiency, fish tapeworm, metformin, omeprazole), $\downarrow$intake (vegans), abnormal metabolism (congenital tanscobalamin II deficiency, inactivation of B_{12} by nitrous oxide).

Folate: $\downarrow$ Intake (alcoholics, elderly, anorexia), $\uparrow$ demand: (pregnancy, lactation, malignancy, chronic inflammation, chronic haemolysis, exfoliative dermatitis), $\downarrow$ absorption: (jejunal disease, e.g. coeliac disease, tropical sprue), drugs (e.g. phenytoin, trimethoprim, methotrexate).

Drugs: Methotrexate (inhibition of dihydrofolate reductase), hydroxyurea (inhibition of ribonucleotide reductase), azathioprine, zidovudine.

Non-megaloblastic: Alcohol excess, liver disease, myelodysplasia, multiple myeloma, hypothyroidism, haemolysis (shift to immature red cells: 'reticulocytosis'), drugs (e.g. tyrosine kinase inhibitors: imatinib, sunitinib).

EPIDEMIOLOGY   More common in the elderly and females. Annual worldwide incidence of pernicious anaemia in those >40 years old is ~25 in 100,000 (most common cause of vitamin B_{12} deficiency in the West).

HISTORY
Non-specific signs of anaemia: Tiredness, lethargy, dyspnoea.

Family history of autoimmune disease. Previous history of gastrointestinal surgery. Symptoms of the cause, e.g. weight loss, diarrhoea, steatorrhoea in coeliac disease.

EXAMINATION
Sign of anaemia: E.g. pallor, tachycardia. There may be signs of the cause, e.g. malnutrition, jaundice, hypothyroid appearance.

Signs of pernicious anaemia: Lemon-tinted skin (mild jaundice), glossitis (red sore tongue), angular stomatitis (cheilitis), weight loss.

Signs of vitamin B_{12} deficiency: Peripheral neuropathy, ataxia, subacute combined degeneration of the spinal cord,[2] optic atrophy, dementia.

INVESTIGATIONS
Blood: FBC ($\uparrow$ MCV, pancytopenia in megaloblastic anaemia, varying degrees of cytopenia in myelodysplasia, exclude reticulocytosis), LFT ($\uparrow$ bilirubin as a result of ineffective erythropoiesis or haemolysis), ESR, TFT, serum vitamin B_{12}, red cell folate, antibodies against parietal cells or intrinsic factor (IF), serum protein electrophoresis (exclude myeloma).

Blood film: Large erythrocytes (macrocytes).

In megaloblastic anaemia: Macroovalocytes, hypersegmented neutrophil nuclei (>5 lobes).

Schilling's test: Part I: radiolabelled vitamin B_{12} is given orally and IM non-radioactive B_{12} is given to saturate vitamin B_{12}-binding proteins. $\downarrow$ Radiolabelled vitamin B_{12} in a 24-h urine collection indicates $\downarrow$ absorption. Part II: Part I repeated with oral IF. If radiolabelled vitamin B_{12} is now detected in urine, the cause is likely to be IF deficiency from pernicious anaemia

---

[1]Pernicious anaemia is caused by autoimmune damage to gastric parietal cells causing atrophic gastritis and consequent $\downarrow$ production of intrinsic factor (IF) needed for vitamin B_{12} absorption in terminal ileum. Pernicious anaemia may be associated with other autoimmune diseases (e.g. vitiligo, hypothyroidism).

[2]Subacute combined degeneration of the spinal cord is the degeneration of the dorsal and lateral columns of the spinal cord causing loss of joint and position sense, ataxia and UMN weakness. Partially or completely relieved by restoring vitamin B_{12} levels.

Anaemia, macrocytic (continued)

or gastrectomy. Potential usefulness only when more simple tests (e.g. anti-IF antibodies) are normal and the diagnosis is in doubt. Measurement of the metabolites methylmalonate and total homocysteine have superior sensitivity to Schilling's test (both ↑ in vitamin B_{12} deficiency).

Bone marrow biopsy (rarely necessary): Megaloblasts (nucleated red cells) or myelodysplastic changes.

Investigations for the suspected cause.

MANAGEMENT

Pernicious anaemia: IM hydroxycobalamin (thrice weekly for 2 weeks, then every 3 months for life).

Folate deficiency: Oral folic acid: 5 mg/day for 1–4 months, or until complete haematologic recovery occurs. Vitamin B_{12} deficiency must be treated first if present (folic acid may worsen neurologic complications of untreated vitamin B_{12} deficiency).

COMPLICATIONS   In pernicious anaemia, ↑ risk of gastric cancer. In pregnancy, folate deficiency predisposes to spinal cord anomalies.

PROGNOSIS   Majority are treatable if there are no complications.

Anaemia, microcytic

DEFINITION   Anaemia associated with low MCV (<80 fl).

AETIOLOGY
Iron-deficiency (commonest cause): Blood loss – e.g. gastrointestinal tract, urogenital tract, hookworm infection.

↓ **Absorption:**	Small bowel disease, Post-gastrectomy.
↑ **Demands:**	Growth, Pregnancy.
↓ **Intake**	Vegans

Anaemia of chronic disease:[1] Often normocytic but may be microcytic.
Thalassaemia: *See* Thalassaemias.
Sideroblastic anaemia: Abnormality of haem synthesis. Can be inherited (X-linked), or secondary to alcohol, drugs (e.g. isoniazid, chloramphenicol), lead, myelodysplasia.
Lead poisoning (e.g. in scrap metal or smelting workers): Interferes with globin and haem synthesis.

EPIDEMIOLOGY   Iron-deficiency anaemia is the commonest form of anaemia worldwide.

HISTORY
Non-specific: Tiredness, lethargy, malaise, dyspnoea, pallor. Exacerbation of pre-existing angina or intermittent claudication. Family history of any causative diseases.
Lead poisoning: Anorexia, nausea, vomiting, abdominal pain, constipation, peripheral nerve lesions.

EXAMINATION   Signs of anaemia, e.g. pallor of skin and mucous membranes. Brittle nails and hair. If long-standing and severe, spoon-shaped nails (koilonychia).
Glossitis: Atrophy of tongue papillae.
Cheilitis: Angular stomatitis.
Signs of thalassaemias (*see* Thalassaemias).
Lead poisoning: Blue gumline, peripheral nerve lesions (wrist or foot drop), encephalopathy, convulsions, ↓ consciousness.

INVESTIGATIONS
Blood: FBC (↓ Hb,↓ MCV, reticulocytes), serum iron (↓ in iron deficiency), iron-binding capacity (↑ in iron deficiency), serum ferritin (↓ in iron deficiency), serum lead (if poisoning suspected).
Blood film:
Iron-deficiency anaemia: Microcytic (small), hypochromic (central pallor >one-third cell size), anisocytosis (variable cell size), poikilocytosis (variable cell shapes).
Sideroblastic anaemia: Dimorphic blood film with a population of hypochromic microcytic cells.
Lead poisoning: Basophilic stippling (coarse dots represent condensed RNA in the cytoplasm).
Hb electrophoresis: For haemoglobin variants or thalassaemias.
Sideroblastic anaemia: Ring sideroblasts in the bone marrow (iron deposited in perinuclear mitochondria of erythroblasts, stain blue–green with Perls' stain).

---

[1]Occurs in chronic inflammatory/autoimmune disease, chronic infections, e.g. TB/infective endocarditis, malignancy, chronic renal failure. Serum ferritin is normal/↑. It may be caused by ↓ RBC survival, ↓ erythropoietin response to the anaemia, ↓ iron release from bone marrow to erythroblasts. Treat the underlying condition.

Anaemia, microcytic (continued)

If iron-deficiency anaemia in >40 years and post-menopausal women: Upper GI endoscopy, colonoscopy and investigations for haematuria should be considered if no obvious cause of blood loss.

MANAGEMENT

Iron deficiency: Oral iron supplements (e.g. 200 mg ferrous sulphate tablets containing 65 mg of elemental iron, twice or thrice daily taken with food). If oral iron intolerance or malabsorption, consider parenteral iron supplements (beware risk of anaphylaxis). Monitor Hb and MCV, aiming for Hb rise of 1 g/dL/week.

Sideroblastic anaemia: Treat the cause (e.g. stop causative drugs). Pyridoxine can be used in inherited forms. If no response, consider blood transfusion and iron chelation.

Lead poisoning: Remove the source, dimercaprol, D-penicillamine, Ca2 + EDTA.

COMPLICATIONS   High-output cardiac failure, complications of the cause.

PROGNOSIS   Depends on the underlying cause.

Antiphospholipid syndrome

DEFINITION   Characterized by the presence of antiphospholipid antibodies (APL) in the plasma, venous and arterial thromboses, recurrent foetal loss and thrombocytopenia.

AETIOLOGY   APL are directed against plasma proteins bound to anionic phospholipids (e.g. β2 glycoprotein-I). APL may develop in susceptible individuals (e.g. those with rheumatic diseases such as SLE) following exposure to infectious agents. Once APL are present, a 'second-hit' is needed for the development of the syndrome. The procoagulant actions of APL may be mediated by their effect on β2-GP-I (clotting and platelet aggregation inhibitor), protein C, annexin V, platelets and fibrinolysis. Complement activation is critical for pregnancy complications.

EPIDEMIOLOGY   More common in young ♀. Accounts for 20% of strokes in <45-year-olds and 27% of women with >2 miscarriages.

HISTORY   Recurrent miscarriages, history of arterial thromboses (stroke), venous thromboses (DVT, pulmonary embolism), headaches (migraine), chorea, epilepsy.

EXAMINATION
Livedo reticularis.
Signs of SLE (malar flush, discoid lesions, photosensitivity).
Signs of valvular heart disease.

INVESTIGATIONS
FBC (↓ platelets), ESR (usually normal), U&Es (APL nephropathy), clotting screen (↑ APTT).
Presence of APL may be demonstrated by
-ELISA testing for anticardiolipin and anti-β2-GPI antibodies.
-Lupus anticoagulant assays: Clotting assays showing effects of APL on the phospholipid-dependent factors in the coagulation cascade.
False-positive VDRL test for syphilis may be a clue to the presence of any type of APL.

MANAGEMENT
Treat thrombotic episodes with SC low molecular weight heparin (LMWH), followed by long-term anticoagulation with oral warfarin (INR range: 2–3).
During pregnancy: Close monitoring, antepartum and postpartum thromboprophylaxis for women with prior thrombosis. Add prophylactic low dose aspirin to LMWH in women with history of pregnancy complications.
For patients with SLE and APL but no APS manifestations, the combination of low-dose aspirin and hydroxychloroquine may be considered.
Advice: Avoid oral contraceptives, and modify risk factors for vascular disease (smoking, hypertension, hyperlipidaemia). Warn patient about risk of miscarriage and thrombosis in pregnancies.

COMPLICATIONS
Foetal miscarriages. Sites for thrombosis include:
arteries: cerebral, coronary, retinal and visceral;
veins: deep or superficial leg, subclavian, axillary, renal, hepatic, portal or retinal veins and cerebral sinuses. Thrombotic episodes causing Addison's disease (when adrenals are involved), or Budd–Chiari syndrome (when hepatic vein is involved). Thrombosis can occur even in the presence of thrombocytopenia. Other neurological syndromes: cognitive deficits, white matter lesions.

PROGNOSIS   Morbidity and mortality associated with antiphospholipid syndrome is high as effective treatment is not yet known. However, successful pregnancy rates are now much higher (>80%).

Deep vein thrombosis (DVT)

DEFINITION   Formation of a thrombus within the deep veins (most commonly of the calf or thigh).

AETIOLOGY
Virchow's triad: Venous stasis, vessel wall injury and blood hypercoagulability.
Risk factors Oral contraceptive pill, surgery, prolonged immobility, long bone fractures, obesity, pregnancy, dehydration, smoking, polycythaemia, anti-phospholipid syndrome, thrombophilia disorders (e.g. protein C deficiency), active malignancy.

EPIDEMIOLOGY   Common, especially in hospitalised patients; exact incidence unknown. Long-term complications of DVT (venous insufficiency, ulceration) affect 0.5% population. Estimated 145 per 100,000.

HISTORY   Asymptomatic or lower limb swelling or tenderness. May present with signs/ symptoms of a pulmonary embolus.

EXAMINATION   Examine for swelling, calf tenderness.
Severe leg oedema and cyanosis (phlegmasia cerulea dolens) is rare.
Respiratory examination for signs of a pulmonary embolus.

Wells Clinical Prediction Score	Score
Lower limb trauma or surgery or immobilisation in a plaster cast	+1
Bedridden for >3 days or surgery within the last 4 weeks	+1
Tenderness along deep venous system	+1
Entire limb swollen	+1
Calf >3 cm bigger circumference; 10 cm below tibial tuberosity	+1
Pitting oedema	+1
Dilated collateral superficial veins (non-varicose)	+1
Malignancy (including treatment up to 6 months previously)	+1
Alternative diagnosis more likely than DVT	−2
Clinical probability of DVT	High >3
	Moderate 1–2
	Low <1

INVESTIGATIONS
Doppler ultrasound: Gold standard. Good sensitivity for femoral veins; less sensitive for calf veins.
Bloods: D-dimers (fibrinogen degradation products) are sensitive but very non-specific and only useful as a negative predictor in low-risk patients. If indicated (e.g. recurrent episodes), a thrombophilia screen should be sent, prior to starting anticoagulation. FBC (platelet count prior to starting heparin), U&E and clotting.
ECG, CXR and ABG: If there is suggestion that there might be PE.

MANAGEMENT
Anticoagulation: Patients should be treated with heparin while awaiting therapeutic INR from warfarin anticoagulation. DVTs not extending above the knee treated with anticoagulation for 3 months, while those extending beyond the knee require anticoagulation for 6 months. Recurrent DVTs may require long-term warfarin. If active anticoagulation is contraindicated and/or high risk of embolisation, placement of an IVC filter, e.g. Greenfield filter, by interventional radiology is indicated to prevent embolus to the lungs.
Prevention: Use of graduated compression stockings. Mobilisation if possible. At-risk groups (immobilised hospital patients) should have prophylactic heparin, e.g. low-molecular-weight heparin if no contraindications.

COMPLICATIONS

Of the disease: Pulmonary embolus, damage to vein valves and chronic venous insufficiency of the lower limb (post-thrombotic syndrome). Rare: Venous infarction (phlegmasia cerulea dolens).

Of the treatment: Heparin-induced thrombocytopaenia, bleeding.

PROGNOSIS   Depends on extent of DVT; below-knee DVTs lower risk of embolus; more proximal DVTs have higher risk of propagation and embolisation, which, if large, may be fatal.

Disseminated intravascular coagulation (DIC)

DEFINITION A disorder of the clotting cascade that can complicate a serious illness. DIC may occur in two forms.
1. Acute overt form where there is bleeding and depletion of platelets and clotting factors.
2. Chronic non-overt form where thromboembolism is accompanied by generalized activation of the coagulation system.

AETIOLOGY
Infection: Particularly Gram-negative sepsis.
Obstetric complications: Missed miscarriage, severe pre-eclampsia, placental abruption, amniotic emboli.
Malignancy: Acute promyelocytic leukaemia (acute DIC); lung, breast, GI malignancy (chronic DIC).
Severe trauma or surgery.
Others: Haemolytic transfusion reaction, burns, severe liver disease, aortic aneurysms, haemangiomas.
Acute DIC: Activation of coagulation is a consequence of endothelial damage and ↑ release of granulocyte/macrophage procoagulant substances e.g. tissue factor (secondary to endotoxin, membrane lipopolysaccharides, cytokines such as IL-6 and TNF-α). Explosive thrombin generation depletes clotting factors and platelets, while simultaneously activating the fibrinolytic system. This leads to bleeding into the subcutaneous tissues, skin and mucous membranes. Occlusion of blood vessels by fibrin in the microcirculation results in microangiopathic haemolytic anaemia and ischaemic organ damage.
Chronic DIC: The process is identical, but at a slower rate with time for compensatory responses, which diminish the likelihood of bleeding but give rise to a hypercoagulable state and thrombosis can occur.

EPIDEMIOLOGY Seen in any severely ill patient.

HISTORY The patient is severely unwell with symptoms of the underlying disease, confusion, dyspnoea and evidence of bleeding.

EXAMINATION Signs of the underlying aetiology, fever, evidence of shock (hypotension, tachycardia).
Acute DIC: Petechiae, purpura, ecchymoses, epistaxis, mucosal bleeding, overt haemorrhage. Signs of end organ damage (e.g. local infarction or gangrene), respiratory distress, oliguria caused by renal failure.
Chronic DIC: Signs of deep venous or arterial thrombosis or embolism, superficial venous thrombosis, especially without varicose veins.

INVESTIGATIONS
Blood: FBC (↓ platelets, ↓ Hb. *Clotting:* ↑ APTT/PT/TT, ↓ fibrinogen, ↑ fibrin degradation products and D-dimers).
Peripheral blood film: Red blood cell fragments (schistocytes). Other investigations according to aetiology.

MANAGEMENT
Treat the underlying disease: Avoid delay and treat vigorously in ITU setting with specialist input.
Acute DIC: Treatment with platelets and coagulation factors in actively bleeding patients or those at high risk for bleeding (e.g. requiring/after invasive procedures/surgery). Platelet transfusions (1–2 units/10 kg/day if platelets $<50 \times 10^9$/L). Fresh frozen plasma or cryoprecipitate if ↑ INR/PT or fibrinogen <50 mg/dL (target fibrinogen >100 mg/dL).
Chronic DIC: If there is thromboembolism, anticoagulate. It is important to be sure that antithrombin level is >80 % for heparin to be effective.

COMPLICATIONS Shock, acute renal failure, ARDS, life-threatening haemorrhage or thrombosis with organ ischaemia/infarction, death.

PROGNOSIS Mortality is high. Prognosis depends on the underlying disease and the severity of the coagulopathy.

Essential thrombocythaemia

DEFINITION   A myeloproliferative disorder characterized by persistently elevated platelet count, not attributable to secondary causes i.e. infection, inflammation, malignancy, haemorrhage, iron deficiency, hyposplenism or trauma.

AETIOLOGY   The cause of proliferation of megakaryocytes and overproduction of platelets is unknown. Very rare familial variants, some associated with mutations in thrombopoietin gene.

EPIDEMIOLOGY   Rare. UK annual incidence ~1 in 100,000. Mean age is 50–60 years but 20 % are <40 years.

HISTORY   May be asymptomatic and diagnosed on routine blood count (20 %).
Venous or arterial thrombosis: e.g. MI, stroke, superficial thrombophlebitis, DVT (Present in 20–50 % at presentation).
Spontaneous haemorrhage: e.g. GI bleeding, epistaxis, bruising.
Headaches, visual disturbance, lightheadedness, atypical chest pain, acral paraesthesia, pruritus (rare).
Erythromelalgia: Characteristic burning sensation felt in the hands or feet, promptly relieved by aspirin.

EXAMINATION   Splenomegaly is present in 30 %, but often the spleen has atrophied because of repeated thrombosis and infarction.
Livedo reticularis.

INVESTIGATIONS   Diagnosis based on exclusion of secondary causes and other myeloproliferative disorders.
Blood: FBC (persistently ↑ platelets > 450 × 10^9/L. About one-third have ↑ red cell count and ↑ WCC, normal MCV). Normal serum ferritin. ↑ Urate and LDH.
Blood film: Platelet anisocytosis (variation in size) with circulating megakaryocyte fragments. There may be signs of hyposplenism (e.g. Howell–Jolly bodies, target cells).
Bone marrow biopsy: Megakaryocytic hyperplasia, absence of bone marrow evidence for a myelodysplastic disorder.
Tests of platelet function: Aggregation in response to adenosine diphosphate, is consistently abnormal and may help distinguish between primary and secondary causes.
Cytogenetics: For Philadelphia chromosome or *BCR-ABL* fusion gene (to exclude myeloid leukaemia).

MANAGEMENT   Treatment strategies are based primarily on the presence or absence of risk factors for thrombosis.
For high-risk patients: Platelet-lowering agents (e.g. hydroxyurea) in combination with low dose aspirin.
High-risk pregnant patient with essential thrombocythaemia are treated with interferon.
Advice: Stop smoking and control obesity, if present.

COMPLICATIONS   Thrombosis, haemorrhage, development of another myeloproliferative disease or transformation to acute leukaemia. For women, ↑ risk of miscarriage and intrauterine growth retardation during pregnancy.

PROGNOSIS   A chronic disease that is often stable for 10–20 years. Risk (<5 %) of transformation to myelofibrosis or acute leukaemia.

Haemolytic uraemic syndrome and thrombotic thrombocytopenic purpura

DEFINITION Triad of microangiopathic haemolytic anaemia, acute renal failure and thrombocytopaenia. There are two forms:
1. D+ (diarrhoea-associated form); and
2. D− (no prodromal illness identified).

Haemolytic uraemic syndrome overlaps with thrombotic thrombocytopenic purpura (TTP) which has the additional features of fever and fluctuating CNS signs.

AETIOLOGY An aetiological factor causing endothelial injury resulting in platelet aggregation, release of unusually large vWF multimers and activation of platelets and the clotting cascade. This results in small vessel thrombosis, particularly the glomerular-afferent arteriole and capillaries, which undergo fibrinoid necrosis. This is followed by renal ischaemia and acute renal failure. The thrombi also promote intravascular haemolysis.

Infection: Verotoxin-producing *Escherichia coli* 0157 (from contaminated water, meat, dairy products), *Shigella*, neuraminidase-producing infections (e.g. pneumococcal respiratory tract infection), HIV.

Drugs: Oral contraceptive pill, ciclosporin, mitomycin, 5-fluorouracil.

Others: Malignant hypertension, malignancy, pregnancy, SLE, scleroderma.

EPIDEMIOLOGY Uncommon, D+ haemolytic uraemic syndrome often affects young children, occurs more often in summer in epidemics and is the most common cause of acute renal failure in children. TTP mainly affects adult females.

HISTORY
GI: Severe abdominal colic, watery diarrhoea that becomes bloodstained.
General: Malaise, fatigue, nausea, fever <38 °C (D+ form).
Renal: Oliguria or anuria, haematuria.

EXAMINATION
General: Pallor (from anaemia), slight jaundice (from haemolysis), bruising (severe thrombocytopaenia), generalized oedema, hypertension and retinopathy.
GI: Abdominal tenderness.
CNS signs: Especially in TTP (weakness, ↓ vision, fits, ↓ consciousness).

INVESTIGATIONS
Blood:
FBC: Normocytic anaemia, ↑ neutrophils, ↓↓ platelets.
U&E: ↑ Urea, creatinine, urate, K+, ↓ Na+.
Clotting: Normal Plt, APTT and fibrinogen levels, abnormality may indicate DIC.
LFT: ↑ Unconjugated bilirubin, ↑ LDH from haemolysis.
Blood cultures
ABG: ↓ pH, ↓ bicarbonate, ↓ PaCO2, normal anion gap.
Blood film: Fragmented red blood cells, ↑ reticulocytes, spherocytes.

Urine: >1 g protein/24 h, haematuria, fractional excretion Na+ >1 %.
Stool samples: Light and electron microscopy, culture.
Renal biopsy: Contraindicated in severe thrombocytopaenia. In cases of diagnostic doubt:
D+ form: Arteriolar necrosis, glomerular capillary thrombosis.
D − form: Intimal proliferation in arterioles.

MANAGEMENT Requires specialist supportive management.
Medical: Treat hypovolaemia (from diarrhoea, vomiting, capillary leak), control hypertension, IV fluids and furosemide (frusemide) may establish diuresis and prevent the need for dialysis. Haemodialysis if severe uraemia, hyperkalaemia, acidosis. Blood transfusion for anaemia. Plasma exchange and FFP infusions may be required.

Haemolytic uraemic syndrome and thrombotic thrombocytopenic purpura (continued)

TTP: Plasma exchange and FFP infusions have clinical efficacy; For refractory cases, consider steroids, vincristine, splenectomy and antiplatelet agents.

COMPLICATIONS   Neurological complications, hyperkalaemia.

D+ form: GI infarction, acute tubular necrosis, acute or chronic renal failure.

D− form: Cardiomyopathy, malignant hypertension.

PROGNOSIS   Most children with D+ form recover. Adults have a poorer outcome with 70 % having complete recovery; $\sim$ 17% remain dialysis-dependent; 7% overall mortality (often with CNS involvement). Mortality is higher in TTP.

Haemophilia

DEFINITION   Bleeding diatheses resulting from an inherited deficiency of a clotting factor. Three subtypes:
1. **Haemophilia A**: (most common). Caused by a deficiency in factor VIII.
2. **Haemophilia B**: Caused by a deficiency in factor IX (Christmas disease).
3. **Haemophilia C**: (rare). Caused by a deficiency in factor XI.

AETIOLOGY   Haemophilia A and B exhibit X-linked recessive inheritance. A variety of genetic mutations in the factor VIII and XI genes have been described. 30 % of cases are new mutations.
Factor VIII is a vital co-factor in the intrinsic pathway of the coagulation cascade. Activated factor IX activates factor X (converts factor X → Xa).

EPIDEMIOLOGY   Incidence of haemophilia A is ~1 in 5–10,000 males and for haemophilia B is 1 in 25–30,000 males. Haemophilia C is more common in Ashkenazi Jews.

HISTORY   Symptoms usually begin from early childhood.
Swollen painful joints occurring spontaneously or with minimal trauma (haemarthroses). Painful bleeding into muscles. Haematuria. Excessive bruising or bleeding after surgery or trauma.
Female carriers usually asymptomatic, but may have low-enough levels to cause excess bleeding after trauma.

EXAMINATION
Multiple bruises.
Muscle haematomas. Haemarthroses. Joint deformity.
Nerve palsies (nerve compression by haematoma).
Signs of iron-deficiency anaemia.

INVESTIGATIONS   Clotting screen (↑ APTT, reflects the activity of the intrinsic and the common pathway), coagulation factor assays (↓ factor VIII, IX or XI depending on condition; *see* Definition).
Other investigations according to complications (e.g. arthroscopy).

MANAGEMENT   Specialist management and follow-up at a haemophilia centre.
Mild haemophilia A (factor VIII ≥ 10 % of normal)**:** Intranasal or IV DDAVP (vasopressin analogue) ↑ circulating factor VIII levels via release from endothelial storage sites. Alternatively, oral transexamic acid (a fibrinolytic inhibitor) can be used.
Moderate to severe haemophilia: Transfusion with factor VIII or IX concentrate (depending on haemophilia subtype) is needed to maintain levels at 20–50 % of normal.
Following haemorrhage, the desired factor level depends on the severity and location of the bleeding episode e.g. early joint or muscle bleeding episodes are treated to achieve factor levels of 30–40 %. In severe bleeding, intracranial or intra-abdominal haemorrhage or bleeding in face, neck, and hip, or preoperatively, more rigorous transfusion to 80–100% of normal is necessary.
Treatment of complications: Specialist referral for complications. A short course of prednisolone may be used to reduce the pain and swelling associated with joint haemorrhage.
Advice: Avoid antiplatelet drugs (e.g. aspirin), IM injections and contact sports. Hepatitis A and B vaccination. Medicalert card or bracelet.
Genetic counselling for patient and family.

COMPLICATIONS   Severe and fatal haemorrhage. Crippling joint deformity.
10–15 % of patients develop antibodies to the clotting factor (particularly recipients of factor VIII). Hepatitis C and HIV infection in patients who received clotting concentrates before 1985 in developed countries.

PROGNOSIS   The availability of safer blood products and home treatment programmes mean that most people with haemophilia can lead a relatively normal life.

Immune thrombocytopenic purpura (ITP)

DEFINITION Syndrome characterized by immune destruction of platelets resulting in bruising or a bleeding tendency.

AETIOLOGY Often idiopathic. Acute ITP is usually seen after a viral infection in children, while the chronic form is more common in adults. May be associated with infections (malaria, EBV, HIV), autoimmune diseases (e.g. SLE, thyroid disease), malignancies and drugs (e.g. quinine). Autoantibodies that bind to platelet membrane proteins (glycoprotein IIb/IIIa and Ib/IX) results in thrombocytopaenia.

EPIDEMIOLOGY Acute ITP presents in children between 2 and 7 years. Chronic ITP is seen in adults, four times more common in women.

HISTORY Easy bruising, mucosal bleeding, menorrhagia, epistaxis.

EXAMINATION Visible petechiae, bruises (purpura or ecchymoses).
Typically, signs of other illness (e.g. infections, wasting, splenomegaly) would suggest other causes.

INVESTIGATIONS
Diagnosis of exclusion: Exclude myelodysplasia, acute leukaemia, marrow infiltration.
Blood: FBC ($\downarrow$ platelets), clotting screen (normal PT, APTT, fibrinogen), autoantibodies (antiplatelet antibody may be present but not used routinely for diagnosis, anticardiolipin antibody, antinuclear antibody).
Blood film: To rule out 'pseudothrombocytopaenia' caused by platelet clumping giving falsely low counts.
Bone marrow: To exclude other pathology. Normal or $\uparrow$ megakaryocytes.

MANAGEMENT
Oral corticosteroids.
Second-line therapy: IV infusion of immunoglobulin (IVIG). Platelet transfusions are usually contraindicated unless there is severe bleeding. In refractory cases, other immunosuppressants (e.g. azathioprine) may be used.
Surgery: Splenectomy has a 60 % cure rate in carefully selected patients.

COMPLICATIONS Mucosal bleeding. Major haemorrhage is rare (<1 %).

PROGNOSIS
Usually self-limiting in children, with platelets recovering within 1–2 months. ITP is less likely to resolve spontaneously in adults, but can be controlled medically in 60–90 % of cases.

Leukaemia, acute lymphoblastic (ALL)

DEFINITION   Malignancy of the bone marrow and blood characterized by the proliferation of lymphoblasts (primitive lymphoid cells).

AETIOLOGY   Lymphoblasts (arrested at an early stage of development with varying cytogenetic abnormalities, gene mutations and chromosome translocations) undergo malignant transformation and proliferation, with subsequent replacement of normal marrow elements, leading to bone marrow failure and infiltration into other tissues.
Associations/Risk factors Environmental (radiation, viruses). Genetic (Down's syndrome, neurofibromatosis type 1, Fanconi's anaemia, achondroplasia, ataxia telangiectasia, xeroderma pigmentosum, X-linked agammaglobulinaemia, ↑ risk in siblings).

EPIDEMIOLOGY   Most common malignancy of childhood. The peak incidence occurs between 2 and 5 years of age. Second peak in the elderly. Annual UK incidence is 1 in 70,000.

HISTORY
Symptoms of bone marrow failure: Anaemia (fatigue, dyspnoea), bleeding (spontaneous bruising, bleeding gums, menorrhagia), opportunistic infections (bacterial, viral, fungal, protozoal).
Symptoms of organ infiltration: Tender bones, enlarged lymph nodes, mediastinal compression (in T-cell ALL), meningeal involvement (headache, visual disturbances, nausea).

EXAMINATION
Signs of bone marrow failure: Pallor, bruising, bleeding, infection (e.g. fever, GI, skin, respiratory systems).
Signs of organ infiltration: Lymphadenopathy, hepatosplenomegaly, cranial nerve palsies, retinal haemorrhage or papilloedema on fundoscopy, leukaemic infiltration of the anterior chamber of the eye (mimics hypopyon), testicular swelling.

INVESTIGATIONS
Blood: FBC (normochromic normocytic anaemia, ↓ platelets, variable WCC), ↑ uric acid, ↑ LDH, clotting screen.
Blood film: Lymphoblasts evident.
Bone marrow aspirate or trephine biopsy: Hypercellular with >30 % lymphoblasts.
Morphologic classification(French–American–British classification):
L_1: Small lymphoblasts, scanty cytoplasm.
L_2: Larger, heterogenous lymphoblasts.
L_3: Large lymphoblasts with blue or vacuolated cytoplasm.
Immunophenotyping: Using antibodies for cell surface antigens e.g. CD20.
Cytogenetics: Karyotyping chromosomal abnormalities or translocations.
Cytochemistry: B- and T-lineage cells show up with PAS stain and acid phosphatase, respectively.
Lumbar puncture (and CSF analysis): For CNS involvement.
CXR: May show mediastinal lymphadenopathy, thymic enlargement, lytic bone lesions.
Bone radiographs: Mottled appearance with 'punched-out' lesions (e.g. skull caused by leukaemic infiltration).

MANAGEMENT   Combination chemotherapy.
Remission induction: Prednisolone, vincristine, L-asparaginase (3–4 weeks).
Intensification or consolidation: Addition of cytosine arabinoside, daunorubicin.
Prophylaxis of CNS involvement: Intrathecal methotrexate, cranial irradiation now rarely used.
Maintenance (2–3 years): 6-Mercaptopurine, methotrexate, vincristine or prednisolone. Stem cell transplantation.

Leukaemia, acute lymphoblastic (ALL) (continued)

Supportive care: Antiemetics, central venous access (many chemotherapy agents need a central vein), blood product replacement, infection prophylaxis, counselling (especially in children, but also family).

COMPLICATIONS

Secondary to treatment: Tumour lysis syndrome (*see* AML, 'Complications').

Long-term sequelae of chemotherapy: Cardiotoxicity, fertility problems, malignancy (intracranial tumours, non-Hodgkin's lymphoma).

PROGNOSIS   Childhood ALL has a cure rate of ~80 %. Adult ALL has a cure rate of ~30%.

Poor prognosis: Age (<2 years, >10 years), males, ↑ WCC (>50×10^9/L), cytogenetics: translocation (4,11), translocation (9,22), T-cell phenotype, CNS involvement at presentation.

Good prognosis: Translocation (12,21).

Leukaemia, acute myeloblastic (AML)

DEFINITION   Malignancy of primitive myeloid lineage white blood cells (myeloblasts) with proliferation in the bone marrow and blood.

Classified using the FAB (French–American–British) system into eight morphological variants M0–M7.

M0 Myeloblastic with no maturation.

M1 Myeloblastic with little maturation.

M2 Myeloblastic with maturation.

M3 Promyelocytic with coarse cytoplasmic granules. Characteristic Auer rods (crystallisation of granules resembling bundle of sticks or 'faggots'). Associated with DIC.

M4 Granulocytic and monocytic differentiation (myelomonocytic).

M5 Monoblastic differentiation.

M6 Erythroblastic differentiation.

M7 Megakaryoblastic.

AETIOLOGY   Myeloblasts, arrested at an early stage of development, with varying cytogenetic abnormalities (e.g. gene mutations and chromosome translocations), undergo malignant transformation and proliferation, with subsequent replacement of normal marrow elements, bone marrow failure.

EPIDEMIOLOGY   Most common acute leukaemia in adults. Incidence ↑ with age.

HISTORY

Symptoms of bone marrow failure: Anaemia (lethargy, dyspnoea), bleeding (thrombocytopaenia or DIC), opportunistic or recurrent infections.

Symptoms of tissue infiltration: Gum swelling or bleeding, CNS involvement (headaches, nausea, diplopia), especially with M4 and M5 variants.

EXAMINATION

Signs of bone marrow failure: Pallor, cardiac flow murmur, ecchymoses, bleeding, opportunistic or recurrent infections (e.g. fever, mouth ulcers, skin infections, PCP).

Signs of tissue infiltration: Skin rashes, gum hypertrophy, deposit of leukaemic blasts may rarely be seen in the eye (chloroma), tongue and bone – in the latter may cause fractures.

INVESTIGATIONS

Blood: FBC (↓ Hb, ↓ platelets, variable WCC).

↑ Uric acid, ↑ LDH, clotting studies, fibrinogen and D-dimers (when DIC is suspected in M3).

Blood film: AML blasts may show cytoplasmic granules or Auer rods.

Bone marrow aspirate or biopsy: Hypercellular with >30 % blasts (immature cells).

Immunophenotyping: Antibodies against surface antigens to classify lineage of abnormal clones.

Cytogenetics: For diagnostic and prognostic information.

Immunocytochemistry: Myeloblasts granules are positive for Sudan black, chloroacetate esterase and myeloperoxidase, monoblasts are positive for non-specific and butyrate esterase.

MANAGEMENT

Emergency (if DIC): FFP and platelet transfusions (*see* Disseminated intravascular coagulation).

Chemotherapy: Combination cytotoxic chemotherapy (e.g. cytosine arabinoside, daunorubicin, etoposide [topoisomerase inhibitor]). In the M3 variant, all *trans*-retinoic acid is given, as it induces differentiation of the cells involved.

Stem cell transplantation.

Supportive care: Central venous access, blood products, treatment and prophylaxis of infection.

Leukaemia, acute myeloblastic (AML) (continued)

COMPLICATIONS Relapse, sequelae of chemotherapy: infertility, cardiotoxicity, malignancy.

Tumour lysis syndrome(TLS): Rapid cell death with initiation of chemotherapy resulting in hyperkalaemia, hyperphosphataemia, secondary hypocalcaemia, hyperuricaemia, and acute renal failure.

TLS prophylaxis: Good hydration.

If at high risk (WCC $> 50 \times 10^9$/L)**:** Rasburicase (recombinant urate-oxidase, which converts uric acid to an inactive metabolite). Screen for G6PD deficiency prior to administration of rasburicase. Allopurinol for intermediate risk (WCC $= 10$–50×10^9/L).

PROGNOSIS Prognosis depends on age. Overall cure rate is 40–50 % in those <60-years-old on chemotherapy, but may be higher with bone marrow transplantation. 5–10 % long-term survival in those >60-years-old.

Good prognosis: t(8,21) in M2, t(15,17) in M3, inversion 16 in M4 (70–90 % cure rate).

Poor prognosis: Monosomy 5, monosomy 7 and complex karyotypes (10–30 % cure rate).

Leukaemia, chronic lymphocytic (CLL)

DEFINITION   Characterized by progressive accumulation of functionally incompetent lymphocytes, which are monoclonal in origin. There is an overlap between CLL and non-Hodgkin's lymphomas.

AETIOLOGY   Malignant cells may accumulate as a result of their inability to undergo apoptosis (partly due to overexpression of *BCL2* and *Fas*-inhibitory molecules e.g. TOSO). Most common chromosomal changes include trisomy 12, 11q and 13q deletions. Both *BCL-2*, a proto-oncogene, and p53, a tumour suppressor gene, contribute to the biologic behavior of B-CLL cells. Overexpression of certain microRNAs (small non-coding RNAs that modulate the expression of genes at the post-transcriptional level) may predispose to CLL.

EPIDEMIOLOGY   90% are >50 years, $\male > \female$. Rare in Asians.

HISTORY
Asymptomatic: Up to 40–50 % diagnosed on routine blood count.
Systemic symptoms: Lethargy, malaise, night sweats.
Symptoms of bone marrow failure: Recurrent infections (bacterial, viral, fungal), herpes zoster, easy bruising or bleeding (e.g. epistaxis). Assess the patient's performance status and comorbidities.

EXAMINATION   Non-tender lymphadenopathy (often symmetrical), hepatomegaly, splenomegaly.
Later stages, signs of bone marrow failure: Pallor, cardiac flow murmur, purpura/ ecchymoses.

INVESTIGATIONS   CLL may be associated with autoimmune phenomena: Haemolytic anaemia (10 %), thrombocytopaenia or a combination of both (Evan's syndrome).
Blood: FBC (gross lymphocytosis, 5–300 × 10^9/L, anaemia, ↓ platelets). Anaemia may be due to bone marrow infiltration, hypersplenism or autoimmune haemolysis. ↓Serum immunoglobulins.
Blood film: Small lymphocytes with thin rims of cytoplasm and smudge/smear cells.
Bone marrow aspirate or biopsy: Lymphocytic replacement (25–95 %) of normal marrow elements. Immunophenotyping shows the malignant cell to be a relatively mature B cell with weak surface expression of monoclonal IgM or IgD (kappa or lambda light chain only). T-cell variants of CLL are much rarer but more aggressive. 'Hairy cell leukaemia' is a low-grade CLL variant with good prognosis showing monoclonal proliferation of 'hairy' B cells in blood, bone marrow and liver.
Cytogenetics: Provides some prognostic information.
CT (chest, abdomen, and pelvis): On the basis of the patient's symptoms.
Staging:
Rai:
0 Lymphocytosis.
I Above, plus lymphadenopathy.
II Above, plus organomegaly (hepatomegaly or splenomegaly).
III Above, plus anaemia (Hb < 10 g/dL).
IV Above, plus thrombocytopaenia (platelets < 100 × 10^9/L).

Binet:
A < 3 lymphoid areas (neck/axilla/groin lymph nodes, liver or spleen involvement).
B > 3 lymphoid areas.
C Anaemia and/or thrombocytopaenia.

MANAGEMENT
Early asymptomatic stage disease: Watch and wait. Therapy is indicated for patients with advanced stage disease, disease-related symptoms, or repeated infections.

Leukaemia, chronic lymphocytic (CLL) (continued)

Chemotherapy: Traditionally, oral chlorambucil (alkylating agent). More recently: fludarabine + rituximab (anti-CD20 monoclonal antibody).

Side effect: ↓ CD4 cell count, hence co-trimoxazole prophylaxis.

Alemtuzumab (anti-CD52 monoclonal antibody) and bendamustine have superior response rates compared with chlorambucil.

Other: Prednisolone for autoimmune phenomena. Immunoglobulin replacement. Antibiotic prophylaxis, blood products, splenectomy (in massive splenomegaly and hypersplenism).

Haematopoietic cell transplantation: May be considered for patients with relapsed disease.

COMPLICATIONS Up to 15 % transform into a localized high-grade non-Hodgkin's lymphoma (Richter's transformation) or prolymphocytic leukaemia.[1] Chemotherapy complications including infusion-related reactions and tumor lysis syndrome.

PROGNOSIS Wide variation in prognosis, best for early stage disease. 11q and 17p deletions are associated with poor survival. Infections with Gram-negative and encapsulated organisms are the most frequent cause of morbidity and mortality in CLL.

---

[1]Prolymphocytic leukaemia is characterized by larger malignant cells with prominent nucleoli, very high lymphocyte count, massive splenomegaly with little lymphadenopathy. Poor response to treatment.

Leukaemia, chronic myeloid (CML)

DEFINITION   Chronic myeloblastic leukaemia is a malignant clonal disease characterized by proliferation of granulocyte precursors in the bone marrow and blood, distinguished from AML by its slower progression.

AETIOLOGY   Malignant proliferation of stem cells with characteristic (95 % of cases) chromosomal translocation t(9;22) resulting in the Philadelphia (Ph) chromosome. Variants include Ph-negative CML, chronic neutrophilic leukaemia and eosinophilic leukaemia.

Pathology/Pathogenesis The Ph chromosome results in the fusion of the genes *BCR* and *ABL*. This results in transcription of a 210-kDa protein (*BCR-ABL*) with enhanced tyrosine kinase activity that drives cell replication.

Three phases: Relatively stable chronic phase of variable duration (average of 4–6 years), which transforms into an accelerated phase (3–9 months) and then an acute leukaemia phase (blast transformation).

EPIDEMIOLOGY   Incidence increases with age, mean 40–60 years. Four times more common in males.

HISTORY   Asymptomatic in up to 40–50 % and is diagnosed on routine blood count.

Hypermetabolic symptoms: Weight loss, malaise, sweating.

Bone marrow failure symptoms: Lethargy, dyspnoea, easy bruising, epistaxis (infection is rare).

Abdominal discomfort and early satiety.

Occasionally presents with gout or hyperviscosity symptoms (visual disturbance, headaches, priapism).

May present during blast crisis with symptoms of AML or ALL.

EXAMINATION

Splenomegaly: Most common physical finding (90 %).

Signs of bone marrow failure: Pallor, cardiac flow murmur, bleeding or ecchymoses.

INVESTIGATIONS

Blood: FBC (grossly ↑ WCC, ↓ Hb, ↑ basophils/eosinophils/neutrophils, ↑ platelets but may be normal or ↓). Also ↑ uric acid, ↓ neutrophil alkaline phosphatase, ↑ vitamin B_{12} and B_{12}-binding protein (transcobalamin I).

Blood film: Shows immature granulocytes in peripheral blood.

Bone marrow aspirate or biopsy: Hypercellular with raised myeloid–erythroid ratio.

Cytogenetics to demonstrate Ph chromosome.

MANAGEMENT

Chronic phase: Hydroxyurea or interferon-α, with allopurinol to prevent hyperuricaemia and gout.

Specific treatment: Imatinib and Dasatinib (tyrosine kinase inhibitors) act as inhibitors of *BCR-ABL*.

Stem cell transplantation: Allogeneic or autogenous.

Acute phase: (*see* Leukaemia, acute myeloblastic and Leukaemia, acute lymphoblastic).

COMPLICATIONS   Transformation into acute leukemia (80 % AML, 20 % ALL).

PROGNOSIS   Prognostic staging system of Sokal distinguishes between good and poor risk groups on the basis of age, spleen size, percentage of blasts in blood and platelet count. Overall mean survival 5–6 years, with main cause of death transformation into acute leukaemia. Up to 20 % survive >10 years.

Hodgkin's lymphoma

DEFINITION   Lymphomas are neoplasms of lymphoid cells, originating in lymph nodes or other lymphoid tissues. Hodgkin's lymphoma (~15% of lymphomas) is diagnosed histo-pathologically by the presence of Reed–Sternberg cells (a cell of B-lymphoid lineage).

AETIOLOGY   Unknown. Likely to be a result of an environmental trigger in a genetically susceptible individual. EBV genome has been detected in ~50% of Hodgkin's lymphomas, but role in pathogenesis unclear.

EPIDEMIOLOGY   Bimodal age distribution, with peaks 20–30 years and >50 years. More common in males. Annual European incidence is 2–5 in 100,000.

HISTORY   Painless enlarging mass (most often in neck, occasionally in axilla or groin). May become painful after alcohol ingestion.
'B' symptoms: Fevers >38 °C (if cyclical referred to as Pel–Ebstein fever).
Night sweats.
Weight loss >10% body weight in last 6 months.
Other: Pruritus, cough or dyspnoea with intrathoracic disease.

EXAMINATION
Non-tender firm rubbery lymphadenopathy: Cervical, axillary or inguinal.
Splenomegaly, occasionally hepatomegaly.
Skin excoriations.
Signs of intrathoracic disease (e.g. pleural effusion, superior vena cava obstruction).

INVESTIGATIONS
Blood:
FBC: Anaemia of chronic disease, leucocytosis, ↑ neutrophils, ↑ eosinophils. Lymphopaenia with advanced disease. ↑ ESR and CRP, LFT (↑ LDH, ↑ transaminases if liver involved).
Lymph node biopsy
Bone marrow aspirate and trephine biopsy: Involvement seen only in very advanced disease.
Imaging: CXR, CT of thorax, abdomen and pelvis, gallium scan, PET scans.
Staging (Ann Arbor):
I Single lymph node region.
II Two or more lymph node regions on one side of the diaphragm.
III Lymph node regions involved on both sides of diaphragm.
IV Extranodal involvement (liver or bone marrow).
A Absence.
B Presence of B symptoms.
E Localized extranodal extension.
S Involvement of spleen.

Histological subtypes:
1. Nodular sclerosing (70%);
2. Mixed cellularity (20%);
3. Lymphocyte predominant (5%);
4. Lymphocyte depleted (5%).

The Reed–Sternberg cell is pathognomonic. It is a large cell with abundant pale cytoplasm and two or more oval lobulated nuclei containing prominent 'owl-eye' eosinophilic nucleoli (can appear as lacunar or 'popcorn' cells).

MANAGEMENT
Stages I and IIA: Radiotherapy (e.g. 'mantle' field above the diaphragm, 'inverted Y' below the diaphragm) with or without adjuvant chemotherapy.

Stages III and IV: Cyclical chemotherapy (e.g. ABVD regimen of Adriamycin, bleomycin, vinblastine and dacarbazine) with or without adjuvant radiotherapy.

Stem cell transplantation for relapsed disease.

COMPLICATIONS

Secondary malignancy after treatment: Acute myeloid leukaemia (1% at 10 years), non-Hodgkin's lymphoma or solid tumours.

Inverted Y irradiation: Infertility, premature menopause, skin cancers.

Mantle irradiation: Adverse effects on thyroid, cardiac (accelerated coronary artery disease), pulmonary function (fibrosis), skin cancer.

PROGNOSIS

Stages I and II: 80–90% cure rate.

Stages III and IV: 50–70% cure rate.

Prognosis less good with B symptoms, older age or lymphocyte-depleted type.

Lymphoma, non-Hodgkin's (NHL)

DEFINITION   Lymphomas are malignancies of lymphoid cells originating in lymph nodes or other lymphoid tissues. Non-Hodgkin's lymphomas (NHL) are a diverse group consisting of 85% B cell, 15% T cell and NK cell forms, ranging from indolent to aggressive disease and referred to as low, intermediate and high grades.

NHL may be classified according to the Revised European-American Lymphoma (REAL) classification on the basis of clinical, biological and histological criteria. The WHO Classification, published in 2001 and updated in 2008, is considered the latest classification of lymphoma.

AETIOLOGY   Complex process involving the accumulation of multiple genetic lesions (activation of oncogenes by chromosomal translocations and inactivation of tumour suppressor genes by chromosomal deletions or mutations). The genome in certain lymphoma subtypes has been altered by the introduction of foreign genes via a number of oncogenic viruses: EBV has been detected in cases of Burkitt's lymphoma and of AIDS-associated lymphomas. HTLV-1 has been implicated in adult T-cell lymphoma/leukaemia (ATLL). HHV-8 infection is detected in body-cavity-based lymphomas.

Other factors associated with the development of NHL include radiotherapy, immunosuppressive agents, chemotherapy, HIV, HBV, HCV, connective tissue diseases e.g. SLE, and inherited and acquired immunodeficiency syndromes.

EPIDEMIOLOGY   Incidence ↑ with age. More common in males. More common in the West.

HISTORY
Painless enlarging mass: Often in neck, axilla or groin.

Systemic symptoms (less frequent than in Hodgkin's)**:** Fever, night sweats, weight loss > 10 % body weight, symptoms of hypercalcaemia.

Symptoms related to organ involvement (extranodal disease is more common in NHL than in Hodgkin's lymphoma)**:** Skin rashes, headache, sore throat, abdominal discomfort, testicular swelling. Establish the performance status of the patient.

EXAMINATION
Painless firm rubbery lymphadenopathy: Cervical, axillary or inguinal. Oropharyngeal (Waldeyer's ring of lymph nodes) involvement.

Skin rashes: Mycosis fungoides (well-defined indurated scaly plaque-like lesions with raised ulcerated nodules caused by cutaneous T-cell lymphoma) and Sezary's syndrome.

Abdominal mass.

Hepatosplenomegaly.

Signs of bone marrow involvement: Anaemia, infections or purpura.

INVESTIGATIONS
Blood: FBC (anaemia, neutropaenia and thrombocytopaenia if bone marrow involved), U&Es, uric acid, ↑ ESR and CRP, ↑ LDH, LFTs (↑ transaminases with liver involvement), Ca^{2+} (may be ↑). HIV, HBV and HCV serology (in select patients).

Blood film: Lymphoma cells may be visible in some patients.

Bone marrow aspiration and biopsy.

Imaging: CXR, CT thorax, abdomen, pelvis. CT plus PET scanning is of particular value for evaluation of extranodal involvement.

Lymph node biopsy: Histopathologic evaluation, immunophenotyping, cytogenetics.

Staging: As for Hodgkin's.

MANAGEMENT   The histology and extent of disease must be known.

Aggressive: *Early stage (stages I or II) or localized:* Short-course (3 cycles) of CHOP plus rituximab (for CD20+ disease) followed by locoregional radiation therapy. CHOP chemotherapy includes cyclophosphamide, hydroxy daunorubicin, oncovincristine and prednisolone. Rituximab is a monoclonal antibody directed against the CD20 antigen on B-lymphocytes, which regulates cell cycle initiation.

Advanced (stage III or IV) or *bulky disease:* 6–8 cycles of CHOP or CHOP-like chemotherapy plus rituximab for CD20+ disease.

Indolent: Conservative approach ('watch and wait'). Single agent chemotherapy, radiotherapy or combined modality treatment.

Relapse: Autologous or allogeneic stem cell transplantation.

Baseline echocardiogram if considering daunorubicin, and pulmonary function studies if considering bleomycin.

Discuss fertility issues prior to treatment. Consider sperm or fertilized ovum banking.

COMPLICATIONS

Resulting from treatment: Bone marrow suppression, nausea and vomiting, mucositis, infertility, tumour lysis syndrome, secondary malignancies.

PROGNOSIS   Dependent on histological type. Other factors include age, stage, extranodal sites and LDH level.

Multiple myeloma

DEFINITION Haematological malignancy characterized by proliferation of plasma cells resulting in bone lesions and production of a monoclonal immunoglobulin (paraprotein, usually IgG or IgA).

AETIOLOGY Unknown. Postulated viral trigger. Chromosomal aberrations are frequent, certain cytokines (e.g. IL-6) act as potent growth factors for plasma cell proliferation. Associated with ionizing radiation, agricultural work or occupational chemical exposures (benzene).

EPIDEMIOLOGY Annual incidence is 4 in 100,000, peak incidence in 70-year-olds. Afro-Caribbeans > white people > Asians.

HISTORY May be diagnosed incidentally on routine blood tests.
Bone pain: Often in back, ribs. Sudden and severe if caused by pathological fracture or vertebral collapse.
Infections: Often recurrent.
General: Tiredness, thirst, polyuria, nausea, constipation, mental change (resulting from hypercalcaemia).
Hyperviscocity: Bleeding, headaches, visual disturbance.

EXAMINATION Pallor, tachycardia, flow murmur, signs of heart failure, dehydration.
Purpura, hepatosplenomegaly, macroglossia, carpal tunnel syndrome and peripheral neuropathies.

INVESTIGATIONS
Blood: FBC ($\downarrow$ Hb, normochromic normocytic), $\uparrow$ ESR, $\uparrow$ CRP (CRP may be normal with elevated ESR), U&E ($\uparrow$ creatinine, $\uparrow$ Ca^{2+} in 45%), typically normal AlkPhos.
Blood film: Rouleaux formation with bluish background ($\uparrow$ protein).
Serum or urine electrophoresis: Serum paraprotein (two-thirds IgG, one-third IgA), Bence–Jones protein (free light chains, $\varkappa$ or λ in 70% cases).
Bone marrow aspirate and trephine: $\uparrow$ Plasma cells (identified as large cells with a perinuclear halo, eccentric nuclei, blue cytoplasm) – usually >20%.
Chest, pelvic or vertebral X-ray: Osteolytic lesions without surrounding sclerosis. Pathological fractures.

MANAGEMENT
Emergency: Rehydration. Consider dialysis and/or plasmapheresis. Radiotherapy if there is bone pain or cord compression. Treat pathological fractures normally.
Medical: Treatment will depend on stage of disease and symptoms. Asymptomatic disease is treated with monitoring and bisphosphonates.
Symptomatic disease may be treated with chemotherapy and renal support. Commonly used regimens:
• Melphalan and prednisolone (50–60% respond),
• VAD regimen (vincristine, adriamycin, dexamethasone), or
• Lenalidomide (thalidomide-analogue) or Bortezomib (proteasome inhibitor) may be suitable for those with relapsed disease.

Interferon-α may prolong remission phase achieved by chemotherapy.
Bone marrow or stem cell transplantation: May be considered in selected patients combined with high-dose chemotherapy.

COMPLICATIONS Pathological fractures, renal failure (in up to one-third of patients), spinal cord compression, carpal tunnel syndrome and polyneuropathies (amyloidosis).

PROGNOSIS Median survival is 4–6 years from diagnosis. Important prognostic parameters are β2-microglobulin, plasma cell labelling index, CRP, creatinine and age. Monosomy of chromosome 13 associated with poor prognosis.

Durie–Salmon staging: Based on serum Hb, immunoglobulin, Ca^{2+}, creatinine levels and number of radiographical bone lesions on the skeletal survey.

---

* **Monoclonal Gammopathy of Undetermined Significance (MGUS)** is distinct from multiple myeloma and is characterised by an accumulation of plasma cells derived from a single abnormal clone with no evidence of bone lesions, renal disease or hypercalcaemia. May progress to multiple myeloma, B-cell lymphoma or Waldenström's macroglobulinaemia.

Myelodysplastic syndromes

DEFINITION A series of haematologic conditions characterized by chronic cytopaenia (anaemia, neutropaenia, thrombocytopaenia) and abnormal cellular maturation.

Five subgroups	% Blasts in bone marrow
Refractory anaemia (RA)	<5
RA with ringed sideroblasts (RARS)	<5 (> 15 % RS)
RA with excess blasts (RAEB)	5–20
Chronic myelomonocytic leukaemia (CMML)	Up to 20% plus peripheral blood monocyte count >1 × 10^9/L
RAEB in transformation (RAEB-t)	21–30

AETIOLOGY May be primary, or arise in patients who have received chemotherapy or radiotherapy for previous malignancies. Patients may have chromosomal abnormalities – deletions (e.g. partial or total loss of chromosomes 5, 7, 20 or Y), monosomy 7, trisomy 8 or complex karyotypes with multiple abnormalities.

EPIDEMIOLOGY Mean age diagnosis is 65–75 years, more common in males. Twice as common as AML.

HISTORY May be asymptomatic and diagnosed after routine blood count (50%).
Symptoms of bone marrow failure: Anaemia (fatigue, dizziness), neutropaenia (recurrent infections), thrombocytopaenia (easy bruising, epistaxis).
Ask about risk factors (occupational exposure to toxic chemicals, prior chemotherapy or radiotherapy).

EXAMINATION
Signs of bone marrow failure: Anaemia (pallor, cardiac flow murmur), neutropaenia (infections), thrombocytopaenia (purpura or ecchymoses). Gum hypertrophy and lymphadenopathy. Spleen not enlarged, except in CMML.

INVESTIGATIONS
Blood: FBC (pancytopaenia).
Blood film: Normocytic or macrocytic red cells, ovalomacrocytosis, variable microcytic red cells in RARS, ↓ granulocytes, granulocytes display ↓ or absent granulation and bilobed ('Pelgeroid') nucleus, ↑ monocytes (CMML), myeloblasts.
Bone marrow aspirate or biopsy: Hypercellularity, ringed sideroblasts (haemosiderin deposits in the mitochondria of erythroid precursors form an apparent ring around the nucleus) with dyserythropoietic features, abnormal granulocyte precursors and mega-karyocytes. 10 % show marrow fibrosis.

MANAGEMENT
Supportive treatment: Red cell and platelet transfusions, antibiotics, haematopoietic growth factors (e.g. erythropoietin, granulocyte colony-stimulating factor).
Immunosuppressive regimen (ciclosporin, antithymocyte globulin)**:** For patients with hypocellular or normocellular bone marrows, particularly those who are HLA– DR2 positive.
Iron chelation: For patients with prolonged red cell transfusion requirements and iron overload.
Chemotherapy: Hypomethylating agents –azacitidine or decitabine in patients with intermediate or high International Prognosis Scoring System (IPSS) scores. High-intensity anti-leukaemic therapy may be used for patients <60, >10% bone marrow blasts, good performance status and normal cytogenetics. Hydroxyurea for CMML.

Allogenic haematopoietic cell transplantation: For patients <60 years with an HLA-matched sibling or unrelated donor (improves survival).

COMPLICATIONS Pancytopaenia may result in opportunistic infections and haemorrhage. Approximately 20 % progress to acute leukaemia. Iron overload can result from repeated transfusion.

PROGNOSIS Survival is adversely affected by ↑ age, cytopaenias, percentage of blasts in the bone marrow and abnormal karyotype (particularly complex karyotypes). Among patients with an abnormal karyotype, the outcome is more favourable for del(5q) or del(20q).

Myelofibrosis

DEFINITION   Disorder of haematopoietic stem cells characterized by progressive marrow fibrosis in association with extramedullary haematopoiesis and splenomegaly.

AETIOLOGY   Primary stem cell defect is not known, but results in increased numbers of abnormal megakaryocytes (platelet precursor cells) with stromal proliferation as a secondary reactive phenomenon to growth factors from the megakaryocytes. ~30% of patients have previous history of polycythaemia rubra vera or essential thrombocythaemia.

EPIDEMIOLOGY   Rare. Annual incidence ~0.4 in 100 000. Peak onset 50–70 years.

HISTORY
Asymptomatic: Diagnosed after abnormal blood count.
Systemic symptoms:
Common: Weight loss, anorexia, fever and night sweats, pruritus.
Uncommon: Left upper quadrant abdominal pain, indigestion (caused by massive splenomegaly).
Bleeding, bone pain and gout are less common complaints.

EXAMINATION   Splenomegaly (massive in 10%) is the main physical finding, hepato-megaly present in 50–60%.

PATHOLOGY/PATHOGENESIS   Abnormal megakaryocytes release cytokines (e.g. PDGF and PF4) which stimulate fibroblast proliferation and collagen deposition in bone marrow, with resulting extramedullary haematopoiesis in liver and spleen. The gain-of-function V617F mutation in the JAK2 gene is associated with disease progression.

INVESTIGATIONS
Blood: FBC (variable Hb, WCC and platelets initially, but later anaemia, leukopaenia and thrombocytopaenia). LFT (abnormal).
Blood film: Leucoerythroblastic changes (circulating red and white cell precursors) with characteristic 'tear drop' poikilocyte red cells.
Bone marrow aspirate or biopsy: Aspiration usually unsuccessful ('dry tap'). Trephine biopsy shows fibrotic hypercellular marrow, with dense reticulin fibres on silver staining.

MANAGEMENT
Supportive therapy: Red cell transfusion, folic acid, allopurinol.
Chemotherapy: Thalidomide in combination with steroids or imatinib has been shown to be helpful in delaying or halting progression. Hydroxyurea for splenomegaly and hyper-metabolic symptoms.
Radiotherapy: Short-term palliation of splenomegaly.
Surgery: Splenectomy for severe cases. Stem cell transplantation can be curative for selected patients.

COMPLICATIONS   Heart failure, infections. Iron overload resulting from blood transfu-sions. Transformation to AML occurs in 10–20%.

PROGNOSIS   Median survival is 3–5 years, with wide variation. The degree of anaemia (Hb < 10 g/dL) is the most important prognostic factor.

Polycythaemia

DEFINITION   An increase in haemoglobin (Hb) concentration above the upper limit of normal for a person's age and sex. Classified into relative polycythaemia (normal red cell mass but ↓ plasma volume) or absolute (true) polycythaemia (↑ red cell mass).

AETIOLOGY
Polycythaemia rubra vera: Characterized by clonal proliferation of myeloid cells with variable morphologic maturity and haematopoietic efficiency. Mutations in JAK2 tyrosine kinase participates in the pathogenesis.
Secondary polycythaemia:
Appropriate ↑ erythropoietin: Caused by chronic hypoxia (e.g. chronic lung disease) leading to upregulation of erythrogenesis.
Inappropriate ↑ erythropoietin: Renal (carcinoma, cysts, hydronephrosis), hepatocellular carcinoma, fibroids, cerebellar haemangioblastoma. Secondary polycythaemia may be a feature of erythropoietin abuse amongst athletes.
Relative polycythaemia: Dehydration (e.g. diuretics, burns, enteropathy), Gaisböck's syndrome (seen in young male smokers with ↑ vasomotor tone and hypertension).

EPIDEMIOLOGY   Annual UK incidence of polycythaemia rubra vera is 1.5 in 100,000. Peak age is 45–60 years.

HISTORY   Headaches, dyspnoea, tinnitus, blurred vision as a result of hyperviscosity. Pruritus after hot bath, night sweats.
Thrombosis (DVT, stroke), pain resulting from peptic ulcer disease, angina, gout, choreiform movements.

EXAMINATION   Plethoric complexion.
Scratch marks as a result of itching, conjunctival suffusion and retinal venous engorgement.
Hypertension.
Splenomegaly (present in 75% of polycythaemia rubra vera).
Signs of underlying aetiology in secondary causes.

INVESTIGATIONS
Required for diagnosis: *FBC:* ↑ Hb (>16.5 g/dL in ♀, >18.5 g/dL in ♂), ↑ haematocrit (>48% in ♀, >52% in ♂), ↓ MCV.
Isotope dilution techniques: Using infusion of radiolabelled albumin (^{131}I) and RBCs (^{51}Cr) allow confirmation of plasma volume and red cell mass (RCM) and distinguish between relative and absolute polycythaemia.[1]
Polycythaemia rubra vera: ↑ WCC, ↑ platelets, ↓ serum erythropoietin. JAK2 mutation (present in almost all, but is not specific to polycythaemia rubra vera). Bone marrow trephine and biopsy shows erythroid hyperplasia and ↑ megakaryoctyes.
Secondary polycythaemia: ↑Serum erythropoietin, exclude chronic lung disease/hypoxia (pulse oximetry, ABG, CXR), look for erythropoietin-secreting tumours (e.g. abdominal CT, brain MRI).

MANAGEMENT
Polycythaemia rubra vera: Regular venesection to ↓ haematocrit below 45% in ♂ and 42% in ♀. Aspirin to ↓ risk of thrombosis. Hydroxyurea in patients who are at high-risk for thrombosis (age >60, prior thrombosis). IFN alpha in refractory pruritus, high-risk women of childbearing potential and in those refractory to hydroxyurea.

---

[1]These tests are rarely necessary as almost all female patients with Hb >16.5 g/dL and all male patients with Hb >18.5 g/dL have been shown to have ↑ RCM. Patients with lower Hb values may require RCM and plasma volume measurements to distinguish absolute polycythaemia from relative polycythaemia.

Polycythaemia (continued)

Symptomatic treatment of complications (e.g. allopurinol for hyperuricaemia, H_2-antagonists for peptic ulcers).

Secondary: Treat underlying disorder.

Relative: Fluid repletion, stop smoking of tobacco, use of caffeine-containing beverages and diuretics.

COMPLICATIONS   Thrombosis (due o hyperviscosity and ↑ platelet) resulting in stroke or MI, haemorrhage (resulting from defective platelet function), gout and renal calculi (hyper-uricaemia), peptic ulceration occurs in 5–10% of patients with polycythaemia rubra vera.

PROGNOSIS   Good prognosis with management. In polycythaemia rubra vera, the mean survival is 16 years. Without treatment median survival ~1–2 years. 30% develop myelo-fibrosis and 5% acute leukaemia.

Sickle cell anaemia

DEFINITION A chronic condition with sickling of red blood cells caused by inheritance of haemoglobin S (Hb S).

Sickle cell anaemia: Homozygosity for Hb S.

Sickle cell trait: Carries one copy of Hb S.

Sickle cell disease: Includes compound heterozygosity for Hb S and C and for Hb S and β-thalassaemia.

AETIOLOGY Autosomally recessive inherited point mutation in the β-globin gene resulting in valine substituting glutamic acid on position 6, producing the abnormal protein, Hb S.

Deoxygenation of Hb S alters the conformation with resulting hydrophobic interactions between adjacent Hb S and formation of insoluble polymers, resulting in sickling of red cells (formation of crescent shape cells) with ↑ fragility and inflexibility. They are prone to:

1. Sequestration and destruction, leading to ↓ RBC survival (~20 days).
2. Occlusion small blood vessels causing hypoxia which, in turn, causes further sickling and occlusion.

Factors precipitating sickling are infection, dehydration, hypoxia and acidosis.

EPIDEMIOLOGY Rarely presents before 4–6 months (because of continuous production of foetal haemoglobin). Common in Africa, Caribbean, Middle East and areas with high prevalence of malaria (carrier frequency in Afro-Caribbeans ~8%).

HISTORY

Symptoms secondary to vaso-occlusion or infarction:

Autosplenectomy (splenic atrophy or infarction): Leading to increased risk of infections with encapsulated organisms (e.g. pneumococcus, *Haemophilus influenzae*, meningococcus, *Salmonella*).

Abdominal pain.

Bones: Painful crises affecting small bones of hands or feet (dactylitis) in children, and ribs, spine, pelvis and long bones in adults. Chronic hip or shoulder pain (avascular necrosis).

Myalgia and arthralgia.

CNS: Can cause fits or strokes (e.g. hemiplegia).

Retina: Visual loss (proliferative retinopathy).

Symptoms of sequestration crises (red cell pooling in various organs)**:** *Spleen.*

Liver: Exacerbation of anaemia.

Lungs: 'Acute chest syndrome': breathlessness, cough, pain, fever.

Corpora cavernosa: Persistent erection (pripiasm) and impotence.

EXAMINATION

Signs secondary to vaso-occlusion, ischaemia or infarction: *Bone*: Joint or muscle tenderness or swelling (caused by avascular necrosis). Short digits (caused by infarction in small bones).

Retina: Cotton wool spots from areas of ischaemic retina.

Signs secondary to sequestration crises:

Organomegaly: Spleen is enlarged in early disease but later reduces in size because of splenic atrophy.

Priapism.

Signs of anaemia.

INVESTIGATIONS

Blood: FBC (anaemia, reticulocytes are ↑ in haemolytic crises and ↓ in aplastic crises), U&E.

Blood film: Sickle cells, anisocytosis, features of hyposplenism (target cells, Howell–Jolly bodies).

Sickle solubility test: Dithionate added to blood causes ↑ turbidity.

Haemoglobin electrophoresis: Shows Hb S, absence of Hb A (in Hb SS) and ↑ levels of Hb F.

Sickle cell anaemia (continued)

Hip X-ray: Common site for avascular necrosis of the femoral head.
MRI or CT head: If there are neurological complications.

MANAGEMENT
Acute (painful crises)**:** Oxygen, IV fluids, strong analgesia (IV opiates), antibiotics.
Infection prophylaxis: Penicillin V. Regular vaccinations (e.g. against pneumococcus).
Folic acid: In severe haemolysis or in pregnancy.
Hydroxyurea: Increases Hb F levels and ↓ frequency and duration of sickle cell crisis.
Red cell transfusion: For severe anaemia. Repeated transfusions with iron chelators may be necessary for those with frequent crises or after CNS crisis.
Exchange transfusion: In severe crises, before surgery, pregnancy.
Advice: Avoid precipitating factors, good hygiene and nutrition, genetic counselling, prenatal screening.
Surgical: Bone marrow transplantation in selected patients, joint replacement for avascular necrosis.

COMPLICATIONS Complications of vaso-occlusion and sequestration (*see* History). Aplastic crises (infection with B19 parvovirus, temporary cessation of erythropoiesis), haemolytic crises, pigment gallstones, cholecystitis, renal papillary necrosis, leg ulcers (local ischaemia), cardiomyopathy.

PROGNOSIS Most of those with sickle cell disease, with good care, survive to ~50 years. Major mortality is usually a result of pulmonary or neurological complications (adults) or infection (children).

Thalassaemias

DEFINITION   Group of genetic disorders characterized by reduced globin chain synthesis.

AETIOLOGY   The autosomal recessive genetic defects result in an imbalance of globin chain production and deposition in erythroblasts and erythrocytes causing ineffective erythropoiesis, haemolysis, anaemia and extramedullary haemopoiesis.

α-Thalassaemia: ↓ α-Globin chain synthesis. Chromosome has 4 α-globin genes.

4 gene deletion: Hb Barts (γ4) and intrauterine death (hydrops fetalis).

3 gene deletion: Microcytic hypochromic anaemia, splenomegaly.

1-2 gene deletion: Microcytic hypochromic red cells; no anaemia.

β-Thalassaemia major (homozygous β -thalassaemia): β-Globin gene mutations on chromosome 11 causes no or minimal β-chain synthesis (β0 or β +).

β-Thalassaemia intermedia: Mild defect in β-chain synthesis causing microcytic anaemia, ↓ α-chain synthesis or ↑ γ-chains.

β-Thalassaemia trait (heterozygous carrier): Asymptomatic, mild microcytic anaemia, ↑ red cell count.

EPIDEMIOLOGY   Worldwide, but more common in the Mediterranean and areas of the Middle East.

HISTORY

β-Thalassaemia major: Anaemia presenting at 3–6 months (when γ-chain synthesis switches to β-chain synthesis). Failure to thrive, prone to infections.

α- or β-Thalassaemia trait: May be asymptomatic. Detected on routine blood tests or from a family history.

EXAMINATION

β-Thalassaemia major: Pallor, malaise, dyspnoea, mild jaundice.

Frontal bossing and thalassaemic facies (marrow hyperplasia).

Hepatosplenomegaly (erythrocyte pooling, extramedullary haemopoiesis).

Patients with β-thalassaemia intermedia may also have the aforementioned signs.

INVESTIGATIONS

Blood: FBC (↓Hb, ↓ MCV, ↓ MCH).

Blood film: Hypochromic, microcytic anaemia, target cells, nucleated red cells and ↑ reticulocyte count.

Hb electrophoresis: Absent or ↓ Hb A and ↑ levels of Hb F (fetal Hb, α2 γ2).

Bone marrow: Hypercellular with erythroid hyperplasia.

Genetic testing: Rarely necessary. For specific mutations.

Skull x-ray: 'Hair-on-end' appearance (caused by expansion of marrow into cortex) in β-thalassaemia major.

MANAGEMENT   α- or β-Thalassaemia trait do not usually require treatment.

β-Thalassaemia major: Regular blood transfusions together with SC desferrioxamine or oral deferiprone (for iron chlelation to prevent of iron overload) 5–7 nights weekly. Bone marrow transplant from an HLA-matched donor in selected individuals.

Surgical: Splenectomy (if requirements for blood transfusion are very high, but delay operation until 5–6 years old), requires vaccination and penicillin prophlaxis.

COMPLICATIONS   Severe thalassamias can cause the following complications.

Iron overload:

Skin: 'Slate-grey' skin pigmentation.

Liver: Secondary haemochromatosis leading to liver damage.

Endocrine organs: Short stature, delayed puberty, diabetes mellitus, hypothyroidism.

Heart: Cardiac failure or arrhythmias.

Thalassaemias (continued)

Infections:
Prone to encapsulated organisms (e.g. meningococcal and pneumococcus) after splenectomy. *Yersinia entercolitica* and *Rhizopus* (rare fungal infection) in those taking desferrioxamine.

Osteoporosis: Secondary to marrow expansion and endocrinological complications, fractures.

PROGNOSIS Normal life expectancy in those with thalassemia trait.

In β-thalassaemia major, regular transfusions and iron chelation improves prognosis. Mortality is mainly caused by heart failure (from iron overload) and infections. Bone marrow transplantation has 90 % success rate.

Acne vulgaris

DEFINITION   Inflammation of the pilosebaceous unit of the skin.

AETIOLOGY   Increased production and impaired normal flow of sebum (caused by follicular hyperkeratinization and obstruction of the pilosebaceous duct) leading to inflammation and formation of closed or open comedones. The bacteria *Propionibacterium acnes*, *Staphylococcus epidermidis* and *Pityrosporum* yeast may be involved in pathogenesis. Associated with polycystic ovarian syndrome, cortisol excess (Cushing's syndrome), prolactinoma and puberty.

EPIDEMIOLOGY   Ubiquitous. Begins in puberty and tends to recede with age.

HISTORY   Usually self-diagnosed, acute onset, greasy skin, may be painful.

EXAMINATION   Open comedones (whiteheads: flesh-coloured papules), closed comedones (blackheads: the black colour is caused by oxidation of melanin pigment), papules, pustules, nodules, cysts and seborrhoea primarily affecting the face, neck, upper torso and back. Three grades: mild, moderate and severe.

INVESTIGATIONS   Normally none required, especially if experiencing puberty.
Blood: LH levels (increased LH: FSH ratio may be seen in PCOS), prolactin, sex-hormone-binding globulin, testosterone, 17-OH-progesterone (9 a.m., follicular phase; if congential adrenal hyperplasia is suspected).
Urine: 24-h urinary cortisol (if Cushing's syndrome suspected).
Imaging: Pelvic ultrasound (if PCOS suspected).

MANAGEMENT: Start treatment early to prevent scarring.
For mild/moderate acne: Over-the-counter preparations containing benzoyl peroxide, azelaic acid.
For moderate/severe acne: Consider topical antibiotics (clindamycin, erythromycin), topical vitamin A derivatives (tretinoin).
For severe inflammatory acne or if failure of topical treatment:
Consider systemic antibiotics (oxytetracycline, minocycline, erythromycin).
For severe acne: Also consider oral vitamin A derivative (isotretinoin) – available only by specialist prescription.
Side effects: Teratogenic, hyperlipidaemia.
For females: Oral contraceptive pill or cyproterone acetate reduces severity.
Advice: Counsel patients that an improvement may not be seen for a couple of months, use of non-greasy cosmetics, wash face daily.

COMPLICATIONS   Facial scarring (atrophic, 'ice pick', hypertrophic, keloidal), hyperpigmentation, secondary infection, psychological morbidity.

PROGNOSIS   Generally improves spontaneously over months or years.

Basal cell carcinoma (skin)

DEFINITION Commonest form of skin malignancy; also known as a 'rodent ulcer'.

AETIOLOGY Prolonged sun exposure or UV radiation.
Associated with abnormalities of the patched/hedgehog intracellular signaling cascade, as seen in Gorlin's syndrome (naevoid basal cell carcinoma syndrome). Other risk factors include photosensitizing pitch, tar and arsenic.

Pathophysiology: Small dark blue staining basal cells growing in well-defined aggregates invading the dermis with the outer layer of cells arranged in palisades. Numerous mitotic and apoptotic bodies are seen. Growth rate is usually slow, but steady and insidious. It does not metastasize, but has the potential to invade and destroy local tissues.

EPIDEMIOLOGY Common in those with fair skin and areas of high sunlight exposure, common in the elderly, rare before the age of 40 years. Lifetime risk in Caucasians is 1:3.

HISTORY A chronic slowly progressive skin lesion usually on the face but also on the scalp, ears or trunk.

EXAMINATION
Nodulo-ulcerative (most common): Small glistening translucent skin over a coloured papule that slowly enlarges (early) or a central ulcer ('rodent ulcer') with raised pearly edges. Fine telangiectatic vessels often run over the tumour surface. Cystic change may be seen in larger more protuberant lesions.

Morphoeic: Expanding, yellow/white waxy plaque with an ill-defined edge (more aggressive).

Superficial: Most often on trunk, multiple pink/brown scaly plaques with a fine 'whipcord' edge expanding slowly; can grow to more than 10 cm in diameter.

Pigmented: Specks of brown or black pigment may be present in any type of basal cell carcinoma.

INVESTIGATIONS Biopsy is rarely necessary (diagnosis is based mainly on clinical suspicion).

MANAGEMENT Cryotherapy, curettage, cauterization and photodynamic therapy are used for small superficial lesions.

Surgical: Excision with a 0.5 cm margin of surrounding normal skin for discrete nodular or cystic nodules in patients under 60 years; Mohs' micrographic surgery, which includes careful review of tissue excised under frozen section, is the treatment of choice for large tumours (1 cm diameter) and lesions near the eyes, nose and ears. Excision and skin flap coverage may be necessary.

Radiotherapy: Useful in basal cell carcinomas involving structures that are difficult to surgically reconstruct (e.g. eyelids, tearducts). Repeated treatments may be necessary as there is risk of side effects such as radiation dermatitis, ulceration or depilation.

COMPLICATIONS The tumour has a slow but relentless course. Can become disfiguring on the face. Has the potential to invade, lead to loss of vision in the orbital region.

PROGNOSIS Good with appropriate treatment. If left, may continue to grow, invade and ulcerate. Regular follow-up is necessary to detect local recurrence or other lesions.

Eczema

DEFINITION A pruritic papulovesicular skin reaction to endogenous or exogenous agents.

AETIOLOGY Numerous varieties caused by a diversity of triggers.

Exogenous: Irritant, contact, phototoxic.

Endogenous: Atopic, seborrhoeic, pompholyx, varicose, lichen simplex.[1]

Irritant: Prolonged skin contact with a cell-damaging irritant (e.g. ammonia in nappy rash).

Contact: Type IV delayed hypersensitivity to allergen (e.g. nickel, chromate, perfumes, latex and plants).

Atopic: Two major models currently exist to explain the pathogenesis:

1 Impaired epidermal barrier function due to intrinsic structural and functional skin abnormalities (predominant model).

2 Immune function disorder in which Langerhans cells, T cells and immune effector cells modulate an inflammatory response to environmental factors (traditional model).

Seborrhoeic: *Pityrosporum* yeast seems to have a central role.

Varicose: Increased venous pressure in lower limbs.

EPIDEMIOLOGY

Contact: Prevalence 4 %.

Atopic: Onset is commonly in the first year of life. Childhood incidence 10–20 %.

HISTORY Itching (can be severe), heat, tenderness, redness, weeping, crusting.

Enquire into occupational exposures or irritants used at home (e.g. bleach). Enquire into family/personal history of atopy (e.g. asthma, hay fever, rhinitis).

EXAMINATION

Acute: Poorly demarcated erythematous oedematous dry scaling patches. Papules, vesicles with exudation and crusting, excoriation marks.

Chronic: Thickened epidermis, skin lichenification, fissures, change in pigmentation.

By type:

Contact and irritant: Eczema reaction occurs where irritant/allergen comes into contact with the skin. In some cases, autosensitization (spread to other sites) can occur in contact eczema.

Atopic: Particularly affects face and flexures.

Seborrhoeic: Yellow greasy scales on erythematous plaques, particularly in the nasolabial folds, eyebrows, scalp and presternal area.

Pompholyx: Acute and often recurrent painful vesiculobullous eruption on palms and soles.

Varicose: Eczema of lower legs, usually associated with marked varicose veins.

Nummular: Coin shaped, on legs and trunk.

Asteatotic: Dry, 'crazy paring' pattern.

INVESTIGATIONS

Contact:

Skin patch testing: Disc containing postulated allergen is diluted and applied to back for 48 h. Positive if allergen induces a red raised lesion.

Atopic: Laboratory testing, including IgE levels, are not used routinely and are not currently recommended.

Swab for infected lesions (bacteria, fungi and viruses).

---

[1] Lichen simplex is the thickening of skin secondary to a cycle of itch – scratch – itch, and is characterized by well-demarcated hyperpigmented lichenified plaques.

Eczema (continued)

MANAGEMENT

Irritant or contact: Avoid precipitant. Barrier protection (e.g. gloves, barrier cream).

Atopic: Avoid precipitants. Topical steroids. Low potency steroids are used for face and skin folds (areas at high risk for atrophy). The use of potent steroids in these areas should be prescribed by a dermatologist. Tacrolimus (calcineurin inhibitor) ointment for moderate to severe eczema not responding to potent steroids. Systemic immunosuppressants or phototherapy may be helpful in very severe cases.

Topical or systemic antibiotics for secondary infection. Medicated bandages (e.g. zinc paste for severe limb eczema). For pruritus, antihistamines. Emollients (in bath water, as soap substitute or by direct application to affected area).

Seborrhoeic: Topical 1 % hydrocortisone and antifungal. Ketoconazole shampoo for scalp involvement.

Pompholyx: Potent topical steroids, potassium permanganate salts, systemic steroids in severe attacks.

COMPLICATIONS   Secondary infection, particularly from *Staphylococcus aureus* and HSV. HSV superinfection can be life-threatening. ↑ predisposition to *Molluscum contagiosum*.[2]

PROGNOSIS   Good prognosis for irritant eczema if the relevant agent is identified and avoided. Endogenous eczema may have a chronic relapsing course. Of all patients, 90 % with atopic eczema recover by puberty.

Wiskott–Aldrich syndrome: Association of eczema, thrombocytopaenia, immunological abnormalities and a predisposition to lymphoma and leukaemia.

---

[2] *Molluscum contagiosum* is a common childhood skin infection with multiple small translucent vesicle-like papules that have a central punctum. It is caused by a contact-transmissible pox virus. In adults, suspect HIV.

Erythema multiforme

DEFINITION   An acute hypersensitivity reaction of the skin and mucous membranes. Stevens–Johnson syndrome is a severe form with bullous lesions and necrotic ulcers.

AETIOLOGY   Degeneration of basal epidermal cells and development of vesicles between the cells and the underlying basement membrane; lymphocytic infiltrate is seen around the blood vessels and at the dermal – epidermal junction. Immune complex deposition is variable and non-specific. Precipitating factor identified in only 50 % of cases.

Drugs	Sulphonamides, penicillin, phenytoin, barbiturates
Infection	*Viral:* HSV, EBV, coxsackie, adenovirus, ORF *Bacterial:* Mycoplasma pneumoniae, Chlamydiae *Fungal:* Histoplasmosis
Inflammatory	Rheumatoid arthritis, SLE, sarcoidosis, ulcerative colitis, systemic vasculitis
Malignancy	Lymphomas, leukaemia, myeloma
Radiotherapy	

EPIDEMIOLOGY   Any age group, but most commonly children and young adults. $\male : \female \sim 2:1$.

HISTORY   Non-specific prodromal symptoms of upper respiratory tract infection.
Sudden appearance of itching/burning/painful skin lesions (*see* EXAMINATION), which may fade, leaving behind pigmentation.

EXAMINATION   Classic target ('bull's eye') lesions with a rim of erythema surrounding a paler area, vesicles/bullae, urticarial plaques. The lesions are often symmetrical, distributed over the arms and legs including the palms, soles and the extensor surfaces.
Stevens–Johnson syndrome is characterized by:
- *Affecting >2 mucous membranes*: Conjunctiva, cornea, lips (haemorrhagic crusts), mouth, genitalia.
- *Systemic symptoms*: Sore throat, cough, fever, headache, myalgia, arthralgia, diarrhoea and vomiting.
- *Shock*: Hypotension, tachycardia.

INVESTIGATIONS   Usually unnecessary as erythema multiforme and Stevens–Johnson syndrome are clinical diagnoses. Investigations may be necessary to determine the precipitating factor.
Blood: ↑ WCC, eosinophils, ESR, CRP, throat swab, serology, albumin (↓ in extensive exudation), ↑ urea (as a result of catabolic state and dehydration), autoantibodies.
Imaging: CXR (to exclude sarcoidosis and atypical pneumonias).
Skin biopsy: Histology and direct immunofluorescence may be indicated in cases of diagnostic doubt.

MANAGEMENT   Symptomatic. Antihistamines (for itching) and NSAIDs (analgesia). Treat underlying cause, e.g. stop the implicated drug, treat the infection. Use of systemic corticosteroids is controversial. Oral aciclovir for recurrent episodes.
Stevens–Johnson syndrome: Nurse in ITU. Close attention to fluid and electrolyes balance, heat loss, analgesia and the risk of secondary infections. Denuded areas are treated like burns. Mouth ulceration may be so severe that total parenteral nutrition is required. If the urethra is involved, catheterization is necessary.

Erythema multiforme (continued)

COMPLICATIONS Blindness in 3–10 % (if cornea affected), secondary infection of denuded areas, renal failure.

Stevens–Johnson syndrome: Lesions of respiratory tract can be complicated by pneumonia and respiratory failure.

PROGNOSIS   Most cases of erythema multiforme resolve within 2–5 weeks. There may be recurrence in a small minority, usually triggered by HSV. Cases caused by drugs and Mycoplasma are more likely to progress to Stevens–Johnson syndrome. Mortality of Stevens–Johnson syndrome ~ 5–15 %.

Toxic epidermal necrolysis: Widespread skin erythema leading to epidermal necrosis. Eventually, there is desquamation of epidermis in large sheets, leaving denuded shiny dermis underneath. High mortality (> 30 %). Can be a reaction to drugs, e.g. penicillin, anticonvulsants, sulphonamides, NSAIDs, allopurinol.

Erythema nodosum

DEFINITION   Panniculitis (inflammation of the subcutaneous fat tissue) presenting as red or violet subcutaneous nodules.

AETIOLOGY   Delayed hypersensitivity reaction to antigens associated with various infectious agents, drugs, and other diseases.

Infection: *Bacterial* (Streptococcus, TB, *Yersinia*, rickettsia, *Chlamydia*, leprosy), *viral* (EBV), *fungal* (histoplasmosis, blastomycosis, coccidioidomycosis), *protozoal* (toxoplasmosis).

Systemic disease: Sarcoidosis, IBD, Behçet's disease.

Malignancy: Leukaemia, Hodgkin's disease.

Drugs: Sulphonamides, penicillin, oral contraceptive pills.

Pregnancy.

25 % of cases have no underlying cause identified.

EPIDEMIOLOGY   Usually affects young adults. $\female : \male \sim 3: 1$.

HISTORY   Tender red or violet nodules develop bilaterally on the shins and occasionally on the thighs and forearms. Fatigue, fever, anorexia, weight loss and arthralgia are often also present.

Symptoms of the underlying aetiology.

EXAMINATION   Crops of red or violet dome-shaped nodules usually present on both shins (occasionally involving thighs or forearms) which are tender to palpation.

Low-grade pyrexia. Joints may be tender and painful on movement.

Signs of the underlying aetiology.

INVESTIGATIONS   To determine the underlying aetiology.

Blood: Anti-streptolysin-O titre at diagnosis and 2–4 weeks later to assess for antecedent streptococcal infection. FBC, U&Es, CRP, ESR, LFTs, serum ACE ($\uparrow$ in sarcoidosis).

Throat swab and culture.

Mantoux/Heaf skin testing: For TB.

CXR: To look for hilar adenopathy or other evidence of pulmonary sarcoidosis, TB and fungal infections.

MANAGEMENT   Treat the cause. In most cases, manage conservatively.

NSAIDs or potassium iodide may be given for relief of the discomfort associated with the rash.

Persistent cases may require corticosteroids, colchicine, azathioprine or dapsone. When considering corticosteroids, clinicians should assess the possibility of masking an underlying malignant, inflammatory, or infectious condition.

COMPLICATIONS   None. Complications of the underlying cause.

PROGNOSIS   The majority of cases resolve over 3–6 weeks leaving bruise marks.

Occasionally, nodules may persist or recur over several months, but they never ulcerate.

Erythroderma

DEFINITION   Non-specific intense widespread reddening of the skin often preceded by exfoliation.

AETIOLOGY
Pre-existing skin conditions: Eczema, psoriasis.
Malignancy: Cutaneous T-cell lymphoma, lymphoma, leukaemia.
Adverse drug reaction.
Infection: HIV, toxic shock syndrome.
Idiopathic.

EPIDEMIOLOGY   Incidence: 1–2 in 100,000/year. 1 % of dermatological admissions. Age usually > 40 years. $\male : \female = 2.5 : 1$.

HISTORY   The skin feels hot and tight. Pruritus, erythema, scaling and shedding, fever and shivering. Symptoms of cardiac failure. The history should also be directed towards establishing aetiology.

EXAMINATION   The patient may be pyrexial or hypothermic.
Erythema and scaling of ≥ 90 % of the skin. Evidence of skin shedding.
The skin is hot and radiates warmth to the surroundings, can $\rightarrow$ hypothermia.
Peripheral oedema, signs of volume depletion including $\downarrow$ BP and tachycardia.
Signs of cardiac failure.
Signs of the underlying condition, e.g. psoriatic plaques.

PATHOLOGY/PATHOGENESIS   Interaction of cytokines and cellular adhesion molecules $\rightarrow \uparrow$ epidermal turnover rate $\rightarrow$ severe scaling and shedding $\rightarrow$ loss of fluid, electrolytes and albumin. There is increased blood flow through the skin, which may cause temperature dysregulation and high-output cardiac failure.

INVESTIGATIONS
Skin biopsy: In order to make a definitive diagnosis $\pm$ lymph node biopsy if significant lymphadenopathy.
Blood:
FBC: $\downarrow$ Hb, $\uparrow$ WBC if secondary infection, may reveal underlying haematological dyscrasia.
ESR, U&E: May have $\downarrow$ Na$^+$, $\downarrow$ K$^+$, $\uparrow$ urea if lost through skin.
LFT: $\downarrow$ Albumin loss through the skin $\pm$ leakage to extracellular space from leaky capillaries.
Immunoglobulins: Hypergammaglobulinaemia, $\uparrow$ IgE.
Blood film: For Sezary cells typical of T-cell lymphomas.

ABGs: For renal failure (metabolic acidosis) and ARDS.
Imaging: ECG, CXR or echocardiogram may show signs of cardiac failure.

MANAGEMENT   This is a dermatological emergency.
1. Nurse the patient in a warm room.
2. Regularly monitor vital signs.
3. Catheterize and close fluid balance monitoring.
4. Treat the underlying cause if identified.
5. Continue only vital medications.
6. Swab the skin for secondary infection.
7. Ensure topical steroid and bandaging. Consider systemic steroid (controversial and never used in cases of psoriatic erythroderma).
8. Use antihistamine for pruritus and sedative effect.
9. Manage complications.

COMPLICATIONS   Cardiac failure, renal failure, hypothermia, secondary infection, ARDS.

PROGNOSIS   Mortality $\sim$ 20–40 %.

Malignant melanoma

DEFINITION   Malignancy arising from neoplastic transformation of melanocytes, the pigment-forming cells of the skin. The leading cause of death from skin disease.

AETIOLOGY   DNA damage in melanocytes caused by ultraviolet radiation results in neoplastic transformation. 50 % arise in pre-existing naevi, 50 % in previously normal skin. Four histopathological types:
1. *Superficial spreading (70 %)*: Typically arises in a pre-existing naevus, expands in radial fashion before vertical growth phase.
2. *Nodular (15 %)*: Arises de novo, aggressive, no radial growth phase.
3. *Lentigo maligna (10 %)*: More common in elderly with sun damage, large flat lesions, follow an indolent growth course. Usually on the face.
4. *Acral lentiginous (5 %)*: Arise on palms, soles and subungual areas. Most common type in non-white populations.

EPIDEMIOLOGY   Steadily increasing incidence, 6,000/year diagnosed in the United Kingdom, lifetime risk 1 in 80 in the USA. White races have 20 times increased risk to non-white races.

HISTORY   Change in size, shape or colour of a pigmented skin lesion, redness, bleeding, crusting, ulceration.

EXAMINATION   ABCD criteria for examining moles:
A   Asymmetry.
B   Border irregularity/bleeding.
C   Colour variation.
D   Diameter > 6 mm.
E   Elevation.

INVESTIGATIONS
Excisional biopsy: For histological diagnosis and determination of Clark's levels or Breslow thickness.
Lymphoscintigraphy: Radioactive compound is injected around lesion and dynamic images are taken over the course of 30 min to trace the lymph drainage and the sentinel node(s).
Sentinel lymph node biopsy (if primary and < 1 mm depth): Sentinal lymph nodes are dissected and histologically examined for metastatic involvement.
Staging: Imaging by ultrasound, CT or MRI, CXR.
Blood: LFT (liver is a common site of metastases).

MANAGEMENT
Primary prevention: Limit sun overexposure, avoid sunburn.
Wide local excision, margin dependent on depth of invasion (< 1 mm: 1 cm, 1–4 mm: 2 cm margin). Skin grafting may be required.
Chemotherapy: May be necessary as adjunctive treatment or in metastatic disease. Commonly used agents used are dacarbazine (∼ 20 % respond), cisplatin, temozolomide and vinblastine.
Biological therapy: Interferon α-2b, IL-2, and bevacizumab (unlicensed) have been shown to potentially beneficial.

COMPLICATIONS   Lymphoedema may result after block dissection of lymph nodes.

PROGNOSIS   5-year survival 90–95 % for lesions < 1.4 mm, 40 % with node-positive disease and mean survival of 9 months with metastatic disease.
Poorer prognostic indicators: Ulceration, ↑ mitotic rate, trunk lesions compared with limb. Males poorer prognosis than females.

Pemphigoid

DEFINITION   An autoimmune subepidermal blistering (bullous) disease of the skin.

AETIOLOGY   Autoantibodies are formed against the basement membrane hemidesmo-somal glycoproteins BP180 and BP230. Serum levels of anti-BP180 antibodies (present in 65 % patients) correlate with disease activity. MHC class II allele DQB1*0301 is a marker for enhanced susceptibility to this disorder, possibly by facilitating presentation of BP180 proteins to T cells. Anti-BP230 antibodies may form as a consequence of keratinocyte injury. Deposits of polyclonal IgG and complement at the junction of the dermis and epidermis result in activation of the complement cascade, release of proteolytic enzymes and destruction of the basement membrane. Mast cells appear to play an integral role in this process.

Drug-induced bullous pemphigoid may be caused by penicillamine, furosemide, captopril, penicillin, sulfasalazine. Most causative drugs contain sulfhydryl groups that cleave epidermal intercellular substance, resulting in the production of the antibodies.

EPIDEMIOLOGY   Incidence of 4.3 per 100,000 person-years was found in a population-based study from the United Kingdom. Median age at presentation was 80 years. More cases occur in women than men (60 % versus 40 %).

HISTORY   Acute onset. The tense blisters are tender and can be very itchy.
New blisters can keep developing without adequate treatment.

EXAMINATION   Primary lesions are often erythematous and eczematous plaques, gen-eralized on trunk and limbs. Large tense blisters then develop on these sites. ('*Cicatricial*' *pemphigoid:* Heals with scarring and may affect the eye and orogenital mucous membranes.)

INVESTIGATIONS
Skin biopsy:
A delicate 4-mm punch biopsy from the edge of an intact bulla: for light microscopy, to reveal the 'subepiderma'l blister.
A second biopsy for direct immunofluorescence (plus a biopsy of normal skin taken a few millimeters from an involved area placed in Michel's fixative). Deposits of IgG and complement are seen in a linear pattern along the basement membrane zone.

MANAGEMENT   Topical corticosteroid therapy e.g. clobetasol propionate cream.
Patients with disease affecting mucous membranes who cannot be treated topically are treated with oral corticosteroids and steroid-sparing agents.
In patients with extensive involvement: management of fluid loss, pain, temperature control, and septicemia.

COMPLICATIONS   Fluid and electrolyte loss, secondary infections, complications of ster-oids (diabetes mellitus, hypertension, gastric ulceration, osteoporosis).

PROGNOSIS   Good. Control of pemphigoid is easier than that of pemphigus. Complete remission after 1 year is common.

Pemphigus

DEFINITION   Autoimmune intra-epidermal blistering disease.

AETIOLOGY   Believed to be caused by autoimmunity against the proteins attaching the epidermal cells to each other (desmosomal proteins, desmoglein 1 and 3). The trigger is unknown. Rarely, it may be caused by penicillamine or captopril.

EPIDEMIOLOGY   Rare, usually 45–60 years, ♂ = ♀.
Affects all racial groups, more common in Ashkenazi Jews and those from the Indian subcontinent.

HISTORY   Acute onset of sore blisters (*see* Examination).

EXAMINATION   Primary lesions may be confined to the oral mucosa and throat (oral pemphigus). Flaccid blisters rupture readily and leave raw erosions.
Oral involvement may be followed by thin-roofed blisters (e.g. axilla or trunk). Denuding of these blisters produce very tender, red exuding areas.
New lesions appear at the site of lateral sheering forces (Nikolsky's sign, but this is also present in toxic epidermal necrolysis (*see* footnote under Erythema multiforme).
Rarely, large moist verrucous plaques studded with pustules in flexural and intertriginous zones may be seen (pemphigus vegetans).

INVESTIGATIONS
Skin biopsy: Intra-epidermal split and blister formation with separation of individual cells (acantholysis), split may be just above the basal layer (suprabasal blister) leaving an intact layer of basal cells ('row of tombstones') – *pemphigus vulgaris*. In pemphigus foliaceus, there is a superficial epidermal split (only stratum granulosum is involved.) Direct/indirect immunofluorescence will show IgG and C3 localized intercellularly in the epidermis.
Blood: Antidesmosome IgG – positive in ~ 90 % of patients (indirect immunofluorescence), useful for monitoring disease activity.
Monitor FBC and LFT if azathioprine is used.

MANAGEMENT
Medical: High-dose prednisolone (60–120 mg/day orally, smaller doses may have to be continued lifelong). Methotrexate, azathioprine, ciclosporin or cyclophosphamide can be used to avoid steroids. Potent topical steroids can be used for mucocutaneous lesions. Resistant cases may require IV immunoglobulins.
Treat patient as if they had severe burns, thus requiring inpatient care, fluid replacements and wet dressings.
Nasogastric tube feeding may be required with mouth involvement.
Treat secondary infections, analgesia.

COMPLICATIONS   Fluid and electrolyte loss, death, secondary infection, complications of treatment (e.g. prednisolone – osteoporosis, diabetes, hypertension), slight ↑ risk of skin cancer and other malignancies with other immunosuppressants.

PROGNOSIS   High mortality if untreated.

Psoriasis

DEFINITION A chronic inflammatory skin disease, which has characteristic lesions and may be complicated by arthritis.

AETIOLOGY Unknown. Genetic, environmental factors and drugs (e.g. may be triggered by streptococcal infections, antimalarial agents, β-blockers, lithium).

ASSOCIATIONS/RISK FACTORS
- *Guttate psoriasis*: Streptococci sore throat.
- *Palmoplantar pustulosis*: Smoking, middle-aged women, autoimmune thyroid disease, SAPHO (synovitis, acne, palmoplantar pustulosis, hyperostosis seen on radiographs, osteitis – chronic recurrent multifocal inflammation of bones, e.g. sternoclavicular, sacroiliac joint).
- *Generalised pustular*: Hypoparathyroidism.

EPIDEMIOLOGY Affects 1–2 % of the population. Peak age of onset ∼ 20 years.

HISTORY Itching or occasionally tender skin.
Pinpoint bleeding with removing scales (Auspitz phenomenon).
Skin lesions may develop at the site of trauma/scars (Koebner phenomenon).

EXAMINATION
Discoid/nummular psoriasis: Symmetrical well-demarcated erythematous plaques with silvery scales over extensor surface (knee, elbows, scalp, sacrum).
Flexural psoriasis: Less scaly plaques in axilla, groins, perianal and genital skin.
Guttate: Small (∼1 cm) drop-like lesions over trunk, limbs.
Palmoplantar: Erythematous plaques with pustules on palms and soles.
Generalized pustular psoriasis: Pustules distributed over limbs and torso.
Nail: Pitting, onycholysis (lifting off of the nail-plate from the nail-bed), subungual hyperkeratosis, 'salmon patch' on the nail.
Joints: Seronegative arthritis with six possible presentations:
- monoarthritis;
- distal asymmetrical oligoarthritis (distal interphalangeal joints);
- dactylitis (interphalangeal arthritis and flexor tenosynovitis);
- rheumatoid arthritis-like (symmetrical polyarthritis);
- arthritis mutilans (telescoping of the digits); and
- ankylosing spondylitis.

Poor correlation between joint and skin involvement.

PATHOLOGY/PATHOGENESIS Excess proliferation of epidermal cells (rapid cell turnover possibly mediated by cytokines released by lymphocytes in the dermis) and accelerated upward migration of immature keratinocytes.

INVESTIGATIONS Majority of patients do not need any investigations.
Guttate psoriasis: Anti-streptolysin-O titre, throat swab.
Flexural lesions: Skin swabs (exclude candidiasis).
Nail: Analyse nail clippings to exclude onychomycosis (fungal infection).
Joint involvement: Rheumatoid factor (negative), radiographs (distal interphalangeal joints), erosions, periarticular osteoporosis, 'pencil-in-cup' deformity (whittling and cupping of the phalanges); sacroiliitis.

MANAGEMENT
Skin: Emollients for moisturizing skin, moderately potent topical steroids (e.g. Eumovate), dithranol (can irritate/burn the skin), coal tar (↓ DNA synthesis), vitamin D3 analogue (calcipotriol), topical retinoids, PUVA (oral psoralen followed by ultraviolet A light), ultraviolet B (shorter wavelength).

Systemic (severe cases): methotrexate (teratogenic in males and females), retinoids (for pustular psoriasis, avoid in pregnant women), ciclosporin, anti-TNF drugs (infliximab and etanercept) may be promising.

Joints: NSAIDs, intra-articular steroids. Severe cases: methotrexate, ciclosporin (alone or in combination).

Advice: Avoid exacerbating factors for the patient, e.g. smoking, alcohol, etc.

COMPLICATIONS   Arthritis (7 % of cases), anterior uveitis, erythroderma, social complications of the disease if disfiguring.

PROGNOSIS   Chronic disease, which relapses and remits over years. Mortality of generalized pustular psoriasis is improving.

Squamous cell carcinoma (skin)

DEFINITION   Malignancy of the epidermal keratinocytes of the skin. Marjolin's ulcer is a squamous cell carcinoma that arises in an area of chronically inflamed/scarred skin.

AETIOLOGY   The main aetiological risk factor is UV radiation from sunlight exposure, actinic keratoses (sun-induced precancerous lesions). Others include radiation, carcinogens (e.g. tar derivatives, cigarette smoke, soot, industrial oils and arsenic), chronic skin disease (e.g. lupus, leukoplakia), human papilloma virus, long-term immunosuppression (e.g. transplant recipients, HIV) and DNA repair genetic defects (xeroderma pigmentosum).

EPIDEMIOLOGY   Second most common cutaneous malignancy (20% of skin cancers). Often occurring in middle-aged and elderly light-skinned individuals. Annual incidence is about 1/4,000. Male > female (2–3:1).

HISTORY   Skin lesion, ulcerated, recurrent bleeding or non-healing.

EXAMINATION   Variable appearance: ulcerated, hyperkeratotic, crusted or scaly, non-healing lesion, often on sun-exposed areas. Palpate for local lymphadenopathy.

PATHOLOGY/PATHOGENESIS   Bowen's disease is intra-epidermal carcinoma in situ (intra-epidermal proliferation of atypical keratinocytes, basement membrane is intact) and may be seen as solitary or multiple red-brown scaly patches. In squamous cell carcinoma the malignant keratinocytes invade locally into the dermis and can spread to local lymph nodes and distally metastasise e.g. lungs, liver. Staging is based on the TNM system.

INVESTIGATIONS
Skin biopsy: Confirms malignancy and distinguishes it from other skin lesions.
Fine-needle aspiration or lymph node biopsy: Only necessary if suspicion of metastasis.
Staging: CT and/or MRI, PET scanning.

MANAGEMENT
Surgical: For Bowen's disease, curettage and cryotherapy, cauterization or photodynamic therapy can be sufficient to eradicate lesion. Invasive squamous cell carcinomas should be excised with an appropriate margin of 4 or 6 mm (low- or high-risk lesions).
Mohs' micrographic surgery: Excision with close margins and histological examination during surgery to confirm complete excision. Can be used in areas where large excisions are difficult, e.g. lips, near eyes.
Sentinal lymph node biopsy: Can be performed where there is risk of metastatic spread.
Local radiotherapy: For larger lesions or if surgery is difficult (cure rate lower compared with surgery).
Medical: Topical 5-fluorouracil for Bowen's disease or intra-lesional interferons if other options are difficult. Chemotherapy is used for metastatic disease.

COMPLICATIONS   Sun-exposed skin squamous cell carcinomas are usually local at the time of diagnosis, but one-third of those on lips or lingual membranes have spread by the time of diagnosis.

PROGNOSIS   Good if treated appropriately. High-risk factors include:
1. Tumour location (lips, ears, scar).
2. Tumour size > 2 cm (1.5 cm on lips, ear).
3. Deep level of invasion.
4. Poorly differentiated.
5. Perineural invasion.
6. Recurrent tumours.

Glaucoma

DEFINITION Optic neuropathy with typical field defect usually associated with ocular hypertension (intra-ocular pressure, IOP > 21 mmHg).

AETIOLOGY
Primary causes: Acute closed-angle glaucoma (ACAG), primary opened-angle glaucoma (POAG), chronic closed-angle glaucoma.
Secondary causes: Trauma, uveitis, steroids, rubeosis iridis (diabetes, central retinal vein occlusion).
Congenital: Buphthalmos, other inherited ocular disorders.

EPIDEMIOLOGY Prevalence 1 % in over 40 years, 10 % in over 80 years (POAG). Third most common cause of blindness worldwide.

HISTORY
ACAG: Painful red eye, vomiting, impaired vision, haloes around lights.
POAG: Usually asymptomatic, peripheral visual field loss may be noticed.
Congenital: Buphthalmos (ox eye), watering, cloudy cornea.

EXAMINATION (BY SLIT-LAMP)
ACAG: Red eye, hazy cornea, loss of red reflex, fixed and dilated pupil, eye tender and hard on palpation, cupped optic disc, visual field defect (arcuate scotoma), moderately raised IOP.
POAG: Optic disc may be cupped. Usually no signs.

PATHOLOGY/PATHOGENESIS Ocular hypertension compresses and stretches the retinal nerve fibres leaving the optic disc causing scotomas and visual field loss. Ocular hypertension is caused by ↓ outflow of aqueous humour caused by:
* obstruction to outflow by approximation of iris to cornea closing iridocorneal angle and trabecular meshwork/canal of Schlemm causing a rapid and severe rise in IOP (ACAG);
* resistance to outflow through trabecular meshwork (POAG); or
* blockage of trabecular meshwork by blood or inflammatory cells.

INVESTIGATIONS
Goldmann Applanation Tonometry: Standard examination to measure ocular pressure (normal 15 mmHg, POAG 22–40 mmHg, ACAG > 60 mmHg).
Pachymetry: Using ultrasound or optical scanning to measure central corneal thickness (CCT). CCT <590 mm are at higher risk of developing glaucoma.
Fundoscopy: To detect pathologically cupped optic disc (cup – disc ratio > 0.6 or an asymmetry of 0.2). Picture record of optic nerve head is recommended.
Gonioscopy: To assess the iridocorneal angle.
Perimetry (Visual field testing): For arcuate scotoma (early), tunnel vision (late).

MANAGEMENT[1]
ACAG (medical emergency): IV acetazolamide (500 mg), 4% pilocarpine topically, analgesics, antiemetics. May require emergency iridotomy.
Long-term (topical hypotensives)[2]
β-blockers (timolol): ↓ Aqueous humour secretion.
Prostaglandin analogues (Latanoprost): ↑ Flow via uveoscleral drainage.
Carbonic-anhydrase inhibitor (dorzolamide): ↓ Aqueous humour secretion.
Parasympathomimetics: Pilocarpine (constricts pupil, opening up the trabecular meshwork).
Sympathomimetics: Brimonidine (α2-agonist).

---

[1]NICE 2009 guidelines are available on the management of glaucoma at: http://www.nice.org.uk.

[2]The Ocular Hypertension Treatment Study (OHTS) showed that topical hypotensives prevent or delay the development of glaucoma.

Glaucoma (continued)

Surgery:

Laser treatment: Laser trabeculoplasty for POAG; iridotomy for ACAG.

Conventional: Trabeculectomy, canaloplasty or iridectomy facilitates outflow of aqueous humour. 5-fluorouracil or mitomycin may be used to reduce scarring.

COMPLICATIONS

Congenital: Amblyopia and visual loss.

POAG: Visual loss.

ACAG: Visual loss and anterior synechiae.

PROGNOSIS   Poor prognosis for congenital glaucoma caused by amblyopia. Prognosis in acquired glaucoma depends on early diagnosis and treatment.

Retinal vein and artery occlusion

DEFINITION
Retinal artery occlusion (RAO): Occlusion of central or a branch retinal artery.
Retinal vein occlusion (RVO): Occlusion of central or a branch retinal vein.

AETIOLOGY
RVO:
The most common causes are diabetes mellitus, hypertension and glaucoma.
Changes in blood constituents: ↑ Cell adhesiveness (e.g. diabetes mellitus), hyperviscosity syndromes (e.g. multiple myeloma, hyperlipidaemia).
Changes in vessel wall: ↑ Intra-ocular pressure (glaucoma), hypertension causing arteriosclerosis (veins have a common sheath with arteries in the eye and may be compressed by them), primary inflammation (e.g. vasculitis: primary vasculitides, Behçet's syndrome, sarcoidosis).

RAO:
Emboli from carotids arteries (fibrin–platelet or cholesterol emboli) or heart valves (calcific emboli), thrombosis, arteritis.

EPIDEMIOLOGY   Common cause of sudden painless loss of vision (RVO > RAO).

HISTORY
Sudden painless loss of vision.
RAO may be described as a 'descending curtain'. It may be temporary (amaurosis fugax) when the embolus is dislodged.

EXAMINATION   ↓ Visual acuity (when macula is affected), visual field loss and relative afferent pupillary defect (RAPD) may be present in both RAO and RVO. In RAO, visual field loss is usually a unilateral quadrantanopia.
Fundoscopy:
RVO: Flame haemorrhages, cotton wool spots, swollen optic disc (in central RVO).
RAO: Pale oedematous retina with cherry red spot on the macula, narrow truncated arteries, emboli may be seen (white – calcium; yellow – cholesterol).
Tonometry: To measure intraocular pressure (↑ intraocular pressure may be the cause or complication of central RVO).
Signs of the underlying cause: Hypertension, diabetes mellitus, temporal tenderness (temporal arteritis).

INVESTIGATIONS
Exclude other causes of sudden loss of vision (vitreous haemorrhage, retinal detachment, giant cell arteritis, ischaemic optic neuropathy).
Tests to identify the cause/risk factors:
RVO: Blood glucose, ESR, exclude hyperviscosity syndromes and vasculitides, lipid profile and intraocular pressure.
RAO: ESR, carotid doppler ultrasonography, ECG, echocardiogram, lipids.
Fluorescein angiography: Sequential photographs of the fundus are taken following IV injection of fluorescein to identify areas of leakage and poor perfusion to assess risk of rubeosis.

MANAGEMENT
RVO: Treat the underlying condition. Laser may be used to ↓ macular oedema, treat ischaemic areas and prevent neovascularization.
RAO: CO_2 rebreathing (may cause arterial dilatation), IV acetazolamide, anterior chamber paracentesis.

COMPLICATIONS
Loss of vision.

Retinal vein and artery occlusion (continued)

RVO: Macular oedema, neovascularization of the retina and iris (rubeosis) and glaucoma.
RAO: Neovascularization and glaucoma can occur, although uncommon.

PROGNOSIS

RVO: Cotton wool spots and RAPD (indicators of ischaemic retinal damage) are markers of poor prognosis.
RAO: Very poor prognosis even with immediate treatment.

Uveitis, anterior

DEFINITION   Inflammation of the iris and ciliary body (iritis or iridocyclitis).

AETIOLOGY   Anterior uveitis may be caused by infection (e.g. herpes simplex, herpes zoster), or occur as a manifestation of systemic inflammatory conditions e.g. juvenile chronic arthritis, HLA B27-related spondyloarthritides (ankylosing spondylitis, reactive arthritis, inflammatory bowel disease), sarcoidosis, Behçet's disease.

Sympathetic ophthalmia: Inflammation of the contralateral eye weeks/months after penetrating injury (rare).

EPIDEMIOLOGY   Incidence of uveitis is 15 in 100,000 people (75 % are anterior uveitis). Uveitis associated with spondyloarthritis is twice as common in males as in females.

HISTORY   Pain (ciliary spasm and inflammation, pain ↑ on accommodation), photophobia, red eyes, blurred vision, lacrimation. May rarely be associated with tubulointerstitial nephritis (flank pain, haematuria, proteinuria, sterile pyuria and acute renal failure).

EXAMINATION   ↓ Visual acuity, ciliary flush (redness may be confined to the corneoscleral junction), hypopyon (proteinaceous exudate and inflammatory cells in the inferior angle of the anterior chamber), small irregular pupil due to posterior synechiae (adhesions of the iris to the lens).

Slit lamp: Keratic precipitates (deposits of leucocytes on the corneal endothelium).

Fundoscopy: To exclude retinal detachment, posterior inflammation or a tumour that may give rise to anterior uveitis.

Signs of complications: ↑ Intraocular pressure, cataract.

Signs of the underlying aetiology.

INVESTIGATIONS

Investigate for associated systemic conditions depending on associated symptoms: U&Es, spondyloarthritides (sacroiliac joint X-ray, HLA typing), sarcoidosis (CXR, serum calcium, serum ACE), syphilis serology.

MANAGEMENT   Refer to an ophthalmologist.

Treat the underlying infection e.g. antiviral therapy for herpes simplex or herpes zoster.

Anterior uveitis not due to infection: *Topical glucocorticoids* (dexamethasone, prednisolone; drops for daytime and ointment for night-time), systemic steroids and immunosuppressants reserved for severe resistant cases.

Mydriatic drops (antimuscarinics, e.g. cyclopentolate) to ↓ pain caused by ciliary spasm and prevent posterior synechiae formation.

Monitor intraocular pressure.

COMPLICATIONS   Cataract, glaucoma (trabecular meshwork blocked by inflammatory cells or damaged by chronic inflammation), band keratopathy (band of calcium deposited in the cornea), posterior synechiae, rubeosis iridis (new vessels grown on the iris).

PROGNOSIS   Uveitis associated with spondyloarthritides tends to resolve within 3 months of its onset. Recurrences are common. The prognosis for this form of uveitis is generally excellent.

Note: **Posterior uveitis** is chorioretinal inflammation caused by infections, e.g. CMV, toxoplasma, TB, syphilis or systemic inflammatory conditions (e.g. sarcoidosis or vasculitides). Lymphoma may present with bilateral posterior eye inflammation. Posterior uveitis may present with floaters (caused by debris/inflammatory cells in the vitreous) and ↓ vision. Posterior uveitis is treated by observation, periocular and occasionally intraocular glucocorticoid injections, oral glucocorticoid, and/or systemic immunosuppression.

Inflammation of pars plana (the portion of the eye just between the retina and the ciliary body) is associated with multiple sclerosis.

Alcohol dependence

DEFINITION

Alcohol dependence is characterized by three or more of:
- Withdrawal on cessation of alcohol.
- Tolerance.
- Compulsion to drink, difficulty controlling termination or the levels of use.
- Persistent desire to cut down or control use.
- Time is spent obtaining, using, or recovering from alcohol.
- Neglect of other interests (social, occupational, or recreational).
- Continued use despite physical and psychological problems.

Recommended limits for ♀ and ♂ are 14 and 21 units/week, respectively. (1 unit = 8 g alcohol – 1 glass wine or 0.5 pint of beer.)

AETIOLOGY Genetic factors suggested by twin studies and family history (~ 1 in 3 have a parent with alcohol-related problem).

Environmental factors include cultural, parental and peer group influences, availability of alcohol, occupation (e.g. ↑ risk in publicans, doctors, lawyers).

Patients with depressive and anxiety states are at risk.

Alcohol withdrawal: Alcohol enhances inhibitory GABA activity and inhibits excitatory glutamate neurotransmission. Chronic alcohol exposure results in a compensatory reduction in GABA receptor function and upregulation of the glutamate NMDA receptors. Abrupt alcohol cessation leads to overactivation of the excitatory NMDA system relative to the GABA system.

EPIDEMIOLOGY The prevalence of alcohol dependence in primary care populations in the United States was reported as 2–9 % in 2004.

HISTORY

Alcohol history: A drinking diary is useful to record how much, what, when and with whom alcohol is taken.

CAGE screening questions:

Cut-down: '... felt that you should cut-down on intake?

Annoyed: '... felt annoyed by criticism of your drinking?

Guilt: '... felt guilty about how much you drink?

Eye-opener:'... feel that you need a drink when you wake up?

Evaluate for associated comorbidities including smoking, other substance abuse, depression, anxiety and panic attacks.

Acute intoxication: Amnesia, ataxia, dysarthria, disorientation, palpitations, flushing and coma.

Symptoms of withdrawal: Nausea, sweating and tremor, restlessness, agitation, visual hallucination, confusion, seizures.

EXAMINATION

Signs suggestive of chronic alcohol misuse: Dupuytren's contracture, palmar erythema, bruising, spider naevi, telangiectasia, facial mooning, bilateral parotid enlargement, gynaecomastia, smell of alcohol.

Signs of complications: (*See* Complications below and also Alcoholic hepatitis and Liver failure.)

INVESTIGATIONS

Blood: Commonly used markers are MCV (↑), GGT (↑), transaminases (↑). Other less specific markers include ↑ uric acid, ↑ triglycerides or markers of end organ damage (e.g. bilirubin, albumin, PT in liver).

Acute overdose: Blood alcohol, glucose, ABG (risk of ketoacidosis or lactic acidosis), U&E, toxic screen (e.g. barbiturates, paracetamol).

Alcohol dependence (continued)

MANAGEMENT

Acute intoxication: Monitor and support of airway, breathing, circulation. Intubation and ventilation if severe respiratory depression, IV fluids and careful monitoring of urine output, blood glucose (as may ↓), U&E and blood gases.

Withdrawal: IV vitamin B complex (Pabrinex) and reducing doses of chlordiazepoxide. Close attention to dehydration, electrolyte imbalances and infections. Nutritional support important as often malnourished. Lactulose and phosphate enemas may help any encephalopathy.

Advice and intervention: Motivational interviewing techniques, counselling and community-based services, self-help groups (e.g. AA), alcohol treatment units for those with established problems, detoxification period is necessary for those physically dependent.

Medical: Acamprosate reduces craving. Naltrexone (opioid receptor antagonist) may be given to patients who need additional support to maintain abstinence (contraindicated in patients with underlying liver disease, and liver function tests should be monitored). Disulfiram (an aldehyde dehydrogenase inhibitor) causes patient to develop vasomotor symptoms, nausea, abdominal pain when drinking alcohol.

COMPLICATIONS

GI: Oesophagitis, Mallory–Weiss tears, varices, gastritis, peptic ulcers, acute or chronic pancreatitis.

Liver: Fatty change, alcoholic hepatitis, cirrhosis.

Neurological: Acute intoxication.

Withdrawal: Fits, delirium tremens (48–72 h after cessation – coarse tremor, agitation, fever, tachycardia, confusion, delusions and hallucinations). Chronic complications include cerebral atrophy and dementia, cerebellar degeneration, optic atrophy, peripheral neuropathy, myopathy. Indirect effects include hepatic encephalopathy, thiamine deficiency, causing Wernicke's encephalopathy[1] or Korsakoff's psychosis.[2]

Haematological: Anaemia (vitamin B_{12} or folate deficiency, iron deficiency in patients with GI bleeding), thrombocytopaenia (due to enlarged spleen in patient with cirrhosis or direct toxic effect on megakaryocytes), abnormal platelet function.

Respiratory: Depression, inhalation of vomitus.

Cardiac: Hypertension, cardiomyopathy, arrhythmias.

Drug interactions: E.g. oral contraceptive pills (alcohol is a liver enzyme-inhibitor acutely, but chronic abuse induces liver enzymes.)

Teratogenicity: Foetal alcohol syndrome.

Psychosocial: Depression, anxiety, deliberate self-harm. Domestic, employment and financial problems.

PROGNOSIS Depends on complications. Alcoholic fatty liver is reversible on abstinence from alcohol. In general, 5-year survival rates in those with alcoholic cirrhosis who stop drinking are 60–75%, but < 40% in those who continue.

[1] **Wernicke's encephalopathy** is nystagmus, ophthalmoplaegia and ataxia, together with apathy, disorientation and disturbed memory. Treat urgently with thiamine or may progress to Korsakoff's psychosis.

[2] **Korsakoff's psychosis** is characterized by profound impairment of retrograde and anterograde memory with confabulation, as a result of damage to the mammillary bodies and the hippocampus. Irreversible.

Amyloidosis

DEFINITION Heterogeneous group of diseases characterized by extracellular deposition of amyloid fibrils.

AETIOLOGY Amyloid fibrils are polymers comprising low-molecular-weight subunit proteins. These subunits are derived from proteins that undergo conformational changes to adopt a predominantly antiparallel β-pleated sheet configuration. They associate with glycosaminoglycans and serum amyloid P-component (SAP), and their deposition progressively disrupts the structure and function of normal tissue.

Amyloidosis is classified according to fibril subunit proteins.

Type of amyloid	Fibril protein	Underlying disorders
AA	Serum amyloid A protein	Chronic inflammatory diseases (e.g. rheumatoid arthritis, seronegative arthritides, Crohn's disease, familial Mediterranean fever); chronic infections (TB, bronchiectasis, osteomyelitis); malignancy (e.g. Hodgkin's disease, renal cancer)
AL	Monoclonal immuno-globulin light chains	Subtle monoclonal plasma cell dyscrasias, multiple myeloma, Waldenström's macroglobulinaemia, B-cell lymphoma
ATTR (familial amyloid polyneuropath)	Genetic-variant transthyretin	Autosomal dominantly transmitted mutations in the gene for transthyretin (*TTR*). Variable penetrance. Hereditary amyloidosis is also associated with other variant proteins

Amyloidosis can be systemic (generalized) as mentioned earlier or localized e.g. in pancreatic islets of Langerhans (type 2 diabetes), cerebral cortex (Alzheimer's disease), cerebral blood vessels (amyloid angiopathy) and in bones and joints (in long-term dialysis caused by β_2-microglobulin).

EPIDEMIOLOGY:
AA amyloidosis: Lifetime incidence of 1–5 % among patients with chronic inflammatory diseases.
AL amyloidosis: Estimated annual incidence of about 3,000 cases in the United States and 300–600 cases in the United Kingdom.
Hereditary amyloidosis: Present in $\sim$ 5 % of patients with systemic amyloidosis.

HISTORY AND EXAMINATION
Renal: Proteinuria, nephrotic syndrome, renal failure.
Cardiac: Restrictive cardiomyopathy, heart failure, arrhythmia, angina (due to accumulation of amyloid in the coronary arteries).
GI: Macroglossia (characteristic of AL), hepatomegly, splenomegaly, gut dysmotility, malabsorption, bleeding.
Neurological: Sensory and motor neuropathy, autonomic neuropathy (symptoms of bowel or bladder dysfunction, postural hypotension), carpal tunnel syndrome.
Skin: Waxy skin and easy bruising, purpura around eyes (characteristic of AL), plaques and nodules.
Joints: Painful asymmetrical large joints, 'shoulder pad' sign (enlargement of the anterior shoulder).
Haematological: Bleeding diathesis (factor X deficiency due to binding on amyloid fibrils primarily in the liver and spleen; and ↓ synthesis of coagulation factors in patients with advanced liver disease).

Amyloidosis (continued)

INVESTIGATIONS

Tissue biopsy (Congo red stain, immunohistochemistry)**:** To diagnose amyloidosis and identify amyloid fibril protein. Reliable in AA, often poor for AL.

Urine: Proteinuria, free immunoglobulin light chains in AL.

Blood: CRP or ESR, rheumatoid factor, immunoglobulin levels and serum protein electrophoresis, LFTs, U&E. SAA levels for monitoring treatment in AA.

^{123}**I-SAP scan:** Radiolabelled SAP localizes to the deposits enabling quantitative imaging of amyloidotic organs throughout the body.

Bone marrow, echocardiography and other investigations including DNA analysis for underlying disorders.

MANAGEMENT

Medical: Reduction in the supply of the respective amyloid fibril precursor protein (e.g. chemotherapy for monoclonal hyperimmunoglobulinaemia, colchicine in familial Mediterranean fever, anti-inflammatory drugs in rheumatoid arthritis). Dialysis. Management of hypertension, arrhythmias and symptomatic treatment.

Surgical: Organ transplantation in selected cases. Liver transplantation is effective in hereditary ATTR because this particular genetically variant precursor protein is produced in hepatocytes.

COMPLICATIONS   Failure of single or multiple organ systems, most commonly kidneys and heart (in AL type).

PROGNOSIS   Without effective treatment:

AA: 50 % die within 10 years of diagnosis.

AL: 80 % die within 2 years. Survival can be prolonged substantially by treatment in at least 50 % of patients.

Anaphylaxis

DEFINITION Acute life-threatening multisystem syndrome caused by sudden release of mast cell- and basophil-derived mediators into the circulation.

AETIOLOGY Can be classified as:

Immunologic: IgE-mediated or immune complex/complement-mediated. **Non-immunologic:** mast cell or basophil degranulation without the involvement of antibodies (e.g. reactions caused by vancomycin, codeine, ACE inhibitors).

Inflammatory mediators such as histamine, tryptase, chymase, histamine-releasing factor, PAF, prostaglandins and leucotrienes cause bronchospasm, ↑ capillary permeability and ↓ vascular tone, resulting in tissue oedema.

Common allergens include drugs (e.g. penicillin), radiological contrast agents, latex, insect stings, egg, peanuts, shellfish and fish. Anaphylaxis may occur following repeated administration of blood products in patients with selective IgA deficiency (as a result of formation of anti-IgA antibodies). Anaphylaxis can also be induced by exercise.

EPIDEMIOLOGY Relatively common. Anaphylaxis occurs in $\sim$ 1 in 5,000 exposures to parenteral penicillin or cephalosporins.

1–2 % of patients receiving IV radiocontrast experience a hypersensitivity reaction (often minor). 0.5–1 % of children suffer from peanut allergy. 1 in 700 patients have selective IgA deficiency.

HISTORY Acute onset of symptoms on exposure to allergen:
- Wheeze, shortness of breath or sensation of choking.
- Swelling of lips and face.
- Pruritus, rash.

The severity of previous reactions does not predict the severity of future reactions. Patients may have a history of other allergic hypersensitivity disorders e.g. asthma, allergic rhinitis.

Biphasic reactions occur 1–72 h after the first reaction in up to 20% of patients.

EXAMINATION Tachypnoea, wheeze, cyanosis.

Swollen upper airways and eyes, rhinitis, conjunctival injection.

Urticarial rash (erythematous wheals).

Hypotension, tachycardia.

INVESTIGATIONS The diagnosis of anaphylaxis is made clinically.

Serum tryptase (measured within 15 min–3 h after onset of symptoms), or histamine levels (measured preferably within 30 min after symptom onset) and urinary metabolites of histamine (which may remain elevated for several hours after symptom onset) can support the clinical diagnosis. Normal levels of these mediators do not exclude the possibility of anaphylaxis.

After the attack:

Allergen skin testing: Identifies allergen. It should be performed by an allergy specialist, because of the risk of anaphylaxis and the skill required for proper interpretation.

IgE immunoassays: E.g. radioallergosorbent tests (RASTs) to identify food-specific IgE in the serum.

MANAGEMENT Stop any suspected drugs.

Resuscitation according to principles of airway, breathing and circulation.

Secure airway and give 100 % O_2. Intubation and transfer to ITU may be necessary so anaesthetist must be informed early.

Adrenaline IM (0.5 mL of 1:1,000). This can be repeated every 10 min according to response of pulse and BP.

Antihistamine IV (10 mg chlorpheniramine).

Steroids IV (100 mg hydrocortisone).

Anaphylaxis (continued)

IV crystalloid or colloid to maintain blood pressure. If hypotensive, lie patient flat with head tilted down.

Treat bronchospasm with salbutamol ± ipratropium inhaler. Aminophylline IV infusion may be required.

Advice: Educate on use of adrenaline pen for IM administration. Provide Medicalert bracelet. Make note in patient's notes and drug charts. Referral to an allergy specialist for identification of the culprit allergen and education in allergen avoidance.

COMPLICATIONS   Respiratory failure, shock, death.

PROGNOSIS   Good if prompt treatment given.

Arteriovenous fistulae and malformations

DEFINITION

Arteriovenous fistula: An abnormal communication between an artery and vein that bypasses the capillary bed.

Arteriovenous malformations: Malformation with normal endothelium.

Haemangioma/Angioma: Malformation with endothelial hyperplasia.

AETIOLOGY

Congenital: Divided into haemangiomas, (e.g strawberry naevi) and malformations (AVMs). The latter is divided into low flow or high flow (e.g. hepatic or pulmonary AVM).

Hereditary: AVMs and haemangiomas are associated with many different hereditary syndromes, e.g. Klippel–Trénaunay, Kasabach–Merritt, Sturge–Weber, von-Hippel–Lindau and Hereditary Haemorrhagic Telangiectasia (Osler–Weber–Rendu syndrome).

Acquired: Trauma, tumours (e.g. glomus tumour, hypernephroma and sarcomas), infection, inflammation (e.g. aorto-venocaval fistula) or iatrogenic (e.g. Brescia–Cimino fistula for haemodialysis or portocaval shunt in portal hypertension).

EPIDEMIOLOGY   Cutaneous haemangiomas are very common, the others less so.

HISTORY   Presentation is variable, depending on the site and size of the AVM and symptoms may be due to local or systemic effects (*see* Complications).

Congenital cutaneous haemangiomas are often visible from or soon after birth.

Malformations usually grow with age, puberty or pregnancy.

Those within internal organs may only be detected once complications develop.

Other presentations include varicose veins, limb swelling or pain.

EXAMINATION   Cutaneous haemangiomas (Campbell de Morgan spots) are usually scarlet in colour, firm and cannot be emptied of blood on compression.

Internal AVMs may be revealed by an overlying bruit or palpable thrill, possibly with reduced distal pulses and ↑ pulse pressure.

Signs of complications (*see* Complications).

INVESTIGATIONS

Imaging of AVMs: Depends on the site of the lesion. Modalities used include duplex scanning, CT or MRI scanning or invasive angiography.

SPECT scan: Quantification of AV shunting uses radiolabelled microspheres that are introduced into an artery and are too large to pass through capillaries. Those passing through AVMs are trapped in the lungs and quantified using a gamma camera.

MANAGEMENT

Conservative: Cutaneous haemangiomas usually undergo spontaneous regression at the end of the first year of life. Internal organ AVMs may not necessitate treatment and can be monitored.

Interventional radiology: In the case of internal AVMs or fistulae, embolization with metal coils, tissue adhesive or particles can be performed.

Surgery: Often difficult, but excision (after pre-op embolization) may be possible in the case of small and accessible AVMs.

Stereotactic radiosurgery: Useful on small AVMs, may take years for full effect.

COMPLICATIONS

Cutaneous: Cosmetic disfigurement, ulceration, bleeding.

Organ-specific: E.g. brain AVMs can cause focal neurological deficits, seizures or stroke; pulmonary AVMs can cause haemoptysis or parodoxical embolism.

Distal: Ischaemia of peripheral tissues.

Systemic: High-ouput cardiac failure in the case of large AVMs.

PROGNOSIS   Depends on site and aetiology. 90 % of haemangiomas regress by 5–10 years. 1–4 % annual risk of haemorrhage in cerebral AVMs.

Aspirin overdose

DEFINITION   Excessive ingestion of aspirin causing toxicity.

AETIOLOGY   Overdose can occur as a result of deliberate self-harm, suicidal intent or by accident (e.g. in children). Ingestion of 10–20 g can cause moderate-to-severe toxicity in adults.

Aspirin (acetylsalicylate) increases respiratory rate and depth by stimulating the CNS respiratory centre. This hyperventilation produces respiratory alkalosis in the early phase. The body then compensates by increasing urinary bicarbonate and K^+ excretion, causing dehydration and hypokalaemia. Loss of bicarbonate together with the uncoupling of mitochondrial oxidative phosphorylation by salicylic acid and build up of lactic acid can lead to metabolic acidosis.

In severe overdoses, CNS depression and respiratory failure can occur.

EPIDEMIOLOGY   One of the most common drug overdoses.

HISTORY
Ascertain the key facts:
- How much aspirin?
- When?
- Any other drugs?
- Have you had any alcohol?

The patient may be asymptomatic initially.
Early symptoms: Flushed appearance, fever, sweating, hyperventilation, dizziness, tinnitus, deafness.
Late symptoms: Lethargy, confusion, convulsions, drowsiness, respiratory depression, coma.

EXAMINATION   Fever, tachycardia, hyperventilation, epigastric tenderness.

INVESTIGATIONS
Blood: Salicylate levels (500–750 mg/L is a moderate overdose; >750 mg/L is a severe overdose), FBC, U&E (particularly $\downarrow K^+$ if vomiting), LFT ($\uparrow$ AST/ALT), clotting screen ($\uparrow$ PT), glucose and other drug levels (e.g. paracetamol). *ABG:* May show mixed metabolic acidosis and respiratory alkalosis.
ECG: May show signs of hypokalaemia – small T waves, U waves.

MANAGEMENT
Acute: Resuscitate with attention to respiratory rate and blood gases. Treat hypovolaemia (rehydrate), hypokalaemia, hypoglycaemia; vitamin K for hypoprothrombinaemia (occasionally).
If < 12 h after ingestion: Gastric lavage to empty the stomach, and oral activated charcoal to bind to and $\downarrow$ absorption of the drug.
Moderate cases (500–750 mg/L): Urine alkalinization with IV $NaHCO_3$ (with IV potassium chloride for hypokalaemia) aims to $\uparrow$ salicylate excretion (aim for urine pH 7.5–8.5).
Severe cases (> 750 mg/L) or in severe acidosis: Consider haemodialysis.
In all cases, monitor U&E, glucose (may $\uparrow$ or $\downarrow$), temperature, pulse, respiratory rate, BP, urine output.

COMPLICATIONS   Cerebral and pulmonary oedema ($\uparrow$ capillary permeability).
Metabolic disturbances ($\downarrow K^+$, $\downarrow$ or $\uparrow Na^+$, $\downarrow$ or $\uparrow$ glucose).
Acute renal failure.

PROGNOSIS   If treated early, prognosis is good.
Note: In children < 4 years, even low doses of aspirin are associated with an increased risk of developing Reye's syndrome (metabolic acidosis, liver and CNS disturbances). Aspirin can also trigger an asthma attack in certain individuals.

Hyperlipidaemia

DEFINITION   Elevation of one or more plasma lipid fractions.

AETIOLOGY
Primary: Some have molecular genetic basis, but most are unknown.
- *Familial hypercholesterolaemia:* ↓ Functional hepatic LDL receptors.
- *Familial hypertriglyceridaemia:* Unknown. Autosomal dominant.
- *Hypertriglyceridaemia:* Lipoprotein lipase or apo-CII deficiency.
- *Familial combined hyperlipidaemia:* Unknown.
- *Remnant hyperlipidaemia:* Apo-E2 genotype inheritance, accumulation of LDL remnants.

Secondary: Subdivided depending on the predominant abnormality.
- ↑ **Cholesterol**: Hypothyroidism, nephrotic syndrome, cholestatic liver disease, anorexia nervosa.
- ↑ **Triglycerides**: Diabetes mellitus, drugs (β-blockers, thiazides, oestrogens), alcohol, obesity, chronic renal disease, hepatocellular diseases.

Physiology: LDL accumulates in intima of systemic arteries, and is taken up by LDL receptor on macrophage. This forms a foam cell, part of atheromatous plaque. HDL acts as shuttle in periphery for transport of cholesterol esters back to the liver and is therefore cardioprotective.

EPIDEMIOLOGY   50 % of the UK population have a cholesterol level high enough to be a risk for CHD.

HISTORY
Asymptomatic.
Symptoms of CVS complications.
Enquire about other CVS risk factors:
- Diabetes
- Family history
- Smoking
- Hypertension

EXAMINATION   Usually normal. Examine for secondary causes.
Signs of lipid deposits: Around the eyes (xanthelasmas), cornea (arcus), tendons xanthomas (e.g. extensor tendons of the hands, Achilles tendon, patella tendon), tuberous xanthomas on knees and elbows, xanthomas in palmar creases (in remnant hyperlipidaemia), eruptive xanthomas and lipidaemia retinalis (pale retinal vessels) in severe hypertriglyceridaemia.
Signs of complications: E.g. ↓ peripheral pulses, carotid bruit, other cardiovascular risks – associated high BP.

INVESTIGATIONS
Blood: Fasting lipid profile, exclude secondary causes: glucose, TFT, LFT, U&E.
Cardiovascular risk assessment: Assess using various algorithms, e.g. Framingham risk equation, QRISK or ASSIGN.[1]

MANAGEMENT   Treat secondary causes.
Advice: Exercise, lose weight, stop smoking, control BP, control diabetes, ↓ alcohol, dietary modification.

---

[1] Framingham risk score is well validated for estimating 10-year cardiovascular risk (http://hp2010.nhlbihin. net/atpiii/calculator.asp), but it is derived from a North American population. The QRisk and ASSIGN calculators have been developed for an English or Scottish population and can be assessed online at: http:// www.qrisk.org.uk and http://assign-score.com.

Hyperlipidaemia (continued)

Lipid-lowering drugs: Indicated for:

1) *Primary prevention:* Patients with multiple risk factors and no atherosclerosis (primary prevention) when risk for coronary heart disease > 20% in 10 years; and
2) *Secondary prevention:* Patients with established atherosclerosis, e.g. coronary heart disease, carotid artery disease and aortic aneurysms (secondary prevention).

   - Target: total cholesterol < 4 mmol/L, LDL ≤ 2 mmol/L

For ↑ total cholesterol or ↑ LDL:

- *HMG-CoA reductase inhibitors ('statins'):* Potently lowers mortality and CVS morbidity is demonstrated in numerous trials. High dose is recommended as first line (e.g. 40 mg simvastatin).
- *Ezetimibe:* Inhibits cholesterol absorption in the gut. Can be used if a statin is not tolerated, or as an adjunctive agent.

For ↑ tyriglycerides:

- *Fibrates (e.g. bezafibrate):* Stimulates lipoprotein lipase activity via specific transcription factors.
- *Fish oil:* Rich in omega-3 marine trigylcerides, but this is not a recommended method of treating hyperlipidaemia (it can aggravate hypercholesterolaemia.)

Other drugs:

- *Anion-exchange resins (e.g. colestyramine, colestipol):* Binds bile acids and ↓ reabsorption, ↑ hepatic cholesterol conversion to bile acids and ↑ LDL receptor expression on hepatocytes.
- *Nicotinic acid:* ↓ Hepatic VLDL release, ↓ triglycerides, ↓ cholesterol and ↑ HDL. Use is limited by side effects (prostaglandin-mediated vasodilation, flushing, dizziness, palpitations). ↑ Glucose and urate.

COMPLICATIONS   Coronary artery disease, MI, peripheral vascular disease, strokes.

In hypertriglyceridaemia: Pancreatitis and retinal vein thrombosis.

Complication of treatment: Statins are associated with myositis.

PROGNOSIS   Depends on early diagnosis, treatment of hyperlipidaemia and control of other CVS risk factors. There is some evidence that lipid-lowering agents prevent cerebrovascular accidents.

Marfan syndrome

DEFINITION   Autosomal dominant inherited disorder of connective tissue, characterized by abnormalities in musculoskeletal, cardiovascular and ocular systems.

AETIOLOGY   Mutation in fibrillin-1 gene (*FBN1*) located on chromosome 15q. 25 % are spontaneous new mutations and occur anywhere on the gene.
Fibrillin-1 is a main component of extracellular microfibrils, which are abundant in elastic tissue especially of skin, blood vessels, perichondrium and ciliary zonules of the eye. Mutations are predicted to disrupt the structural organization of the microfibrils.
A minority of cases may be due to an inactivating mutation in a gene encoding a receptor for transforming growth factor-β.

EPIDEMIOLOGY   Annual incidence is 1 in 10,000.

HISTORY   Musculoskeletal problems (e.g. frequent joint dislocations).
Visual difficulties (e.g. sudden visual deterioration as a result of lens dislocation).
Cardiovascular complications (e.g. heart failure).
May be asymptomatic and present as a result of family history.

EXAMINATION   Tall stature, long, thin extremities. Arm span > height. Long spidery fingers (arachnodactyly).
Kyphoscoliosis, chest deformities (pectus excavatum or carinatum).
Joint hypermobility common, skin striae. High-arched palate, crowding of teeth.
Lens dislocation.
Signs of mitral valve prolapse or aortic regurgitation (*see* Complications – below and also Mitral regurgitation and Aortic regurgitation).

INVESTIGATIONS   Skeletal examination and family history is often sufficient to diagnose the condition.
Slit lamp examination: To examine for signs of lens dislocation.
Echocardiography: Screens for valve disease.
Genetic analysis: Useful for research purposes and to confirm diagnosis.
Plasma total homocysteine to exclude homocystinuria, which shares some phenotypic features with Marfan syndrome.

MANAGEMENT   Best managed by a specialist centre.
Lifestyle adaptations: Avoidance of strenuous exercise and contact sports, supports when exercising.
Eyes: Annual slit lamp examination.
Musculoskeletal: Orthopaedic assessments.
Cardiac: Regular ECG and echocardiograms to monitor changes in valves and aortic diameter. β-Blockers (e.g. propranolol, atenolol) may slow rate of aortic root dilation by reducing blood pressure (titrate dose to limit heart rate to <110 bpm following submaximal exercise). Calcium channel blocker in those who do not tolerate a β-blocker.
Surgery:
Mitral valve repair. Aortic root surgery when diameter > 5 cm.
Scoliosis that does not respond to physical therapy and bracing.
Severe pectus deformities.
Recurrent pneumothoraces.
Myopia, retinal tears and detachment (treated with photocoagulation).
Genetic counselling and careful monitoring during pregnancy (aortic rupture or dissection can occur at any root size).

Marfan syndrome (continued)

COMPLICATIONS   Heart failure as a result of mitral regurgitation or aortic root dilation and aortic regurgitation, aortic dissection, dysrhythmias, bacterial endocarditis. Spontaneous pneumothorax. Upward dislocation of the lens, myopia and, less commonly, retinal detachment.

PROGNOSIS   Life span is shortened because of cardiovascular complications. Mean survival is in the fourth decade, but may be extended with good care and heart surgery.

Paracetamol overdose

DEFINITION   Excessive ingestion of paracetamol causing toxicity.

AETIOLOGY
Maximum recommended dose: Two 500 mg tablets four times in 24 h. Intake of > 12 g or > 150 mg/kg can cause hepatic necrosis.

ASSOCIATIONS/RISK FACTORS   Chronic alcohol abusers or those on enzyme-inducing drugs (which ↑ cytochrome P450 activity, e.g. anticonvulsants or anti-TB drugs), malnourished, anorexia nervosa, HIV are more susceptible to toxic effects of paracetamol. Overdose of paracetamol is commonly associated with ingestion of other substances, e.g. alcohol.

EPIDEMIOLOGY   Most common intentional drug overdose in the United Kingdom, 70,000/year, ♀ > ♂, causing ∼ 100 deaths/year, this has been reduced by legislation in 1998 restricting pack sizes.

HISTORY   Very important to ascertain timing and quantity of overdose, and presence of risk factors.
0–24 h: Asymptomatic or mild nausea, vomiting, lethargy, malaise.
24–72 h: RUQ abdominal pain, vomiting.
> 72 h: Increasing confusion (encephalopathy), jaundice.

EXAMINATION
0–24 h: No signs are evident.
24–72 h: Liver enlargement and tenderness.
> 72 h: Jaundice, coagulopathy, hypoglycaemia and renal angle pain.

PATHOLOGY/PATHOGENESIS   At therapeutic levels, paracetamol is metabolized in the liver by conjugation with glucuronate or sulphate and excreted by the kidneys. A proportion (< 7 %) is metabolized by cytochrome P450 mixed function oxidases to a toxic highly reactive intermediate N-acetyl-p-benzoquinoneimine (NAPQI), which can be inactivated by conjugation with glutathione. At toxic levels the conjugation pathway and glutathione stores are overwhelmed, leading to NAPQI-induced oxidative damage and acute liver necrosis.

INVESTIGATIONS   Paracetamol levels, 4 h post ingestion (absorbed rapidly, hence peak plasma levels are usually within 4 h). Assess need to treat based on normogram (see UK National Poisons Information Service guidelines). FBC, U&Es, glucose, LFTs, clotting screen, lactate, ABG (for degree of acidosis).

MANAGEMENT   See UK National Poisons Information Service guidelines.
Patient presenting within 8 h of overdose: If level within toxic range, antidote should be given – IV N-acetylcysteine (NAC).
Caution: NAC can cause anaphylactoid reactions (treated with antihistamines). A less effective alternative is oral methionine.
Patient presenting > 8 h after overdose: If dose > 150 mg/kg then start NAC immediately before waiting for levels (efficacy of NAC is more limited after 15 h). Continue NAC until PT is normalized.
Patient with hepatotoxicity: Good supportive care with management of complications.
Liver transplantation indications: Late acidosis (>36h post overdose) with arterial pH < 7.3, PT > 100 sec, creatinine > 300 μM, grade 3 encephalopathy (confused, distressed, barely rousable).

COMPLICATIONS   Acute hepatic failure, hypoglycaemia, cerebral oedema, GI bleeding, coagulation defects, metabolic acidosis, pancreatitis, acute tubular necrosis and renal failure (25 % if severe damage).

PROGNOSIS   Depends on dose ingested and time of presentation. Early treatment with NAC may be lifesaving.

Shorter Topics

Adult Still's disease

An inflammatory disorder characterized by quotidian fevers, arthritis and rash (migratory salmon-coloured rash on trunk or thighs; typically in evening returning to normal in morning). The Koebner phenomenon may be present (cutaneous eruption elicited by stroking the skin). Other manifestations include: pharyngitis, lymphadenopathy, pericarditis, pleural effusions and transient pulmonary infiltrates.

CAUSE   Unknown. An autoimmune disease, possibly triggered by cross-immunity between an infectious agent in a genetically susceptible individual.

INVESTIGATIONS   Exclude infection, malignancy and rheumatic fever. Associated with markedly elevated serum ferritin. FBC (anaemia of chronic disease, ↑ WCC, ↑ platelets), ↑ ESR and CRP. Joint aspiration for microscopy and culture.

MANAGEMENT   NSAIDs (e.g. Ibuprofen) in patients with relatively mild disease. Glucocorticoids from the outset of therapy for patients with high fevers, debilitating joint symptoms or internal organ involvement. TNF-α inhibitors, anakinra, or rituximab if not controlled with NSAIDs and glucocorticoids. Disease-modifying antirheumatic drugs (e.g. methotrexate and cyclosporine) have been also used in the treatment of adult Still's disease.

Alport's syndrome

Haematuric nephritis and sensorineural deafness.

CAUSE   An inherited mutation in the gene coding for collagen type IV.

INVESTIGATIONS   Urine microscopy, 24-h urinary protein, auditory threshold testing and detailed family history ($+$ genetic testing).

MANAGEMENT
Supportive.
In patients with hypertension or overt proteinuria: ACE inhibitor or angiotensin II receptor blocker.
In patients who develop end-stage renal disease: Either dialysis or transplantation.

α_1-Antitrypsin deficiency

↓ Levels of α_1-antitrypsin can lead to lung emphysema or liver cirrhosis.

CAUSE α_1-Antitrypsin is a liver-derived protein which acts as an inhibitor of tissue proteases, in particular neutrophil elastase. ↓ Levels of α_1-antitrypsin results in ↑ elastase activity. In the lung, there is ↑ breakdown of elastin and ↓ mucociliary clearance leading to emphysema and chronic bronchitis. α_1-Antitrypsin accumulation in hepatocytes appears to be responsible for liver damage, but the mechanism is unclear.

INVESTIGATIONS
Blood: LFTs (all enzymes may be ↑).
Plasma electrophoresis: α_1 Band is missing or lowered (< 2 g/L). CXR: bullae may predominate in the lower zones.
Pulmonary function tests: ↓ FEV_1: FVC ratio, ↓ PEF↓, gas transfer coefficient of CO.
Liver biopsy: Staining with PAS to detect α_1-antitrypsin accumulation and assess degree of liver damage.

MANAGEMENT   Stop smoking and ↓ alcohol intake. Genetic counselling.
Lung: Bronchodilators, if severe, assessment for long-term oxygen therapy or single-lung transplantation. IV infusion of α_1-antitrypsin to raise the plasma levels above the protective threshold (Not assessed in randomized trials).
Liver: Transplantation for end-stage disease.
Panniculitis: Dapsone or IV α_1-antitrypsin.

Ataxia-Telangiectasia

Cerebellar ataxia, skin telangiectasias, radiation sensitivity (high risk of malignancies).

CAUSE   An autosomal recessive inherited mutation of the ATM gene.

INVESTIGATIONS   Skin biopsy, cytogenetics, radiation-free screening (e.g. ultrasound).

MANAGEMENT   Regular monitoring for malignancies.

Bacterial overgrowth

Proliferation of abnormal bacterial flora in the small intestine. May present with diarrhoea, steatorrhoea and symptoms/signs of nutrient malabsorption e.g. vitamin B_{12} deficiency.

CAUSE
Motility disorders (e.g. diabetic autonomic neuropathy, amyloidosis).
Anatomical abnormalities (e.g. jejunal diverticulosis).
↓ **Gastric acid production** (gastric resection, vagotomy, chronic atrophic gastritis, pernicious anaemia, PPIs)

INVESTIGATIONS   ↓Hb, ↑MCV, ↓vitamin B_{12}.
Breath test: Detection of exhaled $^{14}CO_2$ (after intake of ^{14}C-labelled bile salts by mouth) or hydrogen (after intake of glucose by mouth).
Proximal small intestinal aspiration: Microbiological culture, analysis of unconjugated bile acid proportion.
Barium follow-through: To detect structural abnormalities.
Small intestinal biopsy: To exclude coeliac disease.

MANAGEMENT
Treat the underlying cause: E.g. surgical correction of the structural abnormality such as a stricture. Rotating antibiotic regimens (e.g. ciprofloxacin, doxycycline and metronidazole). Nutritional support e.g. vitamin B_{12}, vitamin K and calcium.

Behcet's disease

An inflammatory multisystem disease featuring a triad of orogenital ulceration and uveitis.

CAUSE   Unknown, but HLA-B51 and ancestry from Turkey, Greece or central Asia.

INVESTIGATIONS
Pathergy test (needleprick becomes inflamed and a sterile pustule develops within 24–48 h). Complement levels, family history.

MANAGEMENT   Steroids and/or immunosuppression.

Benign paroxysmal positional vertigo (BPPV)

Vertigo lasting seconds to minutes on changing head position (e.g. sitting to lying down, turning head suddenly).

CAUSE   Displacement of otoliths (from degeneration, trauma or post-viral) into the canals (usually posterior canal) resulting in canaliths.

INVESTIGATIONS   Hallpike testing (clinical test).

MANAGEMENT   Epley or Semont manoeuvres for posterior canal BPPV; barbeque manoeuvre for horizontal canal BPPV.

Budd–Chiari syndrome

Obstruction to hepatic venous outflow resulting in abdominal pain, ascites, jaundice, encephalopathy, variceal bleeding and hepato/splenomegaly (due to portal hypertension).

CAUSE Venous thrombosis secondary to a hypercoagulable state or malignancies. Occasionally caused by membranous venous webs in the IVC.

INVESTIGATIONS
Blood: LFT (↑transaminases), FBC, U&Es, clotting and thrombophilia screen.
Doppler ultrasound: ↓ Blood flow in hepatic vein. Hepatic venogram and inferior venacavography. MRI.

MANAGEMENT Medical treatment (supportive care, anticoagulation, and thrombolysis in early stages), radiological procedures (angioplasty, TIPS, and stenting) and surgery (shunting procedures and liver transplantation). Treat complications related to fluid retention, malnutrition, and portal hypertension.

Cysticercosis
Cystic lesions in the brain predisposing to epilepsy.

CAUSE Infestation from eggs of the tapeworm (Taenia solium) transmitted through contaminated water and meat.

INVESTIGATIONS MRI-brain, Plain radiograph of thigh (for calcification).

MANAGEMENT Treatment of epilepsy with anticonvulsants; treatment of lesion is not recommended in most cases as it can provoke an inflammatory reaction. If treatment of lesion is necessary, praziquantel or albendazole and steroids are used. Surgical excision or ventricular shunting may be necessary for lesions causing obstruction.

Familial Mediterranean fever (FMF)/Familial Hibernian fever (FHF)
Periodic fevers, serositis (peritonitis and pleurisy).

CAUSE Mutations in the pyrin protein involved in neutrophil regulation (FMF) and a tumour necrosis factor receptor (FHF).

Friedreich's ataxia
Cerebellar ataxia, peripheral neuropathy, cardiomyopathy and diabetes mellitus.

CAUSE An autosomal recessive inherited mutation of the Frataxin gene.

INVESTIGATIONS Glucose tolerance test, echocardiogram, nerve conduction study, family history, genetic testing.

MANAGEMENT
Supportive.

Kartagener's syndrome
Chronic sinusitis, bronchiectasis, infertility and situs inversus.

CAUSE
Immotile cilia.

Langerhans cell histiocytosis
Proliferation of Langerhans cells affecting multiple systems: Skin (papular rash with brown, red, or crusted areas), lungs (dyspnoea due to fibrosis, bullae, airway obstruction by histiocytomas → restrictive and/or obstructive defects on lung function tests, cysts and nodules on CT), pituitary (*diabetes insipidus:* polydipsia and polyuria), otitis externa, bone pain, radiolucent lesions in skull bones, bone marrow infiltration (pancytopaenia), lymphadenopathy, gingival hypertrophy, weight loss, ataxia, and memory problems.

Langerhans cell histiocytosis (continued)

MANAGEMENT   Purine analogue cladribine is effective for adults with skin, bone, lymph node, and probably pulmonary and CNS disease. Steroids may slow the progression of lung disease in patients with nodular disease.

Lyme disease

Erythema chronicum migrans, any neuropathy (typically facial palsy, multiple mononeuro-pathies) or plexopathy, heart block.

CAUSE
Spirochete (*Borellia bugdoferi*) infection from a tick bite.

INVESTIGATIONS   Lyme serology, Lumbar puncture (elevated CSF protein, high CSF lymphocyte count), nerve conduction study.

MANAGEMENT   In the acute phase, oral doxycycline for 14 days. In the later stages, intravenous ceftriaxone is standard treatment.

Mastocytosis, systemic

Characterized by excessive mast cell proliferation and accumulation in the skin, bone marrow and other tissues. Patients may present with skin findings (pruritus, urticaria pigmentosa: small, hyperpigmented papules that urticate or flush when rubbed [Darier's sign], cutaneous mastocytomas), symptoms due to release of mast cell mediators (allergic reactions and anaphylaxis), symptoms due to mast cell infiltration of various organs (steatorrhoea, mal-absorption, lymphadenopathy, splenomegaly, liver and haematological abnormalities, skel-etal lesions).

CAUSE   ↑ Expression of stem cell factor (required for mast cell development) and activating mutations of its receptor (*c-kit*) have been implicated in the pathogenesis of mastocytosis.

INVESTIGATIONS   FBC, LFTs, ↑ serum tryptase. Punch biopsy of skin lesions with specific histopathologic stains. Bone marrow biopsy and aspiration.

MANAGEMENT   Avoid precipitating factors. Carry an anaphylaxis wallet card and at least 2 doses of adrenaline in a self-injectable form at all times (for treatment of anaphylaxis). One or more drugs to counteract the symptoms caused by ↑ production and release of mast cell mediators: H1 and H2 anti-histamines, cromolyn sodium (prevents the mast cell release of histamine and leukotrienes), anti-leukotriene agents, proton pump inhibitors. 1–5 % progress to a more aggressive form e.g. mast cell leukaemia (treated with polychemotherapy).

Medullary sponge kidney

Characterized by dilation of the terminal collecting ducts in the medulla, causing cysts which contain calcium phosphate stones. May present with renal colic, haematuria and urinary tract infections. Rarely leads to renal insufficiency.

CAUSE   May reflect a developmental abnormality. Underlying defect is not known.

INVESTIGATIONS   Intravenous pyelogram (cystic dilatations appear as a 'brush' radiating outward from the calyces).

MANAGEMENT   Treat urinary tract infections and renal stones. Excellent long-term prognosis.

Ménière's disease

Recurrent episodes of tinnitus, paroxysmal vertigo and unilateral fluctuating hearing loss.

CAUSE   Disturbed homoeostasis of endolymph (fluid within the inner ear).

INVESTIGATIONS   No specific test will confirm the diagnosis. Audiogram, electronystagmography, electrocochleography, vestibular evoked myogenic potential, MRI to rule out other causes.

MANAGEMENT   Limit intake of salt, caffeine, nicotine, and alcohol. Diuretics if diet alone does not control episodes. Vestibular rehabilitation. Hearing aids.
Acute attacks: Antihistamines, benzodiazepines and antiemetics. Surgery for failed medical management (labyrinthectomy, vestibular neurectomy)

Muscular dystrophies

Patterns of muscle atrophy and/or pseudohypertrophy. Examples include Duchenne's muscular dystrophy, Becker muscular dystrophy, limb–girdle muscular dystrophy and fascio-scapulo-humeral dystrophy.

CAUSE   Mutations in various skeletal muscle proteins (e.g. Dystrophin).

INVESTIGATION   CK levels, EMG, muscle biopsy, genetic testing.

MANAGEMENT   Majority of treatment is supportive. Steroids (e.g. prednisolone or deflazacort) have been shown to prolong ambulation and improve respiratory function in Duchenne's muscular dystrophy. No specific treatment for other dystrophies.

Paterson–Brown–Kelly syndrome (Plummer–Vinson syndrome)

Microcytic anaemia and dysphagia due to pharyngeal webs.

Porphyria

Heterogeneous group of inherited disorders of haem biosynthesis. Clinically classified into the following:

Acute attacks (e.g. acute intermittent porphyria): Autonomic dysfunction, abdominal pain, nausea, vomiting, constipation, neuropsychiatric features (motor/sensory neuropathy, seizures, agitation, depression, mania).

Cutaneous (e.g. porphyria cutanea tarda): Skin lesions (e.g. vesicles and bullae) and photosensitivity.

Mixed: Combination of the aforementioned (e.g. variegate porphyria).

CAUSE   Partial deficiency of any of the enzymes in haem biosynthesis pathway e.g. porphobilinogen deaminase in acute intermittent porphyria (autosomal dominant).

INVESTIGATIONS

In acute attacks: Neutrophilia, ↓ Na^+, LFT abnormalities, clotting screen (avoid haem arginate treatment if there is evidence of coagulopathy).

Urine: Turns dark red or brown on standing because of polymerization of porphyrin precursors. Addition of Ehrlich's aldehyde reagent turns urine red. Porphyrin and porphyrin precursors can be measured in urine (↑ ALA and PBG during acute attacks), erythrocytes and faeces (to determine the type of pororphyria). Samples must be protected from light.

MANAGEMENT

Avoid/remove precipitating factors: Drugs (e.g. carbamazepine, oral contraceptives), cocaine, fasting, smoking, alcohol. Medicalert bracelet.

Acute attacks: IV infusion of haem arginate (inhibits ALA synthase and ↓ porphyrin precursor synthesis), 10 % glucose infusion or glucose polymer drink (e.g. Hycal) to maintain high energy intake.

Analgesia: (opiates and chlorpromazine). Seizures (strict fluid restriction, vigabatrine or gabapentin). Hypertension (propranolol).

Cutaneous: Barrier creams. Avoid sunlight, alcohol and oestrogens. Venesection for iron overload, oral chloroquine (↑ urinary porphyrin excretion), β-carotene (quenches active oxygen species). Screen for hepatitis C virus. Encourage family screening.

Refeeding syndrome

Biochemical dysfunction associated with the reinstitution of calorific intake in malnourished patients. May present with respiratory failure, cardiac failure, arrhythmias, rhabdomyolysis, confusion, convulsions, coma and sudden death. Patients may also have ↓ magnesium, calcium, glucose and thiamine. Usually occurs within 4 days of initiation of refeeding.

CAUSE   Refeeding causes a shift from fat to carbohydrate metabolism and increases insulin secretion. Insulin promotes cellular uptake of phosphate and potassium causing hypophosphataemia and hypokalaemia. Many of the clinical manifestations are the result of ↓ ATP in metabolic pathways and ↓ 2,3 diphosphoglycerate in erythrocytes resulting in tissue hypoxia and impairment of myocardial contractility.

MANAGEMENT   Preventative. Measured serum K^+, PO_4, Mg^{2+} and Ca^{2+} and give appropriate IV replacement before refeeding is instituted. Replace thiamine and give a multivitamin daily. Increase calories gradually.

Syringomyelia

Progressive cavitation of the central portion of the spinal cord resulting in lesion of the crossed spinothalamic tracts (loss of pain and temperature sensation) and relative sparing of joint position sense and power.

CAUSE   Unknown, but may be associated with congenital abnormalities like Arnold–Chiari malformation. May be secondary to trauma.

INVESTIGATIONS   MRI of spine. CT myelogram may be necessary.

MANAGEMENT   Neurosurgical intervention in the form of syringostomy.

Tuberous sclerosis

Characterized by hamartomas.
CNS: Cortical tubers, subependymal nodules. Learning disability, epilepsy; yellow retinal phakomas.
Heart: Arrythmias, cardiac failure.
Kidney: Pain or bleeding.
Lung: Pulmonary fibrosis, pneumothorax, cor pulmonale. Periungal fibromas. Shagreen patches (lumpy leathery flesh-coloured plaques over the lower back). Hypopigmented ash leaf-shaped patches over the trunk or buttocks. Adenoma sebaceum (pink/skin-coloured papules over the cheeks, nasolabial folds, forehead, chin). *Café au lait* macules.

CAUSE   Autosomal dominant mutations in *TSC1* (on chromosome 9 coding for hamartin), and *TSC2* (on chromosome 16 coding for tuberin). Hamartin and tuberin may act synergistically in the regulation of cell proliferation and differentiation. 80–90 % arise as new mutations.

INVESTIGATIONS
CNS: CT, MRI, EEG (when initial presentation includes seizures).
Heart: ECG (arrhythmias, e.g. Wolff–Parkinson–White syndrome), echocardiography.
Kidney: Ultrasound (renal cysts/hamartomas/tumours).
Lungs: Pulmonary function test (when there are symptoms), chest CT.

MANAGEMENT   Control epilepsy. Management of learning disability and behaviour disorder. Laser treatment for facial angiofibromas. Evaluation of family members (parents and siblings). Periodic monitoring.

Typhoid and paratyphoid fevers

After an incubation period: 1–4 weeks, present with fever, malaise, headache, dry cough, constipation, confusion, diarrhoea and rash (*Rose spots:* blanching erythematous maculopapular rash), cervical lymphadenopathy, hepato/splenomegaly, abdominal distension and pain.

CAUSE
Bacilli *Salmonella typhi* and *Salmonella paratyphi* types A, B and C, respectively. Transmission is via food or water contaminated by faeces or urine of a sufferer or carrier.

INVESTIGATIONS   Urine and stool culture (usually positive after first week).
Bone marrow aspirate and culture (sensitivity 95 % even during antibiotic administration).
   Blood culture (in the first 2 weeks).

MANAGEMENT   Third-generation cephalosporins. Other options are quinolones and chloramphenicol. Notifiable diseases.

Von Hippel–Lindau disease
CNS and retinal haemangioblastomas, and visceral cysts (kidneys, pancreas) with malignant potential. Associated with phaechromocytoma and renal cell carcinoma.

CAUSE   An autosomal dominant inherited mutation of the *VHL* tumour suppressor gene.

INVESTIGATIONS   MRI brain and spinal cord, retinal photographs, cytogenetics, abdominal ultrasound, urinary catecholamines.

MANAGEMENT   Monitoring for renal cell carcinoma and retinal haemangioblastomas. Anti-angiogenesis drugs are under investigation.

Von Willebrand's disease
Bleeding disorder which may present with mucocutaneous bleeding (mouth, epistaxis, menorrhagia), ↑ bleeding after minor trauma or easy bruising.

CAUSE   Abnormalities in expression or function of von Willebrand's factor (vWF). Usually autosomal dominant and occasionally recessive. There are also acquired forms. vWF is a plasma glycoprotein involved in blood clotting. It acts as an adhesive bridge between platelet receptors (GP-Ib) and damaged subendothelium collagen IV of vessels. It also binds to factor VIII and prevents its degradation.

INVESTIGATIONS   ↑ Bleeding time, ↑ APTT, ↓ factor VIII, ↓ vWF levels. Ristocetin cofactor assay (↓ platelet aggregation by vWF in the presence of ristocetin).

MANAGEMENT   Avoid NSAIDs. DDAVP or tranexamic acid (fibrinolytic inhibitor) for mild bleeding and in minor surgery. Intermediate purity factor VIII concentrate (containing vWF and factor VIII) or specific vWF may be another option.

Wolff–Parkinson–White syndrome
Short PR interval and 'Delta' wave on ECG predisposing to supraventricular tachycardias (SVT).

CAUSE   Accessory pathway (bundle of Kent) bypasses the atrioventricular node causing ventricular pre-excitation.

INVESTIGATIONS   ECG, cardiac electrophysiology, echocardiogram (to detect any associated cardiac anomalies).

MANAGEMENT   Acute treatment of supraventricular tachycardia (adenosine, cardioversion, procainamide). Definitive treatment with radiofrequency ablation of bundle of Kent.

Whipple's disease
May present with fever, lymphadenopathy, migratory arthralgias/arthritis, weight loss, diarrhoea, abdominal pain and CNS manifestations – cognitive dysfunction, oculomasticatory myorhythmia (continuous rhythmic movements of eye convergence with concurrent contractions of the masticatory muscles), cerebellar ataxia, myoclonus, hemiparesis, peripheral neuropathy, seizures.

Whipple's disease (continued)

CAUSE
Infection with *Tropheryma whipplei*, a gram-positive bacillus.

INVESTIGATION   The diagnosis is established by small bowel biopsy – PAS-positive macrophages containing the *Tropheryma whippeli* organism.

MANAGEMENT   Varies with different sites of infection. Initial therapy: IV Ceftriaxone or penicillin G.

Yellow nail syndrome

Characterised by pleural effusion, lymphoedema, yellow dystrophic nails.

CAUSE   Believed to be due to lymphatic system dysfunction.

INVESTIGATIONS   Clinical, CXR, lymphatic Technetium-scintigraphy.

MANAGEMENT   Supportive.

Zollinger–Ellison (ZE) syndrome

Severe peptic ulceration caused by a gastrin-secreting pancreatic islet cell tumour ('gastrinoma'). Steatorrhoea may occur due to $\downarrow$ intestinal pH denaturing pancreatic enzymes. ZE may be associated with hyperparathyroidism. 30 % of cases occur as part of multiple endocrine neoplasia type 1 (MEN 1).

CAUSE   Gastrinomas secrete large amounts of gastrin, a hormone that stimulates acid secretion by the parietal cells in the stomach.

INVESTIGATIONS   FBC (may be anaemic), amylase (to differentiate from pancreatitis), clotting screen and cross-match blood if bleeding ulcers. *Fasting serum gastrin*. Also measure Ca^{2+}, phosphate and PTH if MEN 1 is suspected.
Secretin stimulation test: Dramatic $\uparrow$ in serum gastrin in response to a secretin infusion. Upper GI endoscopy and biopsy (to exclude malignancy).
Localization of tumour: Somatostatin receptor imaging with [111]Indium-pentetreotide (Octreoscan) and SPECT, endoscopic ultrasound, dual phase helical CT scan, MRI, angiography, and arterial stimulation and venous sampling.

MANAGEMENT   High-dose proton pump inhibitor to reduce acid secretion. Regular follow-up endoscopy and biopsy to monitor hyperplasia in the gastric mucosa. Chemotherapy with streptozocin/doxorubicin or temozolomide may be used for metastatic gastrinoma. Surgical removal of the tumour if it has been located.

Differential Diagnoses

Up to 80 % of the diagnosis depends on a good history. The differential diagnosis formed from the history can then be narrowed down by physical examination and investigations. The section on 'History of Presenting Complaint' is a key component of the history. The admitting doctor may divide this section of the history into three subsections to ensure that the most crucial points in the history are dealt with at an early stage:

1. **About the symptom:** What, where (including radiation), when (onset, duration, course), how bad (severity), exacerbating/relieving factors etc.
2. **About the most relevant organ system(s):** For example, questions relating to the respiratory and cardiovascular systems for a patient presenting with breathlessness. Although the 'Systemic Enquiry' section of the history, investigates symptoms related to all systems, it is important to ask about the most relevant organ systems and common 'associated symptoms' at the beginning. See table that follows for a summary of most important questions relating to various organ systems.
3. **Risk factors:** Go through your list of differential diagnoses for the presenting complaint and ask questions about the various differentials and risk factors that increase the likelihood of their development. For example if a patient presents with diarrhoea, the list of differential diagnoses includes infection; therefore, risk factors such as contacts, food history, recent travel etc. should be addressed.

Systemic Enquiry

Cardiovascular
Chest pain, palpitation, breathlessness (exertional, at rest, orthopnoea, paroxysmal nocturnal dyspnoea), ankle swelling, dizziness

Respiratory
Wheeze, breathlessness, cough, sputum, haemoptysis, chest pain, calf pain/swelling

Gastrointestinal
Loss of appetite/weight, nausea/vomiting, dysphagia/odynophagia, indigestion/heartburn, abdominal pain, change of bowel habit (diarrhoea or constipation), bloating, blood/mucus PR, melaena/Haemetemesis, jaundice, pruritus, dark urine, pale stool

Urogential
Urinary frequency, urgency, dysuria, haematuria, loin pain, vaginal/penile discharge, periods/sexual problems

Neurological
Cognitive impairment or reduced consciousness (from collateral history), visual disturbance, hearing loss, speech/swallowing problems, headache, neck/back pain, weakness, paraesthesia, balance/co-ordination problems, bowel/bladder control

Rheumatological
Morning stiffness, joint pain/swelling/stiffness, deformity, malaise/fatigue/weight loss, arthralgia, myalgia, rash, Raynaud's phenomenon, hair loss, red/sore/dry eyes, dry mouth, oral ulcers, gential ulcers

Diabetes & Endocrine
Polyuria, polydipsia, fatigue, weight loss, neck swelling/tenderness, tremor, heat/cold intolerance, sweating, changes in hair, skin, voice, face, hands or feet appearance, pigmentation

Ear, nose, throat
Ear pain/discharge, nasal discharge/crusting, sore throat

General Questions
Fever, sweats, fatigue, malaise, loss of appetite, weight loss, lumps

---

Abdominal pain

Classification by type of pain:
Constant: inflammation, ischaemia
Colicky: obstruction of a viscus
Pain on eating: peptic ulcer, pancreatitis, cholecystitis, mesenteric ischaemia.

Classification by location:

Epigastric

Peptic ulcer
Pancreatitis
Reflux oesophagitis
Acute gastritis
Malignancy: gastric, pancreatic
Pain from adjacent areas: *See* RUQ, central abdominal pain, cardiac/pulmonary/pleural
    pathology, e.g. MI, pericarditis, pneumonia
Functional disorders: non-ulcer dyspepsia, irritable bowel syndrome

Right upper quadrant (RUQ)

Gall bladder pathology: cholecystitis (usually related to gallstones, occasionally may be
    acalculous), biliary colic, cholangitis
Liver pathology: hepatitis, hepatomegaly (congestive, e.g. in congestive cardiac failure,
    Budd–Chiari syndrome), hepatic tumours, hepatic/subphrenic abscess
Pain from adjacent areas: *See* Epigastric (e.g. pancreatitis, peptic ulcer), RIF, Loin pain,
    pulmonary/pleural pathology, e.g. pneumonia, empyema, pulmonary infarction
Appendicitis, e.g. in a pregnant woman
Colonic cancer (hepatic flexure)
Herpes zoster
Fitz–Hugh–Curtis syndromerare (rare complication of pelvic inflammatory disease)

Right iliac fossa (RIF)

Gastrointestinal: appendicitis, mesenteric adenitis (Yersinia, in children), 'Meckel's diverti-
    ulum (in children), inflammatory bowel disease, colonic cancer, constipation, irritable
    bowel syndrome
Reproductive: *Females*: Mittelschmerz (ovulation), ovarian cyst tortion/rupture/haemor-
    rhage, ectopic pregnancy, salpingitis/pelvic inflammatory disease, endometriosis. *Males*:
    seminal vesiculitis, cancer in undescended testis
Renal: UTI, ureteric colic (renal stones)
Pain from adjacent areas: *See* RUQ, suprapubic, central abdominal pain, groin pain, hip
    pathology, psoas abscess, rectus sheath haematoma, right-sided lobar pneumonia

Suprapubic

Urinary retention
Cystitis
Pain from adjacent areas: *See* RIF, LIF

Left iliac fossa (LIF)

Gastrointestinal: diverticulitis, inflammatory bowel disease, colonic cancer, constipation,
    irritable bowel syndrome
Reproductive: *See* RIF
Renal pain: *See* RIF

Abdominal pain (continued)

Pain from adjacent areas: *See* LUQ, suprapubic, central abdominal, hip pathology, psoas abscess, rectus sheath haematoma, left-sided lobar pneumonia

Left upper quadrant (LUQ)

Splenic rupture, splenic infarction (e.g. sickle cell disease), splenomegaly
Subphrenic abscess
Pain from adjacent areas: *See* epigastric (e.g. pancreatitis, peptic ulcer), LIF, loin pain, cardiac/pulmonary/pleural pathology, e.g. MI, pericarditis, pneumonia, empyema, pulmonary infarction
Colonic cancer (splenic flexure)
Herpes zoster

Central abdominal (periumbilical)

Gastrointestinal: intestinal obstruction, early appendicitis, gastroenteritis
Vascular: abdominal aortic aneurysm (leaking, ruptured), mesenteric ischaemia (thrombosis, embolism, vasculitis, e.g. polyarteritis nodosa)
Medical causes, e.g. diabetic ketoacidosis, uraemia
Pain from adjacent areas, e.g. epigastric, iliac fossae

Loin pain

Infection: UTI (pyelonephritis), perinephric abscess/pyonephrosis
Obstruction e.g. renal stones (*See* Urinary tract obstruction)
Renal disease: Tubulointerstitial nephritis, IgA nephropathy, renal vein thrombosis, renal carcinoma, polycystic kidney disease
Haemorrhagic adrenal infarction
Aortic dissection (type B)
Pain from vertebral column

Groin pain

Renal stones (pain radiating from loin to groin)
Testicular pain, e.g. torsion, epididymo-orchitis (pain radiating from scrotum to groin)
Hernia (inguinal)
Hip pathology
Pelvic fractures

Diffuse abdominal pain

Gastroenteritis
Peritonitis
Intestinal obstruction
Inflammatory bowel disease
Mesenteric ischaemia
Medical causes e.g. diabetic ketoacidosis (*see* Medical causes)
Irritable bowel syndrome

Medical causes

CVS/respiratory: MI, pneumonia, Bornholm's disease (Coxsackie B virus infection, rare)
Metabolic: diabetic ketoacidosis, Addisonian crisis, hypercalcaemia, uraemia, porphyria, phaeochromocytoma, lead poisoning, hereditary angioedema (C1-esterase deficiency)
Neurological: herpes zoster, tabes dorsalis
Haematological: sickle cell crisis, retroperitoneal haemorrhage (e.g. anticoagulants), lymphadenopathy
Inflammatory: vasculitis (e.g. Henoch–Schönlein purpura, polyarteritis nodosa), familial Mediterranean fever

Infections: intestinal parasites, tuberculosis, malaria, typhoid fever
Irritable bowel syndrome

Abdominal distension
Fat (obesity)
Fluid (ascites, fluid in the obstructed intestine)
Flatus (intestinal obstruction*), perforated viscus
Faeces
Fetus
Giant organomegaly (e.g. an ovarian cystadenoma, lymphoma)
*Small bowel: adhesions, herniae, intussusception, Crohn's disease, gallstone ileus, foreign
    body, tumour, tuberculosis.
Large bowel: cancer, volvulus, diverticulitis, faeces.

Abdominal masses
See Masses and swellings

Abdominal wall veins, dilated
Caput medusae (portal hypertension)
Inferior vena cava obstruction

Acanthosis nigricans
Malignancy: oesophagus, stomach, large bowel, kidney, bladder
Insulin resistance: diabetes mellitus, PCOS, steroids
Acromegaly
Prader–Willi syndrome

Acanthocytosis
Artifact (blood collected in EDTA tube)
Abetalipoproteinaemia (associated with retinitis pigmentosa, neurological deficits)
Anorexia
Liver failure
Chronic renal failure
Hyposplenism
Hypothyroidism
Chorea–acanthocytosis syndrome

ACE (Angiotensin-converting enzyme), ↑
Sarcoidosis
TB
Lymphoma
Asbestosis
Silicosis

Acidosis
Metabolic
Normal anion gap
↑ GI bicarbonate loss: diarrhoea, fistula (biliary, intestinal, pancreatic), ileostomy,
    ureterosigmoidostomy
Type 1 renal tubular acidosis: ↓ H^+ secretion (distal renal tubules)
Type 2 renal tubular acidosis: ↓ HCO_3^- reabsorption (proximal renal tubules
Type 4 renal tubular acidosis: suppression of ammonia excretion by hyperkalaemia (caused by
    aldosterone deficiency or tubular resistance to the action of aldosterone)
Ammonium chloride ingestion

Acidosis (Continued)

High anion gap

Ketoacidosis: diabetes mellitus, excess alcohol, starvation

Lactic acidosis

  Tissue hypoxia, e.g. shock (haemorrhagic/septic), severe exercise, severe anaemia

  Drugs: metformin, ethanol, methanol, ethylene glycol, zidovudine

  D-Lactic acidosis (short gut syndrome)

  Leukaemia

  Lymphoma

  Liver failure

  Glucose-6-phosphatase deficiency, mitochondrial disorders (e.g. MELAS)

Renal failure

Salicylate poisoning

Respiratory

CNS

Organic disease involving respiratory centre (e.g. vascular, infection, inflammation, trauma, tumour)

Drugs: opiates, benzodiazepines, barbiturates and other anaesthetic agents

Lungs

Severe asthma (uncommonly), COPD, large airway obstruction, obstructive sleep apnoea

Neuromuscular

Motor neurones: Guillain–Barré syndrome, motor neurone disease, poliomyelitis, acute porphyria

Neuromuscular junction/muscle: myasthaenia gravis, muscular dystrophies, muscle relaxants, diaphagmatic paralysis

Chest wall

Severe kyphoscoliosis, severe obesity, traumatic 'flail chest'

Acute confusional state

See Delirium

Alanine-amino transferase (ALT)

See Liver function tests

Alkaline phosphatase

See Liver function tests

Alkalosis

Metabolic

GI loss of H^+

Vomiting, laxative abuse, villous adenoma, VIPoma (Verner–Morrison syndrome)

Renal loss of H^+

Hyperaldosteronism ($\uparrow$ Mineralocorticoid activity stimulates H^+ secretion):

Excess Glucocorticoids: Cushing's syndrome, liquorice (inhibits 11-hydroxysteroid dehydrogenase and $\downarrow$ glucocorticoid metabolism)

$\uparrow$ Na^+ delivery to distal nephron: Diuretics thiazides and loop diuretics (also $\uparrow$ aldosterone secretion). Bartter's syndrome*, Gitelman's syndrome*

Intracellular shift of H^+
Hypokalaemia (also note that the aformentioned causes of GI/renal loss of H^+ also induce K^+ loss)

Other
Compensation for respiratory acidosis
Excessive alkali ingestion (e.g. excess sodium bicarbonate administration in treatment of acidotic states)
Fulminant hepatic failure (failure to synthesize urea and neutralize bicarbonate derived from amino acid metabolism)

*Autosomal recessive disorders. Bartter's syndrome is due to defects in Na-K-2Cl co-transporter in thick ascending limb of Henle. Gitelman's syndrome Na-Cl co-transporter in the distal tubule.

Respiratory
Hyperventilation
Physiological (anxiety, pain, fever, pregnancy, high altitude)
Mechanical overventilation
Respiratory failure (type I): asthma, COPD, pneumonia, pulmonary oedema, pulmonary embolism, ARDS, fibrosing alveolitis, right $\rightarrow$ left shunt
Salicylate poisoning, CO poisoning, theophylline
CNS disease (stroke, infection, tumour, trauma)
Others: liver failure (acute), Gram-negative septicaemia

Alopecia
Non-scarring
Aging (male/female pattern baldness)
Alopecia areata
Traction, trichotillomania
Telogen effluvium: transitory $\uparrow$ in number of hairs in resting phase of the hair growth cycle, associated with stress, (e.g. surgery, febrile illness, childbirth, etc.)
Cutaneous diseases (e.g. psoriasis, eczema)
Drugs (cytotoxics, ciclosporin, OCPs, anticoagulants, antithyroid drugs, vitamin A/retinoids)
Endocrine diseases (hypopituitarism, hypo/hyperthyroidism, diabetes mellitus)
Nutritional deficiency (iron, zinc, biotin, caloric deficiency)
Congenital

Scarring
Trauma/burns
Infection: pyogenic infection, TB (lupus vulgaris), syphilis, viral (varicella, herpes simplex), fungal (e.g. ringworm), protozoal (Leishmaniasis), leprosy
Inflammatory disease: SLE, scleroderma, sarcoidosis
Skin disease: lichen planus, cicatricial pemphigoid, necrobiosis lipoidica, folliculitis decalvans

Ambiguous genitalia
See Pseudohermaphrodite

Amenorrhoea
Non-pathological: pregnancy, lactation, menopause, drugs (e.g. Depo-Provera)
Hypothalamus: starvation, anorexia, excessive exercise, weight loss, GnRH deficiency (isolated or part of Kallmann's syndrome)

Amenorrhoea (continued)

Pituitary: hypopituitarism, hyperprolactinaemia

Ovaries: PCOS, premature ovarian failure, damage to ovaries (infection e.g. mumps, autoimmune, surgery, radiotherapy), ovarian dysgensis *(e.g. Turner's syndrome)*

Uterus/vagina: *absent uterus, imperforate hymen, transverse vaginal septum* Asherman's syndrome: scarring of endometrial lining 2° to infection and instrumentation, e.g. D&C

Thyroid: hypo/hyperthyroidism

Adrenals: adrenal tumours, Cushing's syndrome

Note: The causes in *italics* present only with primary amenorrhoea.

Amnesia
Acute/transient

In the presence of other cognitive deficits: acute confusional state (*See* Delirium)

Trauma (head injury)

Transient global amnesia (may be associated with migraine)

Temporal lobe epilepsy

Migraine

Transient ischaemic attack (TIA), tumours (rare)

Chronic/persistent

In the presence of other cognitive deficits (*See* Dementia)

Medial temporal lobe lesions (bilateral)

Vascular: posterior cerebral artery occlusion (bilateral)

Infection: herpes simplex encephalitis

Inflammation: limbic encephalitis (may be paraneoplastic), sarcoidosis

Tumours: midline (in the region of the third ventricle)

Toxic/metabolic: thiamine deficiency (Korsakoff's psychosis in alcoholism, hyperemesis gravidarum)

Amylase, ↑

Pancreatitis (acute)

Acute abdomen: peptic ulcer, perforation, intestinal obstruction, ruptured ectopic pregnancy

Diabetic ketoacidosis

Renal failure

Salivary gland disorders: calculi, mumps

Morphine (spasm of sphincter of Oddi)

Macroamylasaemia: amylase complexed with another protein, e.g. immunoglobulin and its renal clearance reduced

ANA

SLE (95 %), drug-induced lupus (100 %)

Systemic sclerosis (90 %)

Sjögren's syndrome (80 %)

Rheumatoid arthritis (60 %)

Polymyositis (40 %)

Polyarteritis nodosa (20 %)

Other diseases: chronic active hepatitis, diabetes, Waldenström's macroglobulinaemia, myasthaenia gravis

Normal population (5–8 %)

Anaemia
Macrocytic

Alcohol

Folate/B_{12} deficiency
Haemolytic anaemia
Hypothyroidism
Liver disease
Myelodysplasia
Drugs: methotrexate, hydroxyurea, azathioprine, zidovudine.

Microcytic

Iron deficiency: blood loss (GI [e.g. peptic ulcer, malignancy], urogenital [e.g. menorrhagia, haematuria]), hookworm (Ancylostroma duodenale)↓ absorption (gastrectomy, small bowel disease), ↑ demands (growth, pregnancy), ↓ intake (e.g. vegans)
Thalassaemia
Sideroblastic anaemia: congenital (X-linked), alcohol, drugs (isoniazid, chloramphenicol), lead, myelodysplasia
Lead poisoning
Anaemia of chronic disease (often normocytic, but may be microcytic)

Normocytic

Anaemia of chronic disease (chronic infection, inflammatory/connective tissue diseases, malignancy)
Haemolytic anaemia (may also cause macrocytic anaemia)
Hypothyroidism (may also cause macrocytic anaemia)
Pregnancy
Renal failure
Bone marrow failure

Haemolytic
Hereditary
Haemoglobinopathies: sickle cell anaemia, thalassaemia
Membrane defects: spherocytosis, elliptocytosis
Metabolic defects: pyruvate kinase deficiency, glucose-6-phosphate dehydrogenase deficiency

Acquired
Autoimmune: Warm antibodies (idiopathic, SLE, lymphoma, drugs, e.g. methyldopa), Cold antibodies (idiopathic, infections, e.g. *Mycoplasma* sp., EBV, other viruses, lymphoma)
Alloimmune: Transfusion reaction, haemolytic disease of newborn
Drugs: penicillin, quinidine
Microangiopathic haemolytic anaemia: TTP, HUS, DIC, malignant hypertension, malignancy (widespread adenocarcinoma), pregnancy complications (preeclampsia, HELLP syndrome: haemolysis, ↑ liver enzymes, ↓ platelet count)
Artificial heart valves
March haemoglobinuria
Infection: malaria, clostridia
Paroxysmal nocturnal haemoglobinuria
Secondary to liver and renal disease

Aplastic
Idiopathic
Inherited: Fanconi anaemia, dyskeratosis congenita
Acquired: drugs (cytotoxics, chloramphenicol, gold, methotrexate), chemicals (parathion, benzene), radiation, viral infection (B19 parvovirus, HIV, hepatitis, measles), paroxysmal nocturnal haemoglobinuria, sepsis

ANCA
p-ANCA
Microscopic polyangiitis
Churg–Strauss disease
Others: inflammatory bowel disease, primary sclerosing cholangitis, biliary cirrhosis, auto-
immune hepatitis, rheumatic autoimmune diseases

c-ANCA
Wegener's granulomatosis
Infections, e.g. amoebic colitis

Androgenization
PCOS
Congenital adrenal hyperplasia
Cushing's syndrome
Adrenal tumours

Angioid streaks
Pseudoxanthoma elasticum
Ehlers–Danlos syndrome
Paget's disease of bone
Sickle cell anaemia
Acromegaly, hypercalcaemia, lead poisoning

Angular stomatitis
See Cheilitis

Anisocoria
Physiological inequality
Unilateral miosis (See Miosis) or mydriasis (See Mydriasis)
Prosthetic eyeball

Anisocytosis
Iron deficiency
Thalassaemia
Megaloblastic anaemia

Ankle oedema
See Oedema

Annular skin lesions
Tinea corporis
Urticaria
Pityriasis rosea
Granuloma annulare
Sarcoidosis
Subacute cutaneous lupus erythematosus
Erythema annulare centrifugum
Erythema chronicum migrans
Erythema multiforme
Nummular eczema
Psoriasis
Leprosy

Anosmia

Nasal congestion (rhinitis), nasal polyps

Neurological: tumours on the floor of the anterior fossa (e.g. meningioma), head trauma, neurodegenerative diseases

Congenital: Kallmann's syndrome (anosmia and GnRH deficiency), cleft palate

Aortic regurgitation

Valve leaflet damage/abnormalities: infective endocarditis, rheumatic fever, trauma, bicuspid aortic valve

Aorta and valve ring dilatation: aortic dissection, aortitis (e.g. syphilis), arthritides (rheumatoid arthritis, seronegative arthritides, e.g. ankylosing spondylitis, Reiter's syndrome), ↑ ↑BP

Others: Marfan's syndrome, pseudoxanthoma elasticum, Ehlers–Danlos syndrome, osteogenesis imperfecta, inflammatory bowel disease

Aortic stenosis

Stenosis secondary to rheumatic heart disease

Calcification of a congenital bicuspid AV

Calcification/degeneration of a tricuspid AV in elderly

Apex beat
Heaving (pressure loaded)

Aortic stenosis (*See* Aortic stenosis)

Systemic hypertension

Thrusting (volume loaded)

Mitral regurgitation (*See* Mitral regurgitation)

Aortic regurgitation (*See* Aortic regurgitation)

Tapping

Mitral stenosis (*See* Mitral stenosis)

Apex beat not palpated

Obesity, muscular chest wall

Dextrocardia

COPD

L-sided pneumothorax

L-sided pleural effusion

Large pericardial effusion

Aphasia

See Dysphasia

Appetite, ↓

See Weight loss, ↓ appetite

APTT, ↑

Haemophilia

von Willebrand's disease

Liver disease

Warfarin therapy, vitamin K deficiency

Heparin

DIC

APTT, ↑ (continued)
Antiphospholipid syndrome

Note: APTT monitors the intrinsic pathway i.e. deficiency or inhibition of coagulation factors: XII, XI, IX, VIII, X, V, II and fibrinogen.

Arachnodactyly
Normal finding
Marfan's syndrome
Homocysteinuria
Ehlers–Danlos syndrome

Arm pain
Trauma, strain injury
Arthritis (*See* Monoarthralgia)
Cervical spinal cord compression (prolapsed disc, cervical spondylosis, tumours)
Brachial plexus involvement: apical lung cancer, cervical rib, brachial neuralgia
Peripheral neuropathies
Carpal tunnel syndrome
Vascular: subclavian artery stenosis, arterial/venous thrombosis, embolism
Bone: tumours (primary, secondary: lung, breast, prostate, kidney, thyroid)
Referred cardiac pain
See also Shoulder pain

Arm swelling
Congenital lymphoedema (rare)
Trauma
Cellulitis
Deep venous thrombosis (DVT) (axillary vein may be associated with excessive exercise, cervical rib)
Axillary lymph node involvement: radiotherapy, surgical excision, malignancy, filariasis

Arterial blood gases
Hypoxia, normal or low $P_a CO_2$ (respiratory failure: type 1)
Asthma
COPD
Pulmonary embolism
Pulmonary oedema
Pneumonia
Pulmonary fibrosis
R → L shunt
ARDS

Hypoxia, high $P_a CO_2$ (respiratory failure: type 2)
CNS
Organic disease involving respiratory centre (vascular, infection, inflammation, trauma, tumour)
Drugs: opiates, benzodiazepines, barbiturates and other anaesthetic agents

Lungs
Severe asthma, COPD, large airway obstruction, obstructive sleep apnoea

Neuromuscular
Motor neurones: Guillain–Barré syndrome, motor neurone disease, poliomyelitis, acute porphyria

Neuromuscular junction/muscle: myasthaenia gravis, muscular dystrophies, muscle relaxants, diaphragmatic paralysis

Chest wall
Severe kyphoscoliosis, severe obesity, traumatic 'flail chest'

Arthralgia
See Monoarthralgia and Polyarthralgia

Ascites
Exudate
Malignancy (abdominal, pelvic, peritoneal mesothelioma)
Infection: e.g. TB, pyogenic
Pancreatitis
Myxoedema (hypothyroidism)
Budd–Chiari syndrome (hepatic vein obstruction), portal vein thrombosis
Chylous ascites: obstruction of lymphatics, e.g. surgery, lymphoma
(Characterized by ↑ pH and triglycerides)

Transudate
Cirrohsis
Cardiac failure, constrictive pericarditis
Nephrotic syndrome, renal failure
Rare: Meigs' syndrome (ovarian fibroma, ascites, pleural effusion), ovarian hyperstimulation

Haemorrhagic ascites
Tumour
Trauma
Acute pancreatitis

Aspartate-amino transferase (AST, SGOT)
See Liver function tests

AST
See Liver function tests

Asterixis
Liver failure
CO_2 retention

Ataxia
Cerebellar ataxia
Vascular: infarction, haemorrhage
Infection: varicella, cerebellar abscess, TB, toxoplasmosis, cysticercosis
Inflammation: multiple sclerosis, vasculitis
Trauma
Tumour: cerebellar haemangioblastoma, astrocytoma, metastases, paraneoplastic
Toxic/metabolic: alcohol, phenytoin, myxoedema, B_{12} deficiency
Congenital: cerebellar hypoplasia, Dandy–Walker syndrome, Arnold–Chiari malformation
Degenerative: multiple system atrophy
Hereditary ataxias: autosomal recessive (e.g. Friedreich's ataxia, ataxia telangiectasia), autosomal dominant (e.g. spinocerebellar ataxia)

Ataxia (continued)

Storage diseases, e.g. Niemann–Pick disease, Tay–Sachs disease, ceroid lipofuscinosis, metachromatic leukodystrophy, sialidosis and numerous other genetic/metabolic causes, e.g. Refsum disease, Wilson's disease, etc.

Sensory ataxia

Subacute combined degeneration of the cord (See B_{12} deficiency), syphilis (tabes dorsalis), cervical myelopathy, diabetic pseudotabes

Avascular necrosis

Fracture (e.g. scaphoid, neck of femur)
Radiotherapy
Sickle cell
Steroids
Cushing's syndrome
Connective tissue diseases (e.g. rheumatoid arthritis, SLE)
Pregnancy
Pancreatitis
Alcohol
Other: Fabry's disease, Gaucher's disease; Caisson's disease (in deep-sea divers)

Axillary erythematosus rash

Seborrhoeic dermatitis
Contact dermatitis
Flexural psoriasis
Fungal infection: candidiasis, tinea
Erythrasma (*Corynebacterium* infection)

Axis deviation
Left axis deviation (LAD)

Left anterior hemiblock
MI (inferior wall)
Wolff–Parkinson–White syndrome (some types)
Ventricular tachycardia (left ventricular focus)
Obesity, pregnancy, congenital heart defects (e.g. endocardial cushion defects)

Right axis deviation (RAD)

Right ventricular hypertrophy (e.g. secondary to COPD), pulmonary embolism
MI (antero-lateral)
Wolff–Parkinson–White (left-sided accessory pathway)
Dextrocardia
Left posterior hemiblock (rare)

B₁₂ deficiency
↓ Absorption
↓ Intrinsic factor (pernicious anaemia, gastrectomy)
Terminal ileal surgery/disease (coeliac disease, Crohn's disease, tuberculosis, bacterial overgrowth, lymphoma, tropical sprue, fish tapeworm, pancreatic insufficiency)
Drug-induced malabsorption, e.g. metformin

↓ Intake
Vegans

Other
Transcobalmin deficiency (congenital), nitrous oxide (inactivates B₁₂)

Back pain
Trauma/fractures, strenuous activity

Younger patients (≤40 year)
Prolapsed disc, ankylosing spondylitis, spondylolisthesis, alkaptonuria (rare)

Older patients (≥40 year)
Osteoarthritis, spinal stenosis and spinal claudication, osteoporosis, Paget's disease of bone, herpes zoster

Serious causes
Infection (TB, bacterial osteomyelitis)
Malignancy (metastasis, multiple myeloma)
Cord compression
Fracture

Vascular/GI/pelvic
Aortic aneurysm, peptic ulcer, pancreatic cancer, renal disease, rectal cancer, uterine tumours, pelvic inflammatory disease, endometriosis, ovarian cyst, retroperitoneal fibrosis

Basophilic stippling
Pyrimidine-5'-nucleotidase deficiency
Lead poisoning (inhibition of pyrimidine-5'-nucleotidase)
Sideroblastic anaemia
Thalassaemia

Blackouts
Cardiovascular (transient ↓ blood flow to the brain)
Arrhythmia: bradycardia (heart block), tachycardia
Outflow obstruction: aortic stenosis, Hypertrophic obstructive cardiomyopathy (HOCM), pulmonary embolism, pulmonary stenosis
Postural hypotension: hypovolaemia, autonomic neuropathy (e.g. diabetes), antihypertensive medication (e.g. ACE inhibitors)
MI, aortic dissection, any condition that ↓ cardiac output

Neurological
Epilepsy, stroke/transient ischaemic attack (TIA) (rarely)

Blackouts (Continued)
Vasovagal (reflex bradycardia)
Prolonged standing esp. in warm surroundings, emotion
Other causes of vagal overactivity: micturition, cough, carotid sinus hypersensitivity
   (e.g. on shaving the neck or head turning)
Metabolic: hypoglycaemia

Note: There is no clearcut loss of consciousness in 'drop attacks'.

Blasts
Leukaemia
Myelofibrosis

Bleeding, prolonged
Platelet disorders (*See* Bleeding time)
Coagulation disorders:
Haemophilia
Liver disease
Vitamin K deficiency/warfarin
Disseminated intravascular coagulation

Blood film
Acanthocytes: *See* Acanthocytosis
Anisocytosis: *See* Anisocytosis
Basophilic stippling: *See* Basophilic stippling
Blasts: *See* Blasts
Burr cells: *See* Burr cells
Dimorphic blood film: *See* Dimorphic blood film
Howell–Jolly bodies: *See* Howell–Jolly bodies
Hypochromia: *See* Hypochromia
Leukoerythroblastic anaemia: *See* Leukoerythroblastic anaemia
Leukaemoid reaction: *See* Leukaemoid reaction
Normoblasts: *See* Normoblasts
Pappenheimer bodies: *See* Pappenheimer bodies
Poikilocytosis: *See* Poikilocytosis
Polychromasia: *See* Polychromasia
Reticulocytosis: *See* Reticulocytosis
Spherocytosis: *See* Spherocytosis
Target cells: *See* Target cells
Teardrop cells: *See* Teardrop cells

Blood pressure, ↑ & ↓
See under Hypertension and Hypotension

Bloody diarrhoea
See Diarrhoea

Blue nail(s)
Subungal haematoma
Melanoma
Pseudomonas infection
Wilson's disease

Blue sclerae
Pseudoxanthoma elasticum
Osteogenesis imperfecta
Ehlers–Danlos syndrome
Marfan's syndrome

Bowing of tibia
Paget's disease
Rickets
Treponemal disease: syphilis, yaws
McCune–Albright syndrome
Osteogenesis imperfecta

Bradycardia
Sleep
Physical fitness
Vasovagal attacks
Drugs: amiodarone, β-blocker, Ca^{2+} channel antagonist (e.g. verapamil), digoxin
Acute MI (Sinus node ischaemia), sick sinus syndrome
Atrioventricular block
Cushing's reflex (↑ intracranial pressure)
Hypothyroidism
Hypothermia
Obstructive jaundice

Breath sounds, ↓
Collapse
Pleural effusion
Pneumothorax
Emphysema

Breathlessness
Acute (minutes)
Pulmonary embolism
Pneumothorax
Foreign body
Anaphylaxis
Anxiety

Subacute (hours)
Left ventricular failure (pulmonary oedema)
Asthma
COPD
Chest infection (bacterial, viral, fungal, TB)
Metabolic acidosis

Chronic (days–weeks)
Anaemia
Recurrent pulmonary emboli
Cardiac disease (heart failure, arrhythmias, valvular heart disease)
Asthma
COPD

Breathlessness (continued)

Chest infection, bronchiectasis
Lung cancer
Pulmonary fibrosis (cryptogenic, connective tissue diseases, drugs, environmental/occupational lung disease)
Pulmonary hypertension
Hepatorenal syndrome
Cirrhotic hydrothorax
Neuromuscular disorders, chest wall deformities

Bronchial breathing

Consolidation (pneumonia)
Above pleural effusion
Abscess
Lung cancer
Fibrosis

Bulbar and pseudobulbar palsy
Bulbar palsy: cranial nerves (IX, X, XII) lesions at three different levels

Nuclei (brainstem): vascular, infection (e.g. polio encephalitis), syringobulbia, tumour
Nerve: motor neurone disease, meningeal infiltration, Guillain–Barré syndrome
Muscle: myasthaenia gravis, muscular dystrophy, polymyositis

Pseudobulbar palsy: bilateral UMN lesions to the lower brainstem

Multiple sclerosis
Motor neurone disease
Malignancy
Vascular disease (involving both hemispheres)
Extrapyramidal disease

Bullous skin lesions

Bites (e.g. insect/snake), burns
Infections: impetigo, cellulitis, viral (VZV, HSV, coxsackie), fungal (tinea pedis, 'id' reaction), scabies
Pemphigus, pemphigoid
Pregnancy: herpes gestationis
Porphyria cutanea tarda
Dermatitis herpetiformis (associated with coeliac disease)
Diabetes
Drugs
Eczema (hand and foot)
Erythema multiforme
Epidermolysis bullosa congenita, epidermolysis bullosa acquisita (associated with inflammatory bowel disease, internal malignancy, amyloidosis)

Bundle branch blocks, left and right
Left bundle branch block (LBBB)

Ischaemic heart disease
Cardiomyopathy
Left ventricular hypertrophy (aortic stenosis, hypertension)
Conduction system fibrosis

Right bundle branch block (RBBB)
Ischaemic heart disease
Cardiomyopathy
Massive pulmonary embolism
Atrial septal defect, Ebstein's anomaly

Burr cells
Stomach cancer
Renal failure
Pyruvate kinase deficiency
Post-transfusion

Cachexia
Malnutrition, eating disorders
Malignancy
Infection (e.g. TB, *Cryptosporidium* in AIDS)
Congestive cardiac failure
Alzheimer's disease

Café-au-lait spots
Neurofibromatosis
Tuberous sclerosis
McCune–Albright syndrome
Fanconi anaemia

Calf swelling/pain
Deep venous thrombosis
Cellulitis, necrotizing fasciitis
Baker's cyst rupture
Trauma, compartment syndrome
Ruptured popliteal aneurysm
Ruptured gastrocnemius

Candidiasis
Diabetes mellitus
Drugs: broad-spectrum antibiotics, immunosuppressants, steroids
Extremes of age
HIV
Malignancy
Pregnancy
Iron deficiency (severe)
Chronic mucocutaneous candidiasis

CEA
See Tumour markers

Cerebellar signs
See Ataxia

Charcot's joint
Diabetes mellitus
Syphilis (tabes dorsalis)
Syringomyelia
Leprosy
Others: yaws, progressive sensory neuropathy, Charcot–Marie–Tooth disease, neurofibromatosis (pressure on sensory nerve roots)

Cheilitis (angular stomatitis)
Iron deficiency anaemia
Riboflavin deficiency
Candidiasis

Contact dermatitis (e.g. lipsticks, pen-sucking)
Lip-sucking
Overclosure of the mouth (e.g. without teeth or with dentures)

Cherry red spot

Central retinal artery occlusion (thrombosis, embolus, spasm, giant cell arteritis)
Lysosomal storage diseases: sialidosis, Tay–Sachs disease, Niemann–Pick disease, metachromatic leukodystrophy
CO poisoning

Chest pain

Cardiac/large vessels: angina pectoris, myocardial infarction, pericarditis, aortic dissection, rupture of thoracic aortic aneurysm, bleeding into an atheroma
Respiratory: pulmonary embolism, pneumothorax, pneumonia, connective tissue diseases (e.g. SLE)
Gastrointestinal: reflux oesophagitis, oesophageal spasm, hiatus hernia, peptic ulcer, pancreatitis
Musculoskeletal: Teitze's syndrome (costochondritis), fractured rib, Bornholm's disease (Coxackie B virus infection, rare)
Neurological: herpes zoster, nerve root compression

Pleuritic chest pain

Pulmonary embolism
Pneumothorax
Pneumonia
Pericarditis
Connective tissue disease
Malignancy involving pleura, pathology under the diaphragm

Chest X-ray
Bilateral hilar lymphadenopathy

TB
Sarcoidosis
Lymphoma
Others: bronchial carcinoma, metastatic tumours, recurrent chest infections, AIDS, berylliosis, silicosis

Cavitating lung lesions

Abscess (*Staphylococcus aureus*, Klebsiella, *Pseudomonas aeruginosa*, TB, histoplasmosis)
Tumour (particularly squamous cell carcinoma), lymphoma
Infarct
Inflammatory: Rheumatoid nodule, Wegener's granulomatosis

Coin lesions

Tumours: bronchial carcinoma, metastatic deposit (e.g. breast cancer, renal cell carcinoma, hamartoma, adenoma, fibroma)
Infection: pneumonia, TB, abscess, hydatid cyst
Infarction
Encysted pleural effusion
Rheumatoid nodule
Vasculitides (e.g. Wegener's granulomatosis)
AV malformation

Chest x-ray (Continued)
Airspace/alveolar shadows
Pus (consolidation)
Fluid (pulmonary oedema)
Blood (pulmonary haemorrhage)
Cells (lymphangitis carcinomatosis, alveolar cell carcinoma)

Reticulonodular shadows
Pulmonary fibrosis:
Cryptogenic fibrosing alveolitis
Connective tissue diseases: scleroderma, SLE, sarcoidosis, rheumatoid arthritis, ankylosing spondylitis
Drugs (amiodarone, busulphan, bleomycin, nitrofurantoin), radiation
Extrinsic allergic alveolitis (e.g. farmers' lung, bird fancier's lung, malt worker's lung)
Pneumoconioses (coal workers' pneumoconiosis, asbestosis, silicosis, berylliosis)

Reticulonodular shadows (classified according to the lung zones in which they commonly occur)
Upper zone: TB, allergic bronchopulmonary aspergillosis, radiation, extrinsic allergic alveolitis, ankylosing spondylitis, sarcoidosis.
Middle zone: sarcoidosis
Lower zone: cryptogenic fibrosing alveolitis, drugs, asbestosis, rheumatoid arthritis, scleroderma

White hemithorax
Large pleural effusion
Pneumonectomy
Congenital absence of lung/extensive hypoplasia
Collapse

Cheyne–Stokes respiration
Brainstem lesions or compression (e.g. stroke, ↑ intracranial pressure)
Left ventricular failure
Morphine

Chondrocalcinosis
Osteoarthritis
Excess divalent ions: copper (Wilson's disease), iron (haemochromatosis), calcium (hyperparathyroidism)
Acromegaly
Ochronosis (alkaptonuria)
Hypomagnesaemia
Hypophosphataemia

Chorea
Inherited: Huntington's disease, Wilson's disease, Ataxia telangiectasia, spinocerebellar ataxia
Sydenham's chorea
Pregnancy
Polycythaemia
Inflammatory: SLE, Sarcoidosis

Drugs/toxins: oral contraception, neuroleptics, cocaine, heavy metals, carbon monoxide
Endocrine: Hyperthyroidism, hypoparathyroidism

Choroidoretinitis
Toxoplasmosis
CMV (congenital)
Rubella (congenital)
Sarcoidosis
Diabetes mellitus

CK, ↑
Myocardial infarction, myocarditis
Medications: statins, azathioprine, alcohol
Surgery, trauma, burns, haematoma, IM injections, defibrillation
Rhabdomyolysis, rigorous exercise, seizures
Dermatomyositis, polymyositis, muscular dystrophy
Bowel ischaemia
Myxoedema

Clotting screen
PT: *See* Prothrombin time
APTT: *See* APTT
INR: *See* INR
TT: *See* Thrombin time
DIC: *See* Disseminated intravascular coagulation

Clubbing
Congenital

Acquired
Cardiovascular
Congenital cyanotic heart disease
Infective endocarditis
Atrial myxoma

Respiratory
Cancer: bronchial, mesothelioma
Fibrosis (e.g. cryptogenic fibrosing alveolitis)
Suppurative lung disease (abscess, bronchiectasis, empyema)
Cryptogenic organizing pneumonia (rare)

Gastrointestinal
Cirrhosis
Inflammatory bowel disease
GI lymphoma, malabsorption e.g. coeliac disease
Others: Thyroid acropachy (thyrotoxicosis), unilateral clubbing: axillary artery aneurysm, brachial AV malformations

Cold peripheries
Acute ischaemic limb (thromboembolism)
Raynaud's phenomenon (vasospasm)
Shock
Hypothyroidism
Drugs: β-blockers

Complement deficiency
Congenital e.g. C1 esterase (C1 inhibitor) deficiency (normal C3, ↓ C4)

Acquired
↓ C3 and C4:
  SLE, mixed cryoglobulinaemia
  Subacute bacterial endocarditis
  Serum sickness*
  ↑ Loss/↓ synthesis: malnutrition, nephrotic syndrome, burns, liver failure
↓ C3
  Mesangiocapillary glomerulonephritis, partial lipodystrophy
  Gram-negative (endotoxic) shock
↑ C3 and/or C4
  Acute phase response

Consciousness, ↓
Hypoglycaemia
Hypoxia: cardiac arrest, shock (hypovolaemic, septic), respiratory failure
Vascular: intracranial haemorrhage/infarction
Infection: meningitis, encephalitis
Inflammation (demyelination)
Trauma (head injury)
Tumour (↑ intracranial pressure)
Toxic: drugs e.g. opiates, alcohol, anxiolytics, antidepressants
Metabolic: liver failure, renal failure, electrolyte (Na^+, K^+, Ca^{2+}, Mg^{2+}) disturbances, endocrinopathies e.g. myxoedema coma, vitamin deficiencies (e.g. thiamine, B_{12}), hypothermia
Epilepsy
See also Blackouts

Constipation
Diet: low fibre, inadequate fluid intake
Drugs: opiates, anticholinergics (tricyclics, phenothiazines), iron
Immobility
Old age
Surgical/gastrointestinal:
Anorectal disease (fissure, stricture, rectal prolapse)
Intestinal obstruction (strictures, e.g. IBD, cancers, diverticulosis, pelvic mass, e.g. fibroids)
Irritable bowel syndrome
Post-operative
Endocrine: hypothyroidism, hypercalcaemia, hypokalaemia, porphyria, lead poisoning
Neurological/neuromuscular: autonomic neuropathy, spinal/pelvic nerve injury, scleroderma, Hirschsprung's disease, Chagas' disease

Corneal opacification
Corneal ulcer, keratitis
Acute angle closure glaucoma
Anterior uveitis (iritis)

Corneal ulcer
Bacterial infection (*Staphylococcus aureus/epidermidis*, *Pseudomonas*, *Streptococcus pneumoniae*, *Haemophilus*, coliforms)

---

*Type III (immune complex mediated) hypersensitivity disease, caused by administration of a protein antigen from a non-human species e.g. heterologous anti-toxins, murine/human chimeric monoclonal antibodies.

Viral (herpes simplex, herpes zoster)
Fungal
Acanthamoeba
(Infections may follow corneal abrasion, contact lens wear or topical steroids)

Cottonwool spots
Diabetes (pre-proliferative retinopathy)
Hypertensive retinopathy
Retinal vein occlusion
HIV retinopathy
Haematological disorders: anaemia, leukaemia, hyperviscosity states
SLE, polyarteritis nodosa, dermatomyositis
Papilloedema

Cough
Upper respiratory tract infection
Pulmonary causes:
All lung diseases e.g.
Asthma, COPD, pulmonary emboli, infection (pneumonia, TB, fungal), bronchiectasis, malignancy, interstitial lung disease, sarcoidosis, pneumoconiosis
Other causes:
  Post-nasal drip
  Gastro-oesophageal reflux disease
  ACE inhibitors
  Heart failure
  Psychogenic

Crackles
Fine crackles
Pulmonary fibrosis (*See* Lung function tests, for the causes)
Pulmonary oedema

Coarse crackles
Bronchiectasis
Consolidation (pneumonia)
COPD

Note: Crackles that disappear on coughing are not significant.

Cramp
Idiopathic
Flat feet, hypermobility syndrome, inappropriate leg positioning, prolonged sitting
Extracellular volume/salt depletion (diuretics, excessive sweating, fluid removal during haemodialysis)
Hypomagnesaemia
Hypokalaemia
Hypothyroidism
Drugs: β-agonists, angiotensin II receptor blockers, cisplatin, vincristine
Muscle ischaemia, myopathy, motor neurone disease

Cranial nerve lesions
Pathologies along the course of the nerves:

III
Brainstem: demyelination, infarction, tumour, basilar aneurysm
Posterior communicating artery aneurysm

Cranial nerve lesions (continued)

Inflammation/infiltration of the basal meninges: TB, sarcoidosis, lymphoma, carcinoma, syphilis

Cavernous sinus: aneurysm, thrombosis, tumour

Superior orbital fissure/orbit: tumour, granuloma

Medical third nerve palsy ('pupil spared'): infarction in the nerve trunk secondary to diabetes, hypertension, SLE, polyarteritis nodosa, giant cell arteritis

Migraine

Tentorial herniation ('coning')

IV

Brainstem: demyelination, infarction, tumour

Head trauma

Inflammation/infiltration of the basal meninges: TB, sarcoidosis, lymphoma, carcinoma, syphilis

Cavernous sinus: aneurysm, thrombosis, tumour

Superior orbital fissure/orbit: tumour, granuloma

Infarction in the nerve trunk secondary to diabetes, hypertension, SLE, polyarteritis nodosa, giant cell arteritis

V

Sensory involvement: trigeminal neuralgia, herpes zoster, nasopharyngeal carcinoma

Brainstem: demyelination, infarction, tumour

Cerebellopontine angle: acoustic neuroma, meningioma

Inflammation/infiltration of the basal meninges: TB, sarcoidosis, lymphoma, carcinoma, syphilis

Petrositis (Gradenigo's syndrome)

VI

Damage to the nerve's blood supply (vasa nervosum): diabetes mellitus, hypertension

Wernicke–Korsakoff syndrome (thiamine deficiency)

Brainstem: demyelination, infarction, tumour

False localizing sign of ↑ intracranial pressure

Cerebellopontine angle tumour

Inflammation/infiltration of the basal meninges: TB, sarcoidosis, lymphoma, carcinoma, syphilis

Petrositis (Gradenigo's syndrome)

Orbital tumour

VII

See Facial nerve palsy

Multiple palsies

Brainstem lesions (stroke, tumour)

Basal meningeal infiltration: carcinoma, TB, sarcoid, lymphoma, leukaemia

Trauma

Guillain–Barré syndrome

Botulism

Mononeuritis multiplex

Arnold–Chiari malformation

Paget's disease

See also Bulbar/pseudobulbar palsy and Jugular foramen syndrome for lower cranial nerve lesions.

Creatine kinase
See CK

Creatinine, plasma concentration
↑
↓ GFR (renal failure), high muscle mass, acute muscle damage (rhabdomyolysis)
Transient/minimal increase: after exercise, high meat meal
↓ Tubular secretion: trimethoprim, cimetidine

↓
↑ GFR (pregnancy)
Low muscle mass

Crepitations
See Crackles

CRP, ↑
Infection
Inflammation
Malignancy

Cryoglobulinaemia
Type I: Multiple myeloma, Waldenström's macroglobulinaemia
Type II: Chronic HCV infection, EBV, HBV
Type III: Inflammatory/autoimmune disorders (e.g. SLE, leukocytoclastic vasculitis), lympho-
    proliferative malignancies, HCV

CSF
↑ White cells
Predominantly lymphocytes
Infective meningitis: viral meningitis/meningoencephalitis, TB, fungal (Cryptococcal), listerial,
    syphilis
Inflammatory diseases, e.g. Behçet's disease, sarcoidosis, SLE, multiple sclerosis
Malignancy (meningeal infiltration): lymphoma, leukaemia, other tumours
Drugs: NSAIDs, trimethoprim

Predominantly neutrophils
Bacterial meningitis
Brain abscess eroding into the ventricles
Initial phase of viral meningitis (first 24–48 h)

↓ Glucose
Bacterial meningitis
TB meningitis
Fungal (cryptococcal) meningitis
Occasionally mumps meningitis and herpes encephalitis
Sarcoidosis, CNS vasculitides, carcinomatous meningitis

Normal cells, ↑ protein (cytoalbuminaemic dissociation)
Spinal block (tumour, epidural abscess)
Tumour
Guillain–Barré syndrome

Cyanosis
Central
↓ Oxygen transfer due to lung disease: fibrosing alveolitis, severe pneumonia, COPD, massive pulmonary embolism

R → L shunt (cyanotic congenital heart disease)

Methaemoglobinaemia, sulfhaemoglobinaemia

Acute: asthma, pneumothorax, inhaled foreign body, left ventricular failure

Peripheral
All causes of central cyanosis

Cold exposure

Raynaud's phenomenon

Arterial occlusion

↓ Cardiac output e.g. shock, left ventricular failure

Dactylitis
Psoriatic arthritis
Gonococcal arthritis
Sickle cell (bone marrow infarction)
Sarcoid (bone cysts)

Deafness
Conductive
Wax in the canal
Eardrum: perforation, cholesteatoma (chronic otitis media)
Otosclerosis, ossicular abnormality
Middle ear effusion (secondary to infection or malignancy)

Sensorineural
Infection: measles, mumps, meningitis, syphilis (rare)
Trauma: noise, head injury, surgery
Tumour: acoustic neuroma
Toxic: aminoglycosides, cytotoxic drugs, frusemide
Congenital: maternal rubella, eclampsia, perinatal hypoxia
Genetic: e.g. Alport syndrome, Waardenburg syndrome, DIDMOAD (*See* 'Shorter topics')
Degenerative: presbyacusis
Others: Ménière's disease, Paget's disease of bone

Dehydration
↓ Fluid intake: severe illness, anorexia, malnutrition
Pyrexia/excess sweating
GI loss: diarrhoea, vomiting
Polyuria (e.g. diabetes mellitus, diabetes insipidus, hypercalcaemia)

Delirium (acute confusional state)
Hypoxia (respiratory/cardiac failure)
Hypoglycaemia
Toxic: alcohol (withdrawal, Wernicke's encephalopathy)
Drugs: opiates, anticholinergics, anxiolytics, anticonvulsants, corticosteroids, digoxin, dopa-
    minergic agonists, recreational drugs
Metabolic: liver failure, renal failure, electrolyte imbalances (e.g. hyponatraemia, hypercal-
    caemia), endocrinopathies, nutritional deficiencies (B_{12}, nicotinic acid, thiamine)
Vascular: intracranial bleeding, infarction, venous sinus thrombosis
Infection: *Intracranial* (meningitis, encephalitis, abscess, cerebral malaria, neurocysticercosis),
    Extracranial: chest infection, urinary infection (esp. elderly), surgical wounds, IV lines
Inflammation: vasculitis
Trauma: head injury, subdural haematoma
Tumour: space-occupying lesions
Hypertensive encephalopathy
Epilepsy: status epilepticus, post-ictal states

Dementia
Alzheimer's disease
Vascular: multiple infarctions
Infection: HIV, syphilis, Whipple's disease

Dementia (continued)

Inflammation: vasculitis, SLE, sarcoid, multiple sclerosis

Trauma: head injury, subdural haemorrhage

Tumour: frontal tumours, posterior fossa (causing hydrocephalus), brain metastases, paraneoplastic

Toxic: alcohol, lead, barbiturates

Metabolic: myxoedema, vitamin B_{12} deficiency, hypoglycaemia (repeated)

Inherited: Wilson's disease, Huntington's chorea, some cerebellar ataxias

Degenerative: Parkinson's and other akinetic–rigid syndromes, Pick's disease, prion disease, Lewy body dementia

Desquamating rash

Toxic shock syndrome

Scarlet fever

Drug reaction

Dengue

Measles

Kawasaki's disease

Diarrhoea

Infection: **Viral** (rotavirus, astrovirus, adenovirus, small round structured virus), *Campylobacter, Salmonella, Shigella, Escherichia coli, Yersinia enterocolitica, Staphylococcus aureus, Bacillus cereus, Clostridium botulinum, Clostridium perfringens, Clostridium difficile, Vibrio cholerae, Vibrio parahaemolyticus*, **Parasites** (*Cryptosporidium, Giardia, Entamoeba histolytica*), **AIDS** (AIDS enteropathy, cryptosporidia, microsporidia, *Isospora belli*, CMV)

Inflammatory bowel disease

Malabsorption: small intestine disease/resection, pancreatic insufficiency

Medication: laxatives, antibiotics

Overflow diarrhoea: secondary to constipation

Endocrine: thyrotoxicosis, carcinoid syndrome, diabetes mellitus (autonomic neuropathy), VIPomas

Bloody diarrhoea

Infective colitis: *Campylobacter*, haemorrhagic *E. coli*, *Entamoeba histolytica*, *Salmonella*, *Shigella* (CMV in the immunocompromised)

Inflammatory bowel disease

Ischaemic colitis

Diverticulitis

Malignancy

Digital gangrene

Peripheral vascular disease, diabetes mellitus, Buerger's disease

Vasculitis, e.g. rheumatoid arthritis, polyarteritis nodosa, cryoglobulinaemia

Vasospasm: Raynaud's phenomenon

Emboli (e.g. endocarditis, cholesterol)

Inadvertent intra-arterial injection in IV drug users

Subclavian artery compression (e.g. cervical rib)

Dimorphic blood film

Partially treat iron deficiency

Mixed iron and B_{12}/folate deficiency

Liver disease

Post-transfusion

Post-gastrectomy
Sideroblastic anaemia

Diplopia
Monocular
Originates from cornea or lens, e.g. cataract

Binocular
Cranial nerve palsies (See Cranial nerve lesions: III, IV, VI, multiple palsies)
Orbital fracture
Internuclear ophthalmoplegia (weak adduction of the affected eye and abduction nystagmus of the contralateral eye; resulting from a lesion in the medial longitudinal fasciculus)
Graves' ophthalmopathy
Myasthenia gravis
Miller Fisher variant of Guillain-Barré syndrome (associated with ataxia & areflexia)
Wernicke's syndrome (caused by thiamine deficiency)
Orbital myositis
Tolosa-Hunt syndrome (painful, granulomatous inflammation of the cavernous sinus; responds to corticosteroid therapy)
Tick bite paralysis
Botulism
Ophthalmoplegic migraine
Chronic progressive external ophthalmoplegia (few patients have diplopia since ocular motility defect is typically bilateral and symmetric)

Dizziness
? Vertigo: *See* Vertigo
? Imbalance: *See* Ataxia
? Faintness: anaemia, blackouts (*See* Blackouts)

Dry eyes
↓ Tear production: ↓ Lipid layer (blepharitis), ↓ Aqueous layer (involvement of lacrimal glands: Sjögren's syndrome, rheumatoid arthritis, SLE, surgery, radiation), ↓ Mucin layer (↓ vitamin A, burns, circatricial pemphigoid)
Corneal epitheliopathy: trigeminal dysfunction, contact lens use
Drugs: antihistamines, antidepressants, β-blockers, contraceptive pills, diuretics
↓ Eyelid closure: facial nerve palsy, Graves' disease, prolonged reading

Dry mouth
Drugs: anticholinergics, antidepressants, antihistamines, diuretics, neuroleptics
Dehydration
Systemic disease: Sjögren's syndrome, sarcoidosis, amyloidosis, HIV, uncontrolled diabetes mellitus
Psychogenic: anxiety

Dullness at the lung base
Pleural effusion
Pleural thickening (old TB, empyema, mesothelioma)
Basal collapse
Raised hemidiaphragm (hepatomegaly, phrenic nerve palsy)

Dupuytren's contracture
Familial
↑ Frequency among alcoholics and diabetics

Dysarthria
Cerebellar disease: slurred, scanning speech
Bulbar palsy: nasal speech
Pseudobulbar palsy: slow, indistinct, effortful (spastic speech)
Extrapyramidal disease: soft, monotonous

Dysdiadochokinesis
See Cerebellar signs

Dyspepsia
Oesophagus: gastro-oesophageal reflux, oesophagitis
Stomach/duodenum: peptic ulcer, hiatus hernia, gastritis, duodenitis, gastric cancer
Gall bladder: chronic cholecystitis
Non-ulcer dyspepsia

Dysphagia
Intraluminal
Foreign body

Intramural
Achalasia
Benign stricture: Oesophageal webs or rings
Cancer (oesophageal, gastric, pharyngeal)
Diffuse oesophageal spasm
Oesophagitis: infection, e.g. candidiasis, HSV, CMV, HIV or inflammation, e.g. Gastro-oesophageal reflux disease (GORD), corrosives, radiotherapy
Others: scleroderma, Chagas' disease

Extramural
Lung cancer
Lymphadenopathy
Retrosternal goitre
Pharyngeal pouch
Paraoesophageal hiatus hernia
Aortic aneurysm
Aberrant subclavian artery (dysphagia lusoria)
Atrial (left) enlargement

Neuromuscular
Stroke
Guillain–Barré
Bulbar and pseudobulbar palsy
Myasthaenia gravis
Inflammatory myositis
Motor neurone disease
Syringobulbia

Dysphasia
Broca's (expressive) dysphasia: lesions (e.g. stroke, tumour, trauma) affecting the infero-lateral frontal lobe (dominant)
Wernicke's (receptive) dysphasia: lesions (e.g. stroke, tumour, trauma) affecting the posterior superior temporal lobe (dominant)
Conduction dysphasia

Dyspnoea
See Breathlessness

Dystonia
Idiopathic
Drugs: antipsychotics (phenothiazines, chlorpromazine, haloperidol), antiemetics (metoclo-
    pramide), anticonvulsants
X-linked, e.g. Lesch–Nyhan syndrome
Autosomal dominant, e.g. spinocerebellar degenerations, Huntington's disease
Autosomal recessive, e.g. Wilson's disease
Mitochondrial disease

Dysuria
Urinary tract infection: cystitis, urethritis, acute pyelonephritis (uncommon cause of dysuria)
Urethritis: chlamydial, gonococcal, others: *Trichomonas vaginalis, Candida albicans*, herpes
    simplex
Vaginitis: Candida albicans, Trichomonas vaginalis, bacterial vaginosis
Prostatitis
Interstitial cystitis
Female urethral syndrome

Ear ache
External ear
Trauma/subperichondral haematoma
Boil, furuncle
Otitis externa
Inclusion dermoid
Malignancy (e.g. squamous cell carcinoma, basal cell carcinoma)

Middle ear
Otitis media
Mastoiditis

Referred
Teeth
Tongue (tumour of the posterior third)
Tonsillitis, pharyngitis
Temporomandibular joint
Foreign body

Neurological
Herpes zoster
Glossopharyngeal neuralgia

ECG changes
Axis deviation (left and right): *See* Axis deviation
Bundle branch block (left and right): *See* Bundle branch block
Low voltage complexes: obesity, COPD, pleural effusion, myxoedema
P wave (absent and tall): *See* P wave
ST segment (elevation and depression): *See* ST segment
Tachycardia: *See* Tachycardia
U wave: *See* U wave

Emphysema, surgical
Trauma, surgery, chest drain insertion
Oesophageal injury
Positive pressure ventilation
Obstructive lung disease, e.g. asthma
Gas gangrene

Eosinophilia
See White cell count

Epistaxis
Trauma/irritation: nose picking, forceful blowing, foreign body, chronic intranasal drugs use
   (e.g. cocaine)
Nasal tumours
Anticoagulants, bleeding disorders
Hereditary haemorrhagic telangiectasia

ESR
↑
Infection

Inflammatory/connective tissue diseases
Malignancy
Metabolic, e.g. phaeochromocytoma

↑ESR, normal CRP

SLE
Ulcerative colitis
Myeloma
Recovery from an infection: when CRP has normalized but ESR is still high (has a longer half-life)

Eyelids, swollen

Allergy (contact with cosmetics, chemicals, animals, plants)
Blepharitis (may be associated with rosacea, eczema, psoriasis)
Chalazion, stye, spread of infection from a local lesion e.g. a squeezed comedo
Dacryocytitis

More serious causes

Orbital cellulitis
Herpes zoster ophthalmicus
Herpes simplex

Eye pain

See Painful red eye
Pain on eye movement
Optic neuritis
Orbital myositis

Facial nerve palsy
Unilateral
Bell's palsy (idiopathic) or pathologies along the course of the nerve VII:
Brainstem: infarction, demyelination, tumours
Cerebellopontine angle: acoustic neuroma
Basal meningeal inflammation/infiltration: TB, sarcoidosis, lymphoma
Middle ear: middle ear infection or herpes zoster
Face/parotid: surgery, trauma

Bilateral
Congenital facial diplegia
Guillain–Barré syndrome
Sarcoidosis
Motor nurone disease
Myasthaenia gravis
Muscular dystrophy
Infections: Lyme disease, HIV

Facial pain
Neurological
Giant cell arteritis
Trigeminal neuralgia
Glossopharyngeal neuralgia
Migrainous neuralgia and migraine
Postherpetic neuralgia

Local causes
Post-traumatic
Sinusitis
Orbital and ocular disease, optic neuritis, retro-orbital disease (e.g. posterior communicating
    artery aneurysm)
Dental/oral disease
Temporomandibular joint dysfunction
Ear and parotid disease
Nasopharyngeal tumours
Referred cardiac pain
Atypical facial pain

Facial swelling
Periorbital oedema
Infection: orbital/periorbital cellulitis, trichinosis (rare)
Allergy to insect bites/drugs (including anaphylaxis), C1 inhibitor deficiency
Hypo/hyperthyroidism
Nephrotic syndrome, hypoalbuminaemia
Carotico-cavernous fistula, cavernous sinus thrombosis
Dermatomyositis

Parotid enlargement
See Parotid enlargement

Other causes

Dental/sinus infection
Trauma, burns
Subcutaneous emphysema
SVC thrombosis
Cushing's syndrome, obesity

Faecal incontinence

Diarrhoea (*See* Diarrhoea)
Overflow (faecal impaction, rectal neoplasm)
Pelvic floor abnormality: accidental injury, e.g. pelvic fracture, anorectal surgery, obstetric-traumatic childbirth, rectal prolapse
Neurological: epilepsy, spinal cord compression, stroke, multiple sclerosis, trauma and tumours (brain, spinal cord, cauda equina), peripheral neuropathy (e.g. diabetes), dementia, Parkinson's disease
Congenital: meningomyelocele, anorectal anomalies

Fasciculations

Motor neurone disease
Motor root compression
Polyneuropathy
Primary myopathy
Thyrotoxicosis

Fatigue

Anaemia
Endocrine/metabolic: diabetes mellitus, hypo/hyperthyroidism, Addison's disease, uraemia
Heart failure
Infection
Inflammatory/connective tissue diseases
Malignancy
Drugs, e.g. β-blockers
Depression
Chronic fatigue syndrome

Ferritin ($\uparrow$&$\downarrow$)

$\uparrow$
Acute phase response: infection, inflammation, malignancy
Haemochromatosis
Repeated transfusions in thalassaemia, iron therapy
Still's disease
Sideroblastic anaemia
Anaemia of chronic disease, chronic haemolysis

$\downarrow$
Iron deficiency

Fever in traveller

Hepatitis A
Malaria
Typhoid
Leptospirosis
Dengue
Haemorrhagic fevers

Fever in traveller (Continued)
Longer incubation
Malaria
Typhoid
TB
Brucellosis
Leishmaniasis
Amoebic abscess

Fever of unknown origin
See Pyrexia of unknown origin

Finger pain
Vascular: vasospasm (Raynaud's phenomenon), vasculitis, peripheral vascular disease, emboli
Nerve or nerve root compression: Carpal tunnel syndrome, radiculopathy (e.g. cervical spondylosis)
Infection: paronychia, tendon sheath infection, pulp space infection
Inflammation/Connective tissue disease: rheumatoid arthritis, gout, scleroderma
Trauma: fracture, subungal haematoma
Tumour: bone tumour, glomus tumour

Flaccid paraparesis
Anterior spinal artery syndrome (Acute stages)
Anterior horn cells: poliomyelitis, enterovirus, echovirus, adenovirus, West Nile virus
Nerve root: polyradiculopathy (infection, compression), tabes dorsalis, cauda equina
Peripheral nerves e.g. Guillain–Barré syndrome (*See* Polyneuropathy)
Myoneural junction: Myasthaenia gravis, Lambert–Eaton syndrome
Myopathy

Floaters
Vitreous degeneration/detachment
Vitreous haemorrhage
Posterior uveitis (e.g. toxoplasmosis, sarcoidosis)

Flushing, facial
Physiological: heat, exertion, emotion
Menopause
Phaeochromocytoma
Carcinoid syndrome
Mastocytosis
Drugs: alcohol (particularly with chlorpropamide), testosterone, nitrites
Rosacea

Folate deficiency
↑ Demand: pregnancy/lactation, malignancy, chronic inflammation, chronic haemolytic anaemia, haemodialysis
↓ Absorption: jejunal disease, e.g. coeliac disease, tropical sprue, Whipple's disease, small intestinal resection
↓ Intake: alcoholics, elderly, anorexia
Drugs: phenytoin, trimethoprim, sulphasalazine

Foot drop
Neurological
Common peroneal nerve lesion: mononeuritis multiplex, e.g. diabetes mellitus (*See* Mono-
neuritis multiplex)
L5 root lesion (radiculopathy), e.g. inter-vertebral disc prolapse
Rarer: motor neuron disease, multiple sclerosis, stroke

Muscular
Injury to the dorsiflexors, compartment syndrome

Foot pain
Deformities (e.g. flat feet), strain (muscular, ligamentous strain)
Skin: cellulitis, warts, corns, callosities
Bone: fracture (calcaneal fracture, metatarsal fracture), osteomyelitis, osteochondritis:, e.g.
metatarsal head (Freiberg's disease) and navicular (Köhler's disease), tumours
Joints: septic arthritis, gout, rheumatoid arthritis, osteoarthritis (*See* Monoarthralgia and
Polyarthralgia)
Periarticular: plantar fasciitis, tendonitis (e.g. Achilles tendon, peroneal tendon, tibialis
posterior), bursitis (e.g. retro and infracalcaneal, interMTP)
Vascular: ischaemia, ulcers (*See* Digital gangrene)
Neurological: L4/L5/S1 root pain, Morton's metatarsalgia (plantar nerve neuroma), tarsal
tunnel syndrome

Frequency (urinary), nocturia
Polyuria (*See* Polyuria)
Frequent passage of small amounts of urine: UTI, bladder (stone, tumour, compression by
pelvic mass), prostate enlargement (benign prostatic hyperplasia, cancer), genuine stress
incontinence, detrusor instability, sensory urgency

Frontal bossing
Acromegaly
Paget's disease of the bone
Rickets
Thalassaemia
Hydrocephalus
Rarer causes: Achondroplasia, Gorlin's syndrome

Gait abnormalities
Antalgic gait due to pain
Leg length discrepancies
Waddling: *See* Proximal myopathy
Spastic/scissoring: *See* Spastic paraparesis
Wide-base: *See* Ataxia
Festinant, shuffling gait: Parkinson's disease
Steppage gate: peroneal nerve palsy, Charcot–Marie–Tooth disease, old polio, lead poisoning
Apraxic gaits: frontal lobe lesions

Galactorrhoea
See Hyperprolactinaemia

Gastrointestinal bleeding, upper and lower
Upper GI bleeding (haematemesis)
Peptic ulcer (gastric/duodenal)
Gastritis/gastric erosions, duodenitis, oesophagitis
Gastro-oesophageal varices
Mallory–Weiss tear
Medications: NSAIDs, anticoagulants, steroids, thrombolytics
Oesophageal/gastric cancer

Rare
Bleeding disorders (thrombocytopaenia, haemophilia), hereditary haemorrhagic telangiectasia, Dieulafoy gastric vascular abnormality, aortoduodenal fistulae, angiodysplasia, leiomyoma, Meckel's diverticulum, pseudoxanthoma elasticum

Lower GI bleeding
Anal: haemorrhoids, fissure
Angiodysplasia
Bowel cancer, polyps
Colitis: inflammatory (ulcerative colitis), infective, ischaemic, radiation
Diverticulae (colonic)
Excessive upper GI bleeding
Other: bleeding disorders, aortoenteric fistula, Meckel's diverticulum, solitary rectal ulcer

Gaze palsy
Horizontal
Ipsilateral pontine (pontine paramedian reticular formation) or Contralateral frontal lobe lesions:
Vascular (infarction/haemorrhage, vascular malformations), tumour, demyelination, infection

Vertical
Superior midbrain lesions:
Vascular (infarction/haemorrhage, vascular malformations), tumours (pinealoma/metastatic), demyelination, infection, metabolic (e.g. Niemann–Pick disease, Gaucher's disease, abetalipoproteinaemia), neurodegenerative (Steele–Richardson syndrome: associated with extrapyramidal dysfunction)

Note: In Parinaud's syndrome, paralysis of vertical gaze is associated with large pupils and light–near dissociation.

Genital ulcers
See Ulcers, genital

Gingival hypertrophy
Familial
Drugs: ciclosporin, phenytoin, Ca channel antagonists (nifedipine, diltiazem), oral contraceptive pills
Acute leukaemia
Tuberous sclerosis
Adult Langerhans cell histiocytosis
Pregnancy

Glossitis
Iron deficiency
Deficiency of folate, B_{12}, niacin (B_3), thiamine (B_1), riboflavin, Zn
Candidiasis
Syphilis (rare)

γ–glutamyl transpeptidase (Y-GT, GGT)
Liver disease: cholestasis (*See* under Jaundice), alcohol-induced damage

Glycosuria
Diabetes (1° and 2°: *See* Hyperglycaemia)
Pregnancy
Chronic renal failure
Renal tubular dysfunction/damage (e.g. multiple myeloma, heavy metals, Wilson's disease)

Goitre
Simple goitre (euthyroid): puberty, pregnancy
Thyrotoxicosis: Graves' disease, toxic adenoma, toxic multinodular goitre with one palpable nodule, thyroiditis
Hypothyroidism: Hashimoto's disease
Lithium, anti-thyroid drugs, iodine deficiency/excess, dyshormogenesis
Thyroid cyst
Thyroid carcinoma: papillary, follicular, anaplastic, medullary, lymphoma

γ-GT, ↑
See γ–glutamyl transpeptidase

Groin pain
See Abdominal pain

Gynaecomastia
Physiological: puberty, elderly
Pseudogynaecomastia: e.g. in obese men
Drugs: spirinolactone, cimetidine, cyproterone acetate, chlorpromazine, oestrogens, digoxin, drugs of abuse (heroin, marijuana)
Chronic liver disease
Chronic renal failure

Gynaecomastia (continued)

Hypogonadism
Hyperthyroidism
Tumours: ectopic hCG (e.g. hepatoma and lung), oestrogen-producing (e.g. testicular)

Unilateral

Breast carcinoma
Lipoma, lymphangioma, neurofibroma, haematoma, dermoid cyst

Haematemesis
See Gastrointestinal bleeding

Haemarthrosis
Trauma: iatrogenic, post-operative, fracture, meniscus tear, ligamentous injury (e.g. anterior cruciate)
Haematological: Clotting disorders, sickle cell disease, drugs
Infection: Septic arthritis, TB
Vascular: haemangioma, arteriovenous malformation, aneurysm
Neurological: Charcot's joint
Joint diseases: Osteoarthritis, gout, pseudogout
Scurvy
Tumour: pigmented villonodular synovitis

Haematuria
Kidney, bladder, ureter or urethra
Trauma
Infection: UTI, rarely TB, schistosomiasis
Stones
Tumours
Other causes: glomerulonephritis, IgA nephropathy, interstitial nephritis, cystic renal disease, emboli, renal vein thrombosis, vascular malformation, drugs, e.g. cyclophosphamide, excessive exercise
Prostate: benign prostatic hyperplasia, prostate cancer, prostatitis
General: haematological disorders (haemophilia, thrombocytopaenia, sickle cell disease, leukaemia), anticoagulants

Other causes of urine discoloration
Food: beetroot
Drugs (senna, rifamipcin)
Haemoglobinuria/myoglobinuria
Porphyria (acute intermittent)

Haemoglobin
↓
See Anaemia

↑
See Polycythaemia

Haemoptysis
Lung: infection (TB, pneumonia, abscess, bronchitis, bronchiectasis, fungi, parasites), pulmonary embolism, malignancy, vasculitis (e.g. Wegener's granulomatosis, Goodpasture's disease), trauma, foreign body
Heart: mitral stenosis
General bleeding diathesis
Rarer causes: arteriovenous malformation, amyloidosis, sarcoidosis

Note: Nasal/upper respiratory tract and GI bleeding may be confused with haemoptysis.

Hair loss
See Alopecia

Hallucination
Psychiatric
Schizophrenia/schizoaffective disorder
Mania with psychosis
Severe depression with psychosis
Dementia
Delirium
Puerperal psychosis
Alcoholic hallucinosis

Organic
Cerebrovascular (stroke), infection, toxic/metabolic (e.g. alcohol, hallucinogens, e.g. LSD), drug-induced psychosis (e.g. amphetamine, cocaine)
Sensory organ disease, e.g. retinal ischaemia/optic nerve lesions
Seizures

Hand pain
See Finger pain

Headache
Acute/subacute causes
Head injury
Meningitis/encephalitis
Subarachnoid haemorrhage, intracranial haemorrhage, cerebral venous thrombosis
Carotid/vertebral artery dissection
Acute angle closure glaucoma
Giant cell arteritis
Pituitary apoplexy
Other causes: ↑ ↑ BP, drugs (e.g. GTN, Ca channel antagonists), infections (bacterial, viral illnesses etc.), electrolyte imbalances (e.g. hyponatraemia), hyperviscosity syndromes (e.g. polycythaemia)

Chronic/recurrent
↑ Intracranial pressure (e.g. space occupying lesion, e.g. tumour/abscess, hydrocephalus, benign intracranial hypertension) and ↓ intracranial pressure (e.g. post lumbar puncture)
Migraine
Migrainous neuralgia (cluster headache)
Tension headache, rebound headache (on stopping analgesics)
Sinusitis
Other causes: cervicogenic (referred from cervical spondylosis), hypnic headache, meningeal infiltration (e.g. malignancy, sarcoidosis), refractive errors, Paget's disease of bone, acromegaly, antiphospholipid syndrome
See also Facial pain

Heart sounds
First (S1)
Loud (↑ intensity)
Mitral stenosis, atrial myxoma
Tachycardia, hyperdynamic circulation (e.g. fever, exercise)
↓ PR interval (pre-excitation syndromes)

Soft (↓ intensity)
Mitral regurgitation
Artic regurgitation

Long PR interval
LBBB
Severe heart failure

Variable intensity
Atrial fibrillation
AV block
Nodal or ventricular tachycardia

Second (S2)
Loud
Systemic hypertension, tachycardia ($\uparrow a_2$)
Pulmonary hypertension ($\uparrow p_2$)

Soft
Aortic stenosis ($\downarrow a_2$)
Pulmonary stenosis ($\downarrow p_2$)

Third (S3)
Normal in those <35 years
Ventricular failure
Mitral regurgitation, tricuspid regurgitation, VSD
Constrictive pericarditis, restrictive cardiomyopathy

Fourth (S4)
Aortic stenosis
Hypertensive heart disease
Hypertrophic cardiomyopathy
Myocardial infarction
Pulmonary stenosis

Splitting of S2
Wide
Delayed activation of right ventricle
RBBB, left ventricular pacing, left ventricular pre-excitation (Wolff–Parkinson–White syndrome)

Prolonged right ventricular ejection time
Pulmonary stenosis, pulmonary hypertension

↓ Left ventricular ejection time
Mitral regurgitation, VSD

Wide fixed splitting
ASD

Reversed splitting
Delayed activation of left ventricle
LBBB, right ventricular pacing, right ventricular pre-excitation

Prolonged left ventricular ejection time
Aortic stenosis, HOCM, hypertension, PDA

Heart sounds (Continued)
Single S2
Apparent: obesity, COPD, pericardial effusion
Absent a_2: severe aortic stenosis, severe aortic regurgitation
Absent p_2: absent pulmonary valve, pulmonary atresia, pulmonary stenosis, tetralogy of Fallot
Fusion of a_2 and p_2: Eisenmenger's syndrome

↓ Heart sounds
↓ Conduction of sounds: obesity, COPD, pericardial effusion

Heart murmurs
See Murmurs

Heinz bodies (denatured Hb)
G6PD deficiency
Haemolytic anaemias
Splenectomy

Haemianopia
Bitemporal
Superior temporal quadrants involved first
Pituitary adenoma, meningioma, carotid aneurysm
Nasopharyngeal carcinoma
Sphenoid sinus mucocele

Inferior temporal quadrants involved first
Craniopharyngioma
Third ventricular tumour

Homonymous
Involvement of:
Optic tract, or
Optic radiation (in parietal or temporal lobes), or
Occipital cortex by: stroke/transient ischaemic attack (TIA), space occupying lesions e.g. gliomas, metastasis, abscess

Hemiparesis, hemiplegia
Vascular: stroke (infarction, haemorrhage, TIA)
Infection: brain abscess from local (e.g. middle ear, sinuses) or distant (e.g. lung) infections
Inflammation: multiple sclerosis, cerebral vasculitis
Trauma: extradural or subdural haemorrhage (a history of trauma may not be apparent in the latter)
Tumour
Metabolic: hypoglycaemia can cause transient hemiplegia
Other causes of transient hemiplegia/paresis: epileptic seizures (Todd's paralysis), migraine

Hepatomegaly
Cancer: (2° deposits, hepatoma, liver cell adenoma)
Cirrhosis (early) usually alcoholic, primary biliary cirrhosis
Congestive cardiac failure
Budd–Chiari (hepatic vein thrombosis)
Polycystic liver disease
Infection: hepatitis A, B, C, EBV, CMV, toxoplasmosis, leptospirosis, abscess (amoebic, pyogenic), hydatid cyst

Infiltration: fatty infiltration (alcohol), haemochromatosis, amyloidosis, sarcoidosis, lympho-proliferative diseases

'Apparent hepatomegaly': lowered diaphragm (e.g. in COPD) or Reidle's lobe (an extension of the right lobe)

See also Hepatosplenomegaly

Hepatosplenomegaly
Myeloproliferative disorders*
Lymphoproliferative disorders**
Portal hypertension (*See* Portal hypertension)
Megaloblastic anaemia (e.g. pernicious anaemia)
Infection: hepatitis B or C, EBV, CMV, leptospirosis, toxoplasmosis, tuberculosis, brucellosis
    Worldwide: malaria, schistosomiasis, leishmaniasis
Other: amyloidosis, storage disorders, e.g. Gaucher's disease, infantile polycystic disease

Hiccups
Benign
Gastric distension: over eating, carbonated beverages, aerophagia, gastric insufflation during endoscopy
Excessive alcohol ingestion and tobacco use; sudden changes in ambient or GI temperature, sudden excitement

Phrenic nerve irritation
Neck masses (e.g. goitres), mediastinal masses
Diaphragmatic abnormalities: e.g. gastro-oesophageal reflux, hiatus hernia, intra-operative manipulation
Subdiaphragmatic: e.g. subphrenic abscess

Vagus nerve irritation
Irritation of the recurrent laryngeal nerve by pharyngitis, laryngitis, tumours of the neck
Irritation of the auricular branch of the vagus by foreign bodies touching the tympanic membrane

Toxic/metabolic
Uraemia, alcohol intoxication, general anaesthetic

CNS disorders
Vascular, infective or structural lesions releasing the normal inhibition of the hiccup reflex

Psychogenic
Anxiety, malingering

Hirsutism
Familial, racial (common in some Mediterranean and Indian subcontinent populations)
Ovaries: PCOS, androgen-secreting ovarian tumours
Adrenals: Congenital adrenal hyperplasia, androgen-secreting adrenal tumours, Cushing's syndrome
Drugs: ciclosporin, androgens, minoxidil, phenytoin
Target organ hypersensitivity

---

*Chronic myeloid leukaemia, myelofibrosis, polycythaemia rubra vera, essential thrombocythaemia.
**Lymphoma, CLL, myeloma, Waldenström's macroglobulinaemia, ALL, hairy cell leukaemia.

Hoarse voice

Laryngitis: *Acute* (associated with viral upper respiratory tract infection, acute vocal strain), *Chronic* (associated with chronic vocal cord strain, alcohol, smoking, GORD, postnasal drip, chemical fumes)

Recurrent laryngeal nerve injury: tumours (base of skull, neck, e.g. thyroid, mediastinum, e.g. lung cancer), surgery (thyroid, parathyroid, carotid endarterectomy)

Singer's nodules

Laryngeal trauma (e.g. intubation)

Laryngeal carcinoma

Hypothyroidism

Hysterical aphonia

Homocysteine, ↑

Genetic: Cystathionine β-synthetase deficiency, MTHFR polymorphism

Vitamin deficiency: B_6, B_{12}, folate

Drugs: methotrexate, theophylline, phenytoin

Disease: hypothyroidism, renal failure, breast/ovarian cancer

Lifestyle: aging, smoking, ↑ ↑ coffee consumption

Horner's syndrome

Brain stem/cervical spinal cord: tumour (glioma), infarction, syringomyelia/bulbia

T1 root: brachial plexus lesion, neurofibromatosis

Cervical sympathetic chain: Pancoast tumour (lung apex)

Internal carotid artery: dissection, occlusion

Migraine, cluster headaches

Howell–Jolly bodies

Post-splenectomy

Hyposplenism: sickle cell disease, coeliac disease/dermatitis herpetiformis, ulcerative colitis, tropical sprue, amyloidosis, essential thrombocythaemia

Iron deficiency

Megaloblastic anaemia

Leukaemia

Hyperaldosteronism

1. hyperaldosteronism: adenoma (Conn's syndrome), bilateral adrenal hyperplasia, gluco-corticoid-remediable aldosteronism
2. hyperaldosteronism: ↑ Renin: renin-secreting tumour, renal artery stenosis, cirrhosis, cardiac failure, diuretics, Bartter's syndrome

Hyperbilirubinaemia

Unconjugated: haemolysis (*See* Anaemia, haemolytic), ineffective erythropoiesis, ↓ glucur-onidation (Gilbert's syndrome, Crigler–Najjar syndrome)

Conjugated: *See* Jaundice, hepatocellular and obstructive

Hypercalcaemia

Hyperparathyroidism: primary and tertiary

Malignancy: multiple myeloma, bone metastasis: (prostate, kidney, thyroid, breast, lung), bronchial squamous cell carcinoma, lymphoma

Excess vitamin D: self-administered, sarcoid, TB

Immobility

Other causes

↑ Ca^{2+} intake ('milk alkali syndrome')

Drugs: Lithium, thiazides
Endocrine diseases: hyperthyroidism, phaeochromocytoma, acromegaly, Addison's disease
Familial hypocalciuric hypercalcaemia
Hypercalcaemia can also occur in diuretic phase of acute renal failure

Hypercalciuria
Hypercalcaemia (*See* Hypercalcaemia)
Idiopathic hypercalciuria
↑ Ca^{2+} intake
Renal tubular acidosis
X-linked hypercalciuria (Dent's disease)

Hypergammaglobulinaemia
Polyclonal
Chronic liver disease, primary biliary cirrhosis, autoimmune hepatitis
Chronic inflammatory/connective tissue disease (e.g. Sjögren's syndrome, sarcoidosis, SLE, rheumatoid arthritis, dermatomyositis), inflammatory bowel disease
Chronic infection (e.g. bronchiectasis), TB, brucellosis, leishmaniasis, leprosy, HIV infection

Monoclonal
See Paraproteinaemia

Hyperglycaemia
Stress, e.g. acute/severe illness

Diabetes
Primary (type 1 & 2)
Secondary:
Steroids
Endocrine: Cushing's syndrome, acromegaly, phaeochromocytomas, glucagonomas, somatostatinomas
Pancreatectomy, chronic pancreatitis, haemochromatosis

Hyperhidrosis
Endocrine: thyrotoxicosis, acromegaly, phaeochromocytoma
Chronic infection: TB, brucellosis
Malignancy: lymphoma
Medications: opiates, drugs with cholinergic properties, sympathomimetics
Acute: any acute febrile illness, myocardial infarction, hypoglycaemia, hypotension
Also *See* Night sweats

Hyperkalaemia
Released from cells: acidosis, rhabdomyolysis, suxamethonium
Renal failure
Renal tubular acidosis type 4
ACE inhibitors
Addison's disease
Amiloride and other potassium-sparing diuretics
↑ ↑ Intake
Pseudohyperkalaemia: haemolysis, leucocytosis, thrombocytosis

Hyperkeratosis (palmoplantar)
Friction (e.g. walking barefoot)
Congenital (tylosis, an autosomal dominant condition)
Keratoderma blenorrhagica (Reiter's syndrome)

Hyperkeratosis (palmoplantar) (continued)

Psoriasis
2° syphilis
Toxic/metabolic: drug reaction, arsenic, vitamin A deficiency
Malignancy: gastric adenocarcinoma, bronchial carcinoma

Hyperlipidaemia (2°)

Diabetes (poorly controlled)
Drugs: alcohol, OCP, steroids, thiazides
Myxoedema
Nephrotic syndrome, renal impairment
Obesity
Obstructive jaundice

Hypernatraemia

Dehydration:
↓ Fluid intake: elderly, confused or unconscious
↑ Fluid loss GI: diarrhoea vomiting
Renal: diabetes insipidus, osmotic diuresis (e.g. hyperglycaemia, hypercalcaemia)
Skin: excessive sweating
Hyperosmolar non-ketotic coma
Excess Na$^+$ administration (e.g. sodium bicarbonate)
Excess mineralocortcoids: hyperaldosteronism

Hyperphosphataemia

Renal failure
Hypo and pseudohypoparathyroidism (PTH: phosphate trashing hormone!)
Rhabdomyolysis
Tumour lysis syndrome
Acromegaly
Excessive phosphate intake/administration
Vitamin D intoxication

Hyperpigmentation

Drugs: amiodarone, busulfan, chlorpromazine, phenothiazines
Radiation
Endocrine: Addison's disease, Nelson's syndrome, ectopic ACTH, pregnancy
Liver disease: haemochromatosis, primary biliary cirrhosis
Photosensitive rashes See Photodistributed rash
Post-inflammatory, e.g. after erythroderma
Others: chronic renal failure, chronic wasting (TB, carcinoma), disseminated malignant
    melanomatosis

Hyperprolactinaemia

Physiological: pregnancy, lactation, stress
Prolactinoma, rarely ectopic prolactin (lung, kidney tumours)
↓ Dopamine transport to the anterior pituitary: pituitary tumour compressing pituitary stalk
    (pseudoprolactinoma affect)
Drugs:
Depletion of central dopamine stores: reserpine, methyldopa
Dopamine receptor blockers: (chlorpromazine, haloperidol, sulpiride, metoclopramide,
    domperidone)
↑ TRH secretion stimulates prolactin release (1° hypothyroidism)

Oestrogens: HRT/OCP, PCOS (oestrogen stimulates lactotrophs)
Chest wall injury (stimulation of the reflex pathway normally activated by suckling in lactating women)
Others: liver failure, ↓ dopamine synthesis/release from the hypothalamus (tumour, inflammation, arteriovenous malformations)

Hyperproteinaemia
Haemoconcentration: dehydration, prolonged application of tourniquet
Hypergammaglobulinaemia: *See* Hypergammaglobulinaemia

Hypertension
Essential (idiopathic)
Renal disease: chronic glomerulonephritis, chronic pyelonephritis, cystic kidney disease, renal carcinoma
Drugs: oestrogen-containing OCPs, steroids
Endocrine disease: Cushing's syndrome, Conn's disease, phaeochromocytomas, acromegaly, primary hyperparathyroidism
Vascular: coarctation of aorta, renal artery stenosis
Pre-eclampsia

Hyperthermia*
Heat stroke: impaired thermoregulation or exertional
Neuroleptic malignant syndrome (idiosyncratic reaction to antipsychotics)
Malignant hyperthermia (anaesthetics: succinylcholine and halothane)

Hypertrichosis
Local
Lichen simplex
Melanocytic naevi
Spina bifida

Generalized
Anorexia nervosa
Malnutrition
Medication (minoxidil, ciclosporin, phenytoin),
Malignancy
Porphyria cutanea tarda

Hyperuricaemia
↓ Renal excretion
Idiopathic
Drugs: **c**iclosporin, **a**spirin (low-dose), **n**icotinic acid, **t**hiazides, **l**oop diuretics, **e**thambutol, **a**lcohol, **p**yrizinamide)
Chronic renal disease, e.g. in diabetes mellitus, hypertension

↑ Intake/production
↑ Dietary intake
↑ Synthesis: Lesch–Nyhan syndrome (HGPRT deficiency)
↑ Nucleic acid (purine) turnover: lymphoma, leukaemia, polycythaemia vera, psoriasis

---

* ↑ Core body temperature $> 37.5°C$ due to failure of thermoregulation. It is not synonymous with fever, which is induced by cytokine activation during inflammation and regulated at the level of the hypothalamus.

Hypoalbuminaemia
↓ Synthesis
Acute phase reaction
Liver disease
Malnutrition

↑ Loss
Nephrotic syndrome
Protein-losing enteropathy (coeliac disease, IBD, sprue, Whipple's disease, intestinal lymphoma, intestinal lymphangiectasia)
Burns
Bullous skin lesions

Haemodilution
Sample from IV infusion arm, pregnancy

Rare
Familial idiopathic dysproteinaemia

Hypocalcaemia
Hypoparathyroidism
   Congenital (DiGeorge's syndrome)
   Autoimmune
   Surgical (after thyroidectomy or parathyroidectomy)
   Pseudohypoparathyroidism (resistance to PTH)
   ↓ Mg^{2+}, Fe^{2+} overload, ↑ Cu^{2+} (Wilson's disease)
Vitamin D deficiency
   ↓ Dietary intake/malabsorption
   Lack of sunlight
   Liver disease
   Anticonvulsants (e.g. phenytoin)
   Renal failure
   Vitamin D resistance
↑ Phosphate: chronic renal failure, phosphate therapy
Pancreatitis (acute)
Respiratory alkalosis
Hypoalbuminaemia
Others
   Artifact (collecting blood into an EDTA tube)
   Iatrogenic: bisphosphonates, calcitonin, citrated blood (massive transfusion)

Hypochromia
Iron deficiency anaemia
Thalassaemia
Sideroblastic anaemia

Hypogammaglobulinaemia
Congenital
X-linked, or as part of a combined immunodeficiency state

Acquired
Myeloma
Lymphoma
Leukaemia (CLL)

Nephrotic syndrome, malnutrition, malabsorption, protein-losing enteropathy
Marrow hypoplasia, myeloclerosis
Uraemia, steroids, severe infections

Hypoglycaemia

Excess insulin (or diabetics not having a snack after insulin injection), sulphonylureas, salicylate, pentamidine, quinine
Insulinomas, hepatomas, sarcomas
Alcohol
Addison's disease
Renal failure
Liver failure
Malaria
Post-gastrectomy

Hypokalaemia
Gastrointestinal loss

Vomiting, diarrhoea, villous adenoma, VIPoma, fistulae, ileostomies

Renal loss
Excess mineralocortcoids (→ ↑ K^+ excretion)

Hyperaldosteronism
↑ ↑ Glucocorticoids: Cushing's syndrome, liquorice (inhibits 11 β-hydroxysteroid dehydrogenase and ↓ glucocorticoid metabolism), 11 β-hydroxysteroid dehydrogenase deficiency
Congenital adrenal hyperplasia (11 β-hydroxylase and 17 α-hydroxylase deficiency)

↑ Na^+ delivery to distal nephron (→ ↑ Na^+ absorption and K^+ secretion)

Osmotic diuresis (e.g. in glycosuria)
Diuretics: thiazides and loop diuretics (also ↑ aldosterone secretion)
Bartter's syndrome, Gitelman's syndrome

Others

Hypomagnesaemia
Renal tubular acidosis (type I & II)
Renal tubular damage
Liddle's syndrome (autosomal dominant condition, primary ↑ in collecting tubule sodium reabsorption and often potassium secretion)

Redistribution into the cells

Insulin, β-agonists, alkalosis

Hypomagnesaemia
↓ Intake or GI losses

Malnutrition, alcoholism, diarrhoea, malabsorption, intestinal resection, intestinal fistulae
Renal losses:
Diuretics (loop and thiazides)
Alcohol abuse
Drugs: nephrotoxins, e.g. aminoglycosides, amphotericin B, cyclosporine, cisplatin
Diabetes mellitus, hypercalcaemia, hyperthyroidism, hyperaldosteronism, tubular dysfunction (post-acute tubular necrosis, post-obstructive diuresis, Bartter's or Gitelman's syndrome)
Other
Post-operative, post-parathyroidectomy, pancreatitis (acute), foscarnet

Hyponatraemia
Pseudohyponatraemia:
    Hyperproteinaemia (e.g. multiple myeloma), hypertriglyceridaemia
    Hyperglycaemia
Artifactual: taking blood from the arm into which low sodium solution is infused
Hypervolaemic (oedematous) patients:
Cirrohsis, CCF, nephrotic syndrome, renal failure (urine Na^+ >20)
Hypovolaemic (dehydrated) patients:
Renal loss (urine Na^+ >20): Diuretics (thiazides), renal tubular acidosis, salt-losing nephropathy, adrenal insufficiency
Extra-renal loss (urine Na^+ <20): diarrhoea, vomiting, burns, pancreatitis
Euvolaemic patients:
Hypothyroidism, adrenal insufficiency, SIADH

Hypoparathyroidism
See Hypocalcaemia

Hypophosphataemia
Redistribution into cells
↑ Insulin, e.g. recovery from diabetic ketoacidosis (treatment with insulin stimulates glycolysis and phosphate uptake by the cells), refeeding (e.g. in alcoholics)
Respiratory alkalosis (alkalosis stimulates glycolysis and phosphate uptake by the cells)
Hungry bone syndrome (following parathyroidectomy in patients with pre-existing osteopaenia): due to marked deposition of Ca^{2+} and phosphate in bone

Gastrointestinal
Phosphate binders, e.g. aluminum/magnesium-containing antacids
Diarrhoea (chronic)
↓ Dietary intake

Renal
Hyperparathyroidism (1° and 2°):↑ urinary excretion
Vitamin D deficiency/resistance (both by ↓ GI absorption and by causing hypocalcaemia and 2° hyperparathyroidism)
Hereditary hypophosphataemic rickets (X-linked, autosomal dominant), tumour-induced osteomalacia
Osmotic diuresis, e.g. glycosuria
Fanconi syndrome

Hypopyon
Infection: endophthalmitis, corneal ulcers
Inflammation: anterior uveitis (See Uveitis)
Malignancy: necrosis of intraocular tumours/metastases (e.g. leukaemia, lymphoma, retinoblastoma)
Trauma, surgery

Hypopigmented macules
Post-inflammatory
Vitiligo
Tinea versicolor
Halo naevus
Sarcoidosis
Tuberous sclerosis

T-cell lymphoma (cutaneous)
Leprosy

Hyposplenism
See Howell–Jolly bodies

Hypotension
Septicaemia
Hypovolaemia:
  Haemorrhage
  GI loss
  Renal loss (diuretic, diabetes mellitus, diabetes insipidus, post-obstructive diuresis, acute
    renal failure
  Cutaneous loss (exudative lesions, burns)
Adrenal insufficiency
Cardiovascular:
  Any condition that ↓ cardiac output, e.g. arrhythmias, ↓ diastolic filling (pericardial disease),
    myocardial disease, outflow obstruction

Postural hypotension
Volume depletion
Autonomic neuropathy:
  Metabolic: diabetes mellitus, amyloidosis (rare), drugs (tricyclics, L-dopa)
  Inflammation: Guillain–Barré syndrome
  Infection: HIV, syphilis
  Tumours: paraneoplastic (e.g. small cell lung cancer), hypothalamic
  Degenerative: Parkinson's disease, multiple system atrophy, Shy–Drager syndrome
  Familial dysautonomia (Riley–Day syndrome)
Drugs: Antihypertensives, diuretics, nitrates, antidepressants, sedatives
Leg vein insufficiency

Impotence

Psychological (patients may have morning erections)

Drugs: alcohol, antidepressants, β-blockers, cannabis, diuretics (spirinolactone), major tranquilizers

Endocrine disorders: hypogonadism/androgen deficiency, hyperthyroidism, prolactinomas, acromegaly

Neurological: autonomic neuropathy (e.g. diabetes mellitus, uraemia), nerve damage after bladder neck/prostate surgery, multiple sclerosis

Vascular disease (e.g. atherosclerosis)

Incontinence

Urinary: *See* Urinary incontinence

Faecal: *See* Faecal incontinence

Indigestion

See Dyspepsia

Infertility

Female

Anovulation (1°/2° hypogonadism)

Obstructed fallopian tubes (e.g. post- infection/inflammation/surgery: adhesions)

Uterine cavity abnormalities (e.g. fibroids, endometriosis)

Chromosome abnormalities

Antiphospholipid syndrome

Note: Semen analysis (sperm density, motility etc.) should be performed to exclude male factor infertility.

Male

Hypogonadism (1° or 2°)

Varicocoele

Immotile sperms

Obstruction of epididymis, vas deferens

Coital disorders

Insomnia

Self-limiting: stress, travel etc.

Psychological: depression, mania, anxiety

Medical: drugs, withdrawal of antidepressants/hypnotics, caffeine, pain, pruritus, nocturia, asthma, alcoholism, apnoea, tinnitus, dystonia

Internuclear ophthalmoplegia

Involvement of medial longitudinal fasciculus in the brainstem:

Multiple sclerosis

Vascular: infarction, haemorrhage

Gliomas

Wernicke's encephalopathy

Intracranial pressure, ↑

Vascular: haemorrhage (extradural, subdural, subarachnoid, intracerebral)

Infection: meningitis/encephalitis, abscess

Trauma: head injury

Intracranial pressure, ↑
Tumours
Benign intracranial hypertension, hydrocephalus, cerebral oedema

Iritis
See Uveitis

Iron deficiency
See Anaemia, microcytic

Iron overload
Repeated transfusions, e.g. thalassaemia
Haemochromatosis
Iron therapy

Jaccoud's arthropathy
SLE
Rheumatic fever
Bronchial carcinoma
Hypocomplementaemic urticarial vasculitis

Jaundice
Pre-hepatic
Haemolysis (See Anaemia, haemolytic), ineffective erythropoiesis, ↓ glucuronidation
    (Gilbert's syndrome, Crigler–Najjar syndrome)

Hepatocellular
Viral: A, B, C; (other infections: CMV, EBV, toxoplasmosis, leptospirosis, Q fever)
Drugs (paracetamol, anti-TB drugs, statins, sodium valproate, halothane), toxins, herbal
    medications
Alcoholic hepatitis
Autoimmune hepatitis
Cirrhosis, hepatic metastases, hepatic abscess
Wilson's disease, haemochromatosis, α1-antitrypsin deficiency, Budd–Chiari syndrome
Septicaemia
Dubin–Johnson syndrome, Rotor syndrome

Obstructive
Gallstones (in the common bile duct)
Carcinoma of head of pancreas/ampulla of Vater/bile duct
Lymphadenopathy at the porta hepatic
Benign stricture (following invasive procedures)
Drugs: (antibiotics, OCPs, chlorpromazine, sulphonylureas, gold)
Primary sclerosing cholangitis, primary biliary cirrhosis
Parasites, e.g. schistosomiasis/fasciola, pancreatitis, AIDS cholangiopathy

Jugular foramen syndrome (involving cranial nerves IX, X and XI)
Meningiomata
Metastases
Neurofibroma of nerves IX, X or XII nerves
Other tumours: cerebellopontine angle tumours, cholesteatomas, glomus tumour, carotid
    body tumour
Trauma: fracture at base of skull
Infection from the middle ear spreading into the posterior fossa
Jugular vein thrombosis
Paget's disease

Jugular venous pressure
↑ JVP
Right heart failure
Tricuspid regurgitation
Pericardial effusion, constrictive pericarditis
Fluid overload
Obstruction of superior vena cava

'a' waves (Cannon waves)

Regular: nodal rhythm, paroxysmal nodal tachycardia, partial heart block with very long PR interval

Irregular: complete heart block, multiple ectopic beats

Ketonuria
Diabetes
Starvation
↑ Metabolic requirements: fever, pregnancy, thyrotoxicosis
Glycogen storage diseases

Kidney, enlarged
Cystic kidney
Carcinoma
Hydronephrosis, pyonephrosis
Hypertrophy (following contralateral nephretomy)
Perirenal haematoma
Congenital anomaly

Knee, painful/swollen
See Monoarthralgia

Knee, swelling
Septic arthritis (staphylococci, gonococci, Gram-negative bacilli, TB, Lyme disease)
Trauma, haemarthrosis (in haemophiliacs)
Gout/pseudogout
Rheumatoid arthritis, osteoarthritis
Seronegative arthritides (reactive arthritis, enteropathic arthritis (IBD, Whipple's disease), ankylosing spondylitis, psoriatic arthritis)
Systemic: SLE, Sjögren's syndrome, sarcoidosis, Behçet's disease, vasculitides
Malignancy
Localized swellings:
Anterior
Pre-patellar bursa
Infrapatellar bursa
Osgood–Schlatter disease
Lateral/medial
Lateral/medial meniscus cyst
Exostosis
Posterior:
Semimembranous bursa
Baker's cyst
Popliteal aneurysm

Koebner phenomenon
Psoriasis
Lichen planus
Molluscum contagiosum
Warts
Vitiligo

Kussmaul's breathing
Metabolic acidosis, e.g. diabetic ketoacidosis, uraemia, etc.

Kussmaul's sign
Pericardial effusion
Constrictive pericarditis
Restrictive cardiomyopathy

↑ LDH (Lactate dehydrogenase)
Myocardial infarction
Haemolysis
Hepatocyte damage
Pulmonary embolism
Lymphoma, tumour necrosis

Leg pain
Vascular: arterial occlusion: acute (thromboembolism, trauma, e.g. fracture), chronic (arterosclerosis, arteritis, Buerger's disease) DVT
Neurological: lumbar canal stenosis
    Radiculopathy, plexopathy
    Peripheral neuropathy
Musculoskeletal: soft-tissue (muscle, tendon, ligament) injury, muscle spasm
Arthritis

Leg swelling
Bilateral
Heart failure
Liver failure, other causes of hypoalbuminaemia (malnutrition, malabsorption, nephrotic syndrome, protein-losing enteropathy)
Renal failure
Hypothyroidism
Iatrogenic: oestrogens, calcium channel blockers, fluid overload
Venous insufficiency: acute (prolonged sitting), chronic
Venous obstruction, e.g. pelvic mass, pregnancy, IVC/bilateral iliac vein obstruction

Unilateral
Acute
DVT
Cellulitis
Compartment syndrome, trauma
Baker's cyst rupture

Chronic
Varicose veins
Lymphoedema (non-pitting): primary, lymph node involvement: radiotherapy, infection (filariasis), malignant infiltration, excision
Immobility

Leg weakness
See Weak legs

Leukaemoid reaction
Severe infection, TB
Burns
Malignant bone marrow infiltration
Haemolysis
Haemorrhage

Leukoerythroblastic anaemia
Marrow infiltration: carcinoma, lymphoma, leukaemia, myeloma, tuberculous infiltration,
    sarcoidosis
Hypoxia
Severe anaemia (haemolysis, megaloblastic)
Osteopetrosis

Leukoplakia
Trauma/friction
Infection: HIV, candida, syphilis

Livedo reticularis
Cryoglobulinaemia, systemic lupus erythematosus, antiphospholipid syndrome, polyarteritis
    nodosa
Cholesterol embolus

Lip swellings
Insect bite
Allergic/anaphylactic reaction
Angioneurotic shock (C1 esterase deficiency)
Crohn's disease
Sarcoid
Granulomatous cheilitis

Lip erosions
Herpes simplex
Pemphigus
Erythema multiforme/Stephens–Johnson syndrome
Impetigo

Lipodystrophy
Partial
Congenital
HIV drugs: protease inhibitors
Associated with membranoproliferative glomerulonephritis (type II)

Local
Idiopathic
Injection, e.g. insulin
Pressure
Panniculitis

Liver function tests
AST (SGOT), ↑
Hepatocyte damage (*See* Jaundice)
Haemolysis
Myocardial infarction
Skeletal muscle damage

ALT (SGPT), ↑
Hepatocyte damage
Shock

Liver function tests (Continued)
ALP, ↑
Liver disease: cholestasis (*See* Jaundice, obstructive)
Bone disease (↑ osteoblastic activity): growth in adolescence, healing fracture, Paget's disease of bone, osteomalacia, bone metastases, hyperparathyroidism, renal failure
Placenta: pregnancy
Other: right heart failure, polymyalgia rheumatica, thyrotoxicosis

Loss of consciousness
See Blackouts

Lower motor neurone lesions
Examples include:
Anterior horn cell: motor neurone disease, poliomyelitis
Spinal root: cervical and lumbar disc protrusion
Peripheral nerves: trauma, entrapment, mononeuritis multiplex, polyneuropathy
See also Cranial nerve palsies

Lung function tests
Obstructive defect: FEV$_1$/FVC ratio < 75 %
Asthma
COPD

Restrictive defect: FEV$_1$/FVC ratio > 75 %
Pulmonary fibrosis:
   Idiopathic fibrosing alveolitis
   Connective tissue diseases: scleroderma, SLE, sarcoidosis, rheumatoid arthritis, ankylosing spondylitis
   Drugs (amiodarone, busulphan, bleomycin, nitrofurantoin), radiation
   Extrinsic allergic alveolitis (e.g. Farmers' lung, Bird fancier's lung, Malt worker's lung)
   Pneumoconioses (Coal workers' pneumoconiosis, asbestosis, silicosis, berylliosis)

Interstitial lung disease with preserved lung volume
Lymphangioleiomyomatosis
Tuberous sclerosis
Neurofibromatosis
Sarcoidosis
Eosinophilic granuloma
Chronic hypersensitivity pneumonitis
Idiopathic pulmonary fibrosis with COPD

Transfer factor
↓
Interstitial lung disease (pulmonary fibrosis)
Pulmonary embolus
Emphysema
Anaemia
Arteriovenous malformation

↑
Pulmonary haemorrhage
Polycythaemia
Pneumonectomy
Asthma

L → R shunt
Severe obesity, exercise prior to the test session

Lymphadenopathy

Infection:
   Bacterial, TB, less commonly: brucellosis, syphilis, cat scratch disease
   Viral (e.g. HIV, EBV, CMV, rubella, measles)
   Toxoplasmosis, filariasis, fungal (e.g. coccidiomycosis)
Inflammatory/connective tissue disease: rheumatoid arthritis, sarcoidosis, SLE
Malignancy: metastases, lymphoma, leukaemia
Rare: thyrotoxicosis, histiocytosis, psoriasis, eczema, phenytoin

Lymphocytosis

See White cell count

Lymphopaenia

See White cell count

Macroglossia
Hypothyroidism
Amyloidosis
Acromegaly
Mucopolysaccharidosis
Down's syndrome
Chronic infections, e.g. TB
Space-occupying lesions, e.g. rhabdomyosarcomas

Malar rash
Mitral stenosis
SLE
Rosacea
Seborrhoeic dermatitis

Masses and swellings
Abdomen
Right hypochondrium
Hepatomegaly (See Hepatomegaly)
Enlarged gallbladder (empyema, mucocele, obstruction of the common bile duct e.g. pancreatic cancer, gallbladder mass)
Enlarged kidney (See Kidney, enlarged)
Colonic mass

Epigastrium
Gastric carcinoma
Pancreatic mass: carcinoma, pseudocyst
Liver: left lobe, post-necrotic nodule of a cirrhotic liver
Large recti

Left hypochondrium
Splenomegaly
Enlarged kidney
Pancreatic cancer

Right iliac fossa
Carcinoma of caecum
Crohn's disease
Appendix mass
TB (ileocaecal)
Iliac lymphadenopathy
Ovarian cyst
Transplanted pelvic kidney

Left iliac fossa
Loaded sigmoid colon (esp. in constipation)
Diverticular disease
Colonic cancer
Crohn's disease
Iliac lymphadenopathy

Ovarian cyst
Transplanted pelvic kidney

Suprapubic
Enlarged bladder
Pregnant uterus
Fibroids
Ovarian cyst

Inguinal
Hernias (inguinal, femoral)
Lymphadenopathy
Vascular: saphena varix, femoral aneurysm
Psoas abscess
Ectopic/undescended testis
Lipoma of the cord
Hydrocoele of the cord

Scrotal
Indirect inguinal hernia
Hydrocele
Epididymal cyst
Spermatocoele
Testicular tumour
Gumma
Painful swellings (*See* Testicular pain and swelling)

Megacolon
Inflammatory bowel disease
Ischaemic colitis
Pseudomembranous colitis
Amoebic colitis
CMV colitis (in patients with HIV infection/AIDS)
Trypanosomiasis (South American)
Ogilvie's syndrome (acute colonic pseudo-obstruction)

Memory loss
See Amnesia

Methaemoglobinaemia
Drugs: dapsone, nitrates, nitrites, primaquine, quinolones, sulphasalazine
Congenital

Miosis
Reactive to light
Old age
Horner's syndrome

Non–reactive
Drugs: pilocarpine eye drops, opiates, organophosphates
Argyll Robertson pupil (irregular pupils)
Anterior uveitis (↑ pupil light reflex)
Pontine lesion

Monoarthralgia
Articular
Infection: septic arthritis (staphylococci, gonococci, Gram-negative bacilli, TB, Lyme disease)
Trauma, haemarthrosis (haemophilia)
Gout/pseudogout
Rheumatoid arthritis, osteoarthritis
Seronegative arthritides (reactive arthritis, enteropathic arthritis (IBD, Whipple's disease), ankylosing spondylitis, psoriatic arthritis)
Systemic: SLE, Sjögren's syndrome, sarcoidosis, Behçet's disease, vasculitides
Malignancy

Extra-articular
Bursitis, tenosynovitis, cellulitis

Monocytosis
See White Cell Count

Mononeuritis multiplex
Infection: HIV, herpes zoster, Lyme disease, leprosy
Inflammation: vasculitis (primary, e.g. PAN, Wegener's granulomatosis, Churg–Strauss syndrome, cryoglobulinaemia; secondary: rheumatoid arthritis, SLE), sarcoidosis, Sjögren's syndrome, Behçet's disease
Metabolic: diabetes mellitus
Malignancy: infiltration (lymphoma, carcinoma)
Hereditary neuropathy: prone to pressure palsies

Mouth ulcers
See Ulcers

Murmurs
Systolic
Ejection systolic
Aortic area: aortic stenosis (See Aortic stenosis), aortic sclerosis
Pulmonary area: innocent, atrial septal defect, pulmonary stenosis

Note: In HOCM an ejection systolic murmur is heard at left sternal border, radiating to aortic and mitral areas.

Pansystolic
Mitral regurgitation (See Mitral regurgitation), ventricular septal defect, tricuspid regurgitation (See Tricuspid regurgitation)

Diastolic
Early diastolic: aortic regurgitation (See Aortic regurgitation), pulmonary regurgitation
Mid-systolic: mitral stenosis (See Mitral stenosis), tricuspid stenosis (rare)
Continuous: patent ductus arteriosus

Myalgia
Myopathy: metabolic, inflammatory, infective, drugs, alcohol (See Proximal muscle weakness)
Muscle haematoma, abscess
Infection: systemic
Inflammatory/connective tissue disease
Malignancy

Malignant hyperpyrexia
Parkinson's disease
Polymyalgia rheumatica
Fibromyalgia
Chronic fatigue syndrome

Mydriasis
Drugs: mydriatic eye drops (antimuscarinics, e.g. atropine, cyclopentolate, tropicamide), overdose (cocaine, amphetamine, glutethamide), poisoning, e.g. belladonna, CO, ethylene glycol
Trauma: post-traumatic iridoplegia, iridectomy, lens implant
Third nerve palsy
Holmes–Adie pupil (degeneration of the nerve to the ciliary ganglion)
Acute angle closure glaucoma
Deep coma, cerebral death

Myoclonus
Congenital
Acute metabolic encephalopathy
Creutzfeldt–Jakob disease
Alzheimer's disease
Lysosomal storage diseases, e.g. Gaucher's disease, Tay–Sachs disease
Lewy body dementia

Myoglobinuria
Trauma, surgery
Ischaemia, immobility, coma
Rigorous exercise, seizures
Myositis
Metabolic: hypokalaemia, hypophosphataemia
Drugs/toxins: fibrates, statins, alcohol, CO
Others: malignant hyperthermia, neuroleptic malignant syndrome, inherited muscle disorders

Nail pitting
Psoriasis
Alopecia areata
Eczema
Lichen Planus
Trauma

Nasal discharge
Allergic rhinitis: seasonal/perennial
Vasomotor rhinitis
Infection: viral (acute/chronic), sinusitis
   Rarely: TB, fungal, syphilis, AIDS
Inflammation: polyps (e.g. cystic fibrosis), Wegener's granulomatosis, sarcoidosis, midline
   granuloma
Trauma: foreign body, fracture of anterior fossa (CSF leak)
Tumours (nasopharyngeal, maxillary sinus)

Nausea
See Vomiting

Neck pain
Postural, cold exposure
Trauma: acute flexion-extension injury, fracture, dislocation
Degenerative: cervical spondylosis, diffuse idiopathic skeletal hyperostosis
Inflammatory: rheumatoid arthritis, spondylarthropathy, polymyalgia rheumatica
Neurological: disc prolapse, meningism (meningitis, subarachnoid haemorrhage), vertebral/
   carotid artery dissection, brachial plexus lesions (trauma, thoracic outlet syndrome)
Infection: osteomyelitis (e.g. TB), discitis, general systemic infection (cervical myalgia)
Malignancy: primary and secondary bone tumours, myeloma
Metabolic/endocrine: osteoporosis, osteomalacia, Paget's disease of bone, thyroiditis, hae-
   morrhagic thyroid cyst
Referred pain: temporomandibular/acromioclavicular joint, shoulder, pharynx, heart/vessels,
   lung, diaphragm

Neck swellings
Midline
Thyroid gland swelling
Thyroglossal cyst
Lymph nodes
Rare: sublingual dermoid cyst, pharyngeal pouch, plunging ranula, subhyoid bursa, laryngeal/
   tracheal/oesophageal carcinoma
Manubrium swelling:
Soft: lipoma
Hard: bony tumour or plasmacytoma
Pulsatile: eroding aortic aneurysm

Anterior triangle
Lymph nodes, cold abscess (TB)
Salivary gland (submandibular/parotid) swelling
Branchial cyst

Carotid body tumour
Carotid body aneurysm
Sternomastoid tumour

Posterior triangle
Lymph nodes, cold abscess (TB)
Cystic hygroma
Subclavian artery aneurysm
Tumour of clavicle

Nerve thickening (palpable)
Tuberculoid leprosy
Sarcoidosis
Amyloidosis
Neurofibromatosis
Acromegaly
Hereditary sensorimotor neuropathy type 1
Refsum's disease

Neutropaenia
See White cell count

Neutrophilia
See White cell count

Night sweats
Infections: chronic infections, e.g. TB, subacute bacterial infections (e.g. endocarditis, osteomyelitis), others: HIV, histoplasmosis
Malignancy, e.g. lymphoma, solid tumours
Menopause
Medications: GnRH agonists, antidepressants

Nocturia
See Frequency

Normoblasts
Marrow infiltration
Haemolysis
Hypoxia

Nystagmus
Physiological: at the extreme lateral gaze
Pendular (to-and-fro movements have equal velocity): congenital
Jerky (slow-phase and fast phase are present):
Acute labyrinthitis, other inner ear (labyrinth/vestibular nerve) diseases, e.g. Ménière's disease, benign positional vertigo (otoconial debris in semicircular canals), vestibular neuronitis, acoustic neuroma
Brainstem/vestibular nuclei: vascular (stroke), inflammation (multiple sclerosis, tumour), toxic (alcoholism)
Cerebellar disease (*See* Cerebellar signs)
Drugs (e.g. phenytoin)
Nystagmus is also seen in internuclear ophthalmoplegia ($\downarrow$ adduction on the side of lesion, nystagmus of the contralateral abducting eye)

Nystagmus (continued)

Note: In **A**: hearing loss, tinnitus and vertigo may be present, past phase is to the contralateral side of the lesion. In **C** other cerebellar signs are present, fast phase is to the side of the lesion.

Rotatory nystagmus: a lesion in labyrinth or brainstem.

Vertical nystagmus: drugs or brainstem lesion. If down-beating on downgaze: localizes to the region of the foramen magnum.

O

Ocular pain
Pain on eye movement
Optic neuritis
Orbital myositis
See Painful red eye

Oedema, ankle
Pitting, bilateral
Heart failure
Liver failure, other causes of hypoalbuminaemia: malnutrition, malabsorption, nephrotic
  syndrome, protein-losing enteropathy
Renal failure
Hypothyroidism
Iatrogenic: oestrogens, calcium channel blockers, fluid overload
Venous insufficiency: acute (prolonged sitting), chronic
Venous obstruction, e.g. pelvic mass, pregnancy, IVC/bilateral iliac vein obstruction

Non-pitting
Lymphoedema: primary, lymph node involvement: radiotherapy, infection (filariasis), malignant infiltration, excision

Oliguria
Dehydration
Renal failure (acute, chronic): pre-renal (e.g. shock), renal (acute tubular necrosis), post-renal
  (stones, tumour, retroperitoneal fibrosis)

Onycholysis
Psoriasis
Fungal infection
Thyrotoxicosis
Trauma
Tetracyclines

Ophthalmoplegia
Cranial nerve palsies (See Cranial nerve lesions: III, IV, VI, multiple palsies)
Orbital fracture
Internuclear ophthalmoplegia (weak adduction of the affected eye and abduction nystagmus
  of the contralateral eye; resulting from a lesion in the medial longitudinal fasciculus)
Graves' ophthalmopathy
Myasthenia gravis
Miller Fisher variant of Guillain-Barré syndrome (associated with ataxia & areflexia)
Wernicke's syndrome (caused by thiamine deficiency)
Orbital myositis
Chronic progressive external ophthalmoplegia (few patients have diplopia since ocular
  motility defect is typically bilateral and symmetric)
Tolosa-Hunt syndrome (painful, granulomatous inflammation of the cavernous sinus;
  responds to corticosteroid therapy)
Tick bite paralysis
Botulism
Ophthalmoplegic migraine

Optic disc
Atrophy
Optic neuritis (demyelination)
↑ Intracranial **p**ressure: 2° to long-standing papilloedema (e.g. tumours)
Toxic/metabolic/drugs: tobacco, alcohol, vitamin B$_{12}$ deficiency, diabetes, ethambutol
Infection/infiltration: spread from sinuses, syphilis, sarcoid
Compression: intra-orbital (e.g. optic nerve tumours), tumour of pituitary or sphenoid sinus, carotid aneurysm
Anterior ischaemic optic neuropathy
Trauma: orbital fracture, indirect trauma
Retinal disease: retinitis pigmentosa, macular degeneration
Occlusion of retinal artery
↑ **P**ressure inside the eye (glaucoma)
Hereditary: Leber's optic atrophy, hereditary ataxias, e.g. Friedreich's, DIDMOAD*

Blurred
Papilloedema:
  ↑ Intracranial pressure: Haemorrhage (extradural, subdural, subarachnoid, intracerebral), head injury. Meningitis/encephalitis, tumours, abscesses, benign intracranial hypertension, hydrocephalus, cerebral oedema
  Malignant hypertension
  Retinal vein thrombosis, venous sinus thrombosis
  Hypercapnia
  Hypoparathyroidism
  Hypervitaminosis A
  Lead poisoning
Papillitis (demyelination)

Oral pigmentation
Racial (African, Asian)
Post-trauma/inflammation
Peutz–Jegher's syndrome
Addison's disease
Acanthosis nigricans
Fixed drug eruptions
Heavy metal poisoning

Oral ulcers
See Ulcers

Osler nodes
Subacute bacterial endocarditis
SLE
Haemolytic anaemia
Gonococcal infection

Otorrhoea
Watery: eczema of the ear canal, CSF
Mucoid: chronic suppurative otitis media with a perforation
Purulent: acute otitis externa
Mucopurulent/bloody: trauma, carcinoma of the ear, acute otitis media
Foul smelling: chronic suppurative otitis media with cholasteatoma

*Diabetes insipidus, diabetes mellitus, optic atrophy, deafness.

Oxygen saturation, sources of errors

Hypoperfusion (e.g. shock)
Improper probe placement
Intensive ambient light
Motion artifact
MRI
Nail polish
Skin pigmentation
Abnormal haemoglobins: carboxyhaemoglobin, methaemoglobin
Venous congestion/pulsations: e.g. tricuspid valve incompetence

P wave
Absent
Atrial fibrillation
Hyperkalaemia
Sinoatrial block, junctional (AV nodal) rhythm

Tall
Pulmonary hypertension (primary, secondary to pulmonary emboli, COPD)
Pulmonary stenosis
Tricuspid stenosis

Painful red eye
Scleritis
Anterior uveitis
Acute angle closure glaucoma
Corneal ulcer/bacterial keratitis

Palate, high arched
Marfan's syndrome
Homocytinuria
Multiple endocrine neoplasia type 2b
Turner's syndrome
Noonan's syndrome*
Friedreich's ataxia
Fragile X syndrome

Pallor
Racial, familial
Shock
Syncope
Anaemia
Endocrine: hypothyroidism, hypopituitarism
Other: albinism, vitiligo (widespread), phenylketonuria

Palmar erythema
Liver disease
Alcoholism
Rheumatoid arthritis
Thyrotoxicosis
Pregnancy
Chronic leukaemia

Palmoplantar hyperkeratosis
See Hyperkeratosis

Palmoplantar rash
Palmar erythema (See Palmar erythema)
Pompholyx eczema

---

*Autosomal dominant disorder; 50 % have a mutation in the *PTPN11* gene. Similar features as Turner's syndrome, but have right sided valvular abnormalities and intellectual disability.

Palmoplantar pustulosis (may be associated with synovitis, acne, hyperostosis and osteitis in SAPHO syndrome)
Reiter's syndrome (keratoderma blenorrhagica)
Janeway lesions (infective endocarditis)
Secondary syphilis
Erythema multiforme
Sign of graft-versus-host disease

Palpitations

Fever, exercise, anaemia, pregnancy
Drugs (caffeine, nicotine, salbutamol, anticholinergics, vasodilators, cocaine)
Cardiac: any arrhythmia* (e.g. AF, extrasystoles, SVT, VT), pacemaker, valvular disease, cardiac shunts, cardiomyopathy, atrial myxoma
Endocrine: thyrotoxicosis, phaeochromocytomas, hypoglycaemia, mastocytosis
Psychiatric: panic attacks, generalized anxiety disorder, depression, somatization

Pancytopaenia

Aplastic anaemia
    Congenital: Fanconi's
    Radiation
    Chemicals: benzene, insecticides
    Drugs: chloramphenicol, cytotoxics, gold
    Infection: HIV, viral hepatitis, measles
    Idiopathic
Megaloblastic anaemia
Marrow infiltration
    Lymphoma
    Leukaemia (acute)
    Metastasis
    Myeloma
    Myelofibrosis
SLE, sepsis, hypersplenism, paroxysmal nocturnal haemoglobinuria (PNH)

Papilloedema

See Optic disc

Pappenheimer bodies

Sideroblastic anaemia
Haemolytic anaemia
Post-splenectomy

Paraesthesiae

Peripheral neuropathy, e.g. diabetes mellitus, alcoholism etc. (*See* Polyneuropathy)
Peripheral nerve entrapment/compression, e.g. cervical rib, carpal tunnel syndrome, disc herniation
Spinal cord disease, e.g. cord/nerve root compression, multiple sclerosis
Rarely: cortical/thalamic lesions
Hypocalcaemia, e.g. in respiratory alkalosis, hypomagnesaemia

Paraproteinaemia

Multiple myeloma
Waldenström's macroglobulinaemia

---

* *See* Tachycardia.

Paraproteinaemia (continued)

Primary amyloidosis
Monoclonal gammopathy (benign paraproteinaemia)
Lymphoma, leukaemia
Heavy chain disease

Parotid enlargement
Bilateral

Sjögren's syndrome
Sarcoidosis
Lymphoma
Anorexia
Acromegaly
Alcoholics
Diabetics, hypertriglyceridaemia
Infection: mumps, HIV

Unilateral

Tumours, e.g. benign mixed parotid tumour, Warthin's tumour
Calculi
Cysts
Bacterial infection

Pathological fractures

Congenital: osteogenesis imperfecta, fibrous dysplasia
Malignancy: primary, secondary, myeloma
Osteomyelitis
Osteoporosis
Osteomalacia
Paget's disease of bone
Benign tumours: bone cysts, chondroma

Pelvic girdle pain

Degenerative disc disease (with facet impingement or nuclear prolapse)
Osteoarthritis of hip
Sacroiliitis
Trochanteric bursitis
Meralgia paraesthesia

Percussion note
Dull

Pleural effusion (stony dull)
Collapse
Consolidation
Fibrosis
Pleural thickening

Hyper-resonant

Pneumothorax
COPD (hyperinflation)

Pericarditis

Idiopathic

Infection (viral, e.g. coxsackie, EBV, varicella, mumps, HIV; bacterial, e.g. Streptococci, TB; fungal)
Inflammatory/connective tissue diseases: rheumatoid arthritis, SLE
Myocardial infarction
Malignancy
Myxoedema
Uraemia
Radiotherapy
Surgery/trauma
Drugs: hydralazine, isoniazid

Pericardial effusion
See Pericarditis

Pericardial rub
See Pericarditis

Periorbital oedema
See Facial swelling

Peripheral oedema
See Oedema

Pes cavus
Charcot–Marie–Tooth disease
Friedreich's ataxia
Poliomyelitis
Spina bifida
Syringomyelia
Homocysteinuria

Petechiae
See Purpura

Photodistributed rash
Drugs, e.g. amiodarone, sulphonamides, tetracyclines, griseofulvin, phenothiazines, chloroquine
SLE
Dermatomyositis
Porphyria cutanea tarda
Pellagra
Polymorphous light eruption

Pigmentation
See Hyperpigmentation and Hypopigmented macules

Pins and needles
See Paraesthesiae

Platelets
↓ Production
Bone marrow failure
Myeloma, myelofibrosis, marrow infiltration (lymphoma, carcinoma), anaemia (megaloblastic, aplastic), leukaemia

Platelets (continued)

Drugs: (cytotoxics, chloramphenicol, alcohol), radiotherapy
↓ Megakaryocytes: chemicals, drugs (e.g. co-trimoxazole), viral infection

↑ Destruction/consumption

Autoimmune (ITP)
SLE, CLL, lymphoma
Infections (malaria, viral, e.g. HIV)
Drugs (e.g. analgesics, antibiotics, anticonvulsant, anti-diabetics, heparin, quinine, quinidine)
DIC, TTP, HUS
Sequestration: splenic pooling due to splenomegaly
Dilutional loss (massive transfusion of stored blood)
Artifactual: blood clotting in the sample

Functional disorders

Bernard–Soulier disease
Glanzmann's thrombasthenia
Storage pool disease
Liver disease, myeloproliferative disorders, paraproteinaemia, aspirin, uraemia

↑ Platelets (thrombocytosis)

Secondary
Blood loss
Infection
Inflammation (e.g. Kawasaki's disease)
Mailgnancy (e.g. Hodgkin's disease)
Splenectomy
Trauma/surgery

Primary
Essential thrombocythaemia
Polycythaemia vera
Myelofibrosis (initially, later thrombocytopaenia)
Myelodysplasia
CML

Pleural effusion

Exudate

Infection: TB, bacterial pneumonia
Inflammation/connective tissue disease, e.g. SLE, sarcoidosis
Malignancy: bronchial carcinoma, mesothelioma
Pulmonary infarction
Post-MI
Pancreatitis (acute)

Transudate

Cardiac failure
Hypoproteinaemia
Hypothyroidism
Constrictive pericarditis
Meigs' syndrome

Pleural fluid eosinophilia

Pneumothorax

Haemothorax
Pulmonary infarction (PE)
Malignancy
Benign asbestos pleural effusion
Infection: parasitic e.g. paragonimiasis, fungal infections e.g. coccidioidomycosis, crypto-
coccosis, histoplasmosis
Drug-induced pleural effusion
Idiopathic

Pleuritic chest pain
See Chest pain

Poikilocytosis
Iron deficiency anaemia
Thalassaemia
Myelofibrosis

Polydipsia
See Polyuria

Polyarthralgia
Infection: disseminated septic arthritis (e.g. staphylococcal, gonococcal), viral (e.g. enter-
oviruses, EBV, HIV, Hepatitis B, mumps, rubella), rheumatic fever, Lyme disease, TB
Gout/pseudogout
Rheumatoid arthritis, osteoarthritis (generalized)
Seronegative arthritis: (**R**eactive/Reiter's, **E**nteropathic (Whipple's, IBD), **A**nkylosing spondy-
litis, **P**soriatic arthritis)
Systemic diseases: SLE, sarcoid, Sjögren's, Behçet's, primary vasculitides, polymyalgia
rheumatica
Other: haemochromatosis, sickle cell, malignancy (hypertrophic pulmonary osteoarthropathy)

Migratory polyarthralgia
Gonococcal arthritis
Rheumatic fever

Polychromasia
Haemorrhage
Haematinics (ferrous sulphate, B_{12})
Haemolysis, dyserythropoiesis

Polycythaemia
Relative polycythaemia: dehydration (e.g. alcohol, diuretics), Gaisböck's syndrome
True polycythaemia:

1. Polycythaemia rubra vera
2. Appropriate ↑ in erythropoietin: chronic hypoxia, e.g. high altitude, chronic lung disease,
   cyanotic heart disease. Inappropriate ↑ in erythropoietin, e.g. renal cell carcinoma/cysts,
   hepatoma, cerebellar haemangioblastoma, fibroids

Polyneuropathy
Infection: HIV, Lyme disease, leprosy, diphtheria
Inflammation: Guillain–Barré syndrome, chronic inflammatory demyelinating neuropathy,
Sjögren's syndrome, sarcoidosis, SLE, vasculitides (e.g. polyarteritis nodosa)
Tumours: paraneoplastic, paraproteinaemia

Polyneuropathy (continued)

Toxic: alcohol, heavy metals (e.g. lead), insecticides, drugs (cisplatinum, vincristine, amiodarone, metronidazole, phenytoin, isoniazid, nitrofurantoin, gold)
Metabolic: diabetes mellitus, hypothyroidism, B_{12}/thiamine deficiency, amyloidosis, uraemia
Hereditary: e.g. abetalipoproteinaemia, porphyria, hereditary sensory and motor neuropathy (HSMN or Charcot–Marie–Tooth syndrome), Refsum's syndrome, Tangier disease, lysosomal storage diseases, e.g. Fabry's disease, Niemann–Pick disease

Motor

Porphyria, diphtheria, lead, hereditary motor and sensory neuropathies (HMSN), Guillain–Barré syndrome, chronic inflammatory demyelinating polyneuropathy (CIDP), multifocal motor neuropathy with conduction block

Sensory

Diabetes, vitaminB_{12} deficiency, alcohol, amyloid, HIV, leprosy
Sjögren's, paraneoplastic/paraproteinaemia, isoniazid

Demyelinating

CIPD, Guillain–Barré syndrome, HSMN, HIV, amyloidosis, Refsum's disease, paraproteinaemia

Axonal

Alcohol, diabetes, vasculitides, vitamin deficiencies

Polyuria

Diabetes mellitus (uncontrolled)
Diabetes insipidus:
   Central: tumour, trauma/surgery, infiltration (e.g. TB, sarcoid, histiocytosis X, lymphocytic hypophysitis, DIDMOAD*)
   Nephrogenic: hypercalcaemia, hypokalaemia, Lithium, X-linked
Diuretics
Diuretic phase of acute renal failure, chronic renal failure
Post-obstructive diuresis
Psychogenic polydypsia

Portal hypertension

Prehepatic: portal/splenic vein thrombosis
Hepatic: cirrhosis, granulomata, schistosomiasis
Posthepatic: Budd–Chiari syndrome (hepatic vein thrombosis), congestive cardiac failure, constrictive pericarditis

PR interval
Long

First-degree atrioventricular (AV) block

Short

Wolff–Parkinson–White sndrome
Lown–Ganong–Levine syndrome
Hypertrophic obstructive cardiomyopathy, Duchenne's muscular dystrophy

Priapism

Low flow:
   After normal intercourse
   After self-injection of alprostadil or papaverine for impotence

*Diabetes insipidus, diabetes mellitus, optic atrophy, deafness.

α-Blocking agents, e.g. prazosin
Haematological diseases: sickle cell diseases, leukaemia
Haemodialysis
High flow (rare):
Caused by an injury resulting in an aneurysm of the deep artery of the corpus cavernosum

Proptosis
Unilateral
Orbital tumour (e.g. optic nerve tumour, Hodgkin's lymphoma, etc.), granuloma
Orbital cellulitis

Bilateral
Caroticocavernous fistula
Cavernous sinus thrombosis
Thyrotoxicosis
Orbital abnormalities (craniostenoses)

Prostate-specific antigen (PSA)
See Tumour markers

Proteinuria
Pregnancy
Diabetes mellitus
Hypertension
Infection (UTI)
Inflammation (SLE, glomerulonephritis)
Multiple myeloma
Amyloidosis
Other: fever, exercise, CCF, orthostatic proteinuria, contamination (semen, vaginal discharge)

Prothrombin time (PT), ↑
Warfarin/vitamin K deficiency
Liver disease
DIC
Heparin

Note: PT monitors the extrinsic pathway i.e. deficiency or inhibition of coagulation factors: VII, X, V, II, fibrinogen.

Proximal muscle weakness
Toxic/metabolic: steroids, Cushing's syndrome, thyrotoxicosis, hypothyroidism, osteomalacia, alcohol, heroin
Inflammatory: dermatomyositis, polymyositis
Infection: staphylococcal myositis, parasites (trichinosis, cysticercosis), viral (influenza, coxsackie, echo)
Inherited: muscular dystrophies, metabolic myopathies (e.g. glycogen storage diseases e.g. McArdle's syndrome), mitochondrial myopathies, familial periodic paralysis (associated with hypo/hyperkalaemia), acid maltase deficiency

Pruritus
Cutaneous
Eczema, allergic reactions
Lichen planus

Pruritus (continued)

Scabies
Herpes simplex, herpes zoster, parasites
Dermatitis herpetiformis
Blistering disorders
Psoriasis (occasionally)
Nodular prurigo (following insect bites)
Prurigo of pregnancy

Systemic diseases

Metabolic: liver failure, chronic renal failure
Endocrine: hyperthyroidism, hypothyroidism, diabetes mellitus
Haematological: polycythaemia, iron deficiency anaemia, Hodgkin's lymphoma
Psychological: parasitophobia, anxiety
Tropical infection: filariasis, hookworm
Drugs: alkaloids

Pruritus ani

Incontinence, diarrhoea, poor hygiene
Infection: *Enterobius vermicularis* (threadworm), fungal (candidiasis, tinea cruris), scabies
Anal disease: haemorrhoids, fissure, fistula, wart
Skin disease: contact dermatitis, eczema, psoriasis, lichen sclerosis
Other: anxiety, tight pants

Pseudobulbar palsy

See Bulbar palsy

Pseudohermaphrodite
Female

Excess androgens:
↑ Exposure during the embryonic period: androgen from adrenal/ovarian tumour or luteoma
   of pregnancy, congenital adrenal hyperplasia (CAH), intake of androgens or androgenic
   progestogens taken by the mother
↑ Synthesis in the adrenals: CAH

Male

Leydig cell hypoplasia
Luteinizing hormone (LH) or LH-receptor mutation (autosomal recessive)
Testosterone synthesis defects (autosomal recessive)
5-α Reductase deficiency (autosomal recessive)
Androgen insensitivity: spectrum varies from partial (Reifenstein's syndrome) → complete
   (testicular feminization syndrome)

PT

See Prothrombin time

Ptosis

Third nerve palsy (*See* Cranial nerve palsy)
Horner's syndrome (*See* Horner's syndrome)
Myasthenia gravis
Myotonic dystrophy
Ocular myopathy

Ptosis (continued)

Congenital

Syphilis

Puberty

Delayed

Constitutional growth and puberty delay

Hypogonadism of pre-pubertal onset (*See* Hypogonadism)

Precocious

Complete (central)

Congenital: hydrocephalus, brain malformations

Acquired: tumours (hypothalamic/pituitary: glioma, hamartomas), trauma, radiation, infiltrations

Incomplete

Premature pubic/axillary hair development: excess androgens

Leydig cells stimulated by hCG (which has LH-like activity), e.g. from hepatoma, hepato-blastoma, pineal/hypothalamic teratomas

Leydig cells premature activation (testotoxicosis) due to an activating mutation of the LH receptor

Leydig cell tumour

McCune–Albright syndrome: constitutive activation of the gonadotrophin receptor on Leydig cells

Excess androgens from adrenal tumours, CAH

Exogenous sex steroids

Premature breast development (thelarche): excess oestrogens:

Ovarian cyst (developed possibly due to premature FSH secretion)

Hypothyroidism ($\downarrow$ thyroid hormone $\rightarrow$ $\uparrow$ TSH stimulates FSH secretion: $\uparrow$ FSH $\rightarrow$ ovarian cyst development)

Ovarian neoplasm

McCune–Albright

Pulmonary function tests

See Lung function tests

Pulmonary hypertension

Primary

Secondary:

    Left heart disease (mitral valve disease, LVF, left atrial myxoma/thrombosis)

    Chronic lung disease (COPD)

    Recurrent pulmonary emboli

    $\uparrow$ Pulmonary blood flow (VSD, ASD, patent ductus arteriosus)

    Connective tissue disease (e.g. SLE, scleroderma)

    Drugs: fenfluramine (appetite suppressant)

    HIV

Pulse

Tachycardia: *See* Tachycardia

Bradycardia: *See* Bradycardia

Irregular pulse

Sinus arrhythmia (rate increases with inspiration)

Pulse (continued)

Irregularly irregular: atrial fibrillation, multiple ectopic beats (extrasystoles), atrial flutter with variable block
Regularly irregular: 2° heart block, ventricular bigemini

Bounding pulse

Peripheral vasodilatation: CO_2 retention (e.g. COPD), sepsis, liver failure, thyrotoxicosis
↑ Stroke volume: aortic regurgitation, patent ductus arteriosus, large AV fistulas, thyrotoxicosis, severe anaemia, exercise

Unequal/delayed pulses

Atherosclerosis, thromboembolic disease
Aortic dissection
Aortic aneurysm
Arteritis: Large vessel vasculitis (Takayasu's arteritis, giant cell arteritis, secondary syphilis)
Subclavian steal syndrome
Supravalvular aortic stenosis

Pulse pressure

↑
Aortic regurgitation
Thyrotoxicosis
Pregnancy
Patent ductus arteriosus
High-output cardiac failure (e.g. severe anaemia, beri beri, Paget's disease)
↓
Aortic stenosis
Shock
Pericardial effusion, constrictive pericarditis

Pulsus paradoxicus

Cardiac tamponade, constrictive pericarditis
Asthma (severe)

Pupils

Dilated: See Mydriasis
Constricted: See Miosis
Unequal: See Anisocoria

Purpura

Senile
Steroids (iatrogenic, Cushing's syndrome)
Infection: meningococcal septicaemia/DIC, infective endocarditis
Platelet disorders: quantitative (thrombocytopaenia), qualitative (von Willebrand's disease), coagulopathy (haemophilia, liver disease, anticoagulants)
Vasculitis: e.g.:

1. Henoch–Schönlein purpura, polyarteritis nodosa, Churg–Strauss, Wegener's granulomatosis, cryoglobulinaemia
2. SLE, rheumatoid arthritis

Collagen diseases: scurvy, Ehlers–Danlos syndrome
Others: emboli (e.g. cholesterol), hereditary haemorrhagic telangiectasia, amyloidosis

Pustules
Infection:
  Bacterial: Staphylococcal, Gram-negative bacilli, gonococcal, secondary syphilis
  Viral: HSV, VZV (pustules preceded by vesicles)
  Fungal: (dermatophyte infection inappropriately treated with topical steroids)
  Scabies
Psoriasis (pustular)
Pyoderma gangrenosum
Drugs: steroids, phenytoin, isoniazid
Developing at sites of trauma (pathergy): Behçet's disease, Sweet's syndrome
With other skin signs: acne, rosacea

Pyoderma gangrenosum
Inflammatory bowel disease, autoimmune hepatitis
Rheumatoid arthritis, seronegative arthritides
Haematological: leukaemia, myeloma, polycythaemia rubra vera
Wegener's granulomatosis
Idiopathic (50 %)

Pyrexia of unknown origin (PUO)
Infection: abscesses (subphrenic, liver, pelvis)
  Bacterial: infective endocarditis, osteomyelitis, UTI, biliary infection
  TB, brucellosis, viral infections (HIV, CMV, EBV), malaria
Inflammation/CTD: rheumatoid arthritis, SLE, sarcoidosis, vasculitides, polymyalgia
  rheumatica
Malignancy: lymphomas, leukaemia, renal cell carcinoma, hepatocellular carcinoma, pan-
  creatic carcinoma
Drugs: e.g. sulphonamides, isoniazid, aspirin
Familial Mediterranean fever (FMF), familial periodic fever (FPF)

Pyuria, sterile
TB, inadequately treated UTI, UTI with fastidious culture requirement
Bladder: tumour, chemical cystitis (e.g. cytotoxics)
Calculi
Renal papillary necrosis (e.g. analgesic excess), interstitial nephritis, polycystic kidney disease
Prostatitis
Appendicitis

Q waves
Normal
  If < 25 % of the height of the following R wave or < 2 mm deep
  'Septal' Q waves in the lateral leads
  Common in III, V_5–V_6
Myocardial infarction (> a few hours' duration)
Left ventricular hypertrophy
Bundle branch block

QRS complexes
Axis deviation: *See* Axis deviation
Bundle branch block: *See* Bundle branch blocks
Low voltage QRS complexes
  Incorrect standardization
  Obesity
  COPD
  Pericardial effusion
  Myxoedema
Wide QRS complexes
  Ventricular extrasystoles, ventricular tachycardia, complete AV block
  Bundle branch block: Left and Right
Dominant R waves in V_1: *See* R wave

QT interval
Long
Hypothermia
Hypocalcaemia, hypokalaemia, hypomagnesaemia
Congenital: Romano–Ward syndrome, Jervell–Lange–Nielsen syndrome
Drugs: tricyclic antidepressants, chloroquine, Class Ia anti-arrhythmic drugs
Acute MI, acute myocarditis
Cerebral injury

Short
Hyperthermia
Hypercalcaemia
Digoxin

R wave, dominant in V1
Right ventricular hypertrophy, right BBB, pulmonary embolism
Posterior MI
Myocarditis
Wolff–Parkinson–White syndrome (left-sided accessory pathway)
Misplaced pacemaker! (in left atrium)

Rash
Cutaneous diseases, e.g. eczema, psoriasis, urticaria
Drugs
Infection (bacterial, viral, fungal, parasitic)
Inflammatory/connective tissue diseases
Malignancy
See also Hyperpigmentation, Hypopigmented macules, Malar rash, Photodistributed rash

Raynaud's phenomenon
Idiopathic
Occupational (vibrating tools)
Connective tissue diseases: scleroderma, SLE, Sjögren's syndrome, rheumatoid arthritis, dermatomyositis
Cold agglutinins
Cryoglobulinaemia, macroglobulinaemia (Waldenström's)
Cervical rib
Drugs: β-blockers
Vascular disease

Rectal discharge
Common
Haemorrhoids
Anal fissure
Rectal prolapse
Proctitis
Perianal warts

Occasional
Rectal carcinoma
Anal fistula
Perianal IBD
Solitary rectal ulcer syndrome
Villous adenoma

Rare
Infection: anal TB, gonorrhoea, syphilis, HIV
Anal carcinoma

Red blood cell fragmentation
Artificial heart valve/artificial graft
Microangiopathic haemolytic anaemia: See Anaemia, haemolytic

Red eye
Conjunctivitis (allergic, viral, bacterial, chlamydial)
Episcleritis

Red eye (continued)

Scleritis
Iritis (anterior uveitis)
Acute angle closure glaucoma
Other: inflamed pinguecula, subconjunctival haemorrhage
See also Painful red eye

Red reflex, absent

Cataract
Corneal oedema (acute angle closure glaucoma)
Vitreous hemorrhage
Retinal detachment

Reflexes

Reflexes
↑: See Upper motor neurone lesion
↓: See Lower motor neurone lesion

Absent reflexes with up-going plantars

Conus medullaris lesion
Motor neurone disease
Subacute combined degeneration of the cord (B_{12} deficiency)
Spinal shock
Friedreich's ataxia
Tabes dosalis
Pellagra
Severe hyponatraemia

Relative afferent pupillary defect (RAPD)

Optic neuritis
Optic nerve compression
Central retinal artery occlusion
Retinal detachment
Glaucoma (unilateral)

Respiratory failure

Type 1: See Arterial blood gas
Type 2: See Arterial blood gas

Respiratory rate

↑
Physiological: exercise, anxiety
Lung disease: pneumothorax, pulmonary embolism, obstructive disease, e.g. asthma attack, restrictive disease, infection, inflammation (vasculitis), malignancy
Elevation of diaphragm: ascites, diaphragmatic paralysis
Metabolic acidosis

↓
Physiological: well-conditioned athletes
CNS disease: infection (meningitis, encephalitis), trauma (head injury), tumour (↑ intracranial pressure), drugs (sedatives), coma

Reticulocytosis

Haemolysis
Haemorrhage
After the response to B_{12}/folate/iron treatment given to marrow that lack these

Retinal haemorrhages
Central retinal vein occlusion
Diabetic retinopathy
Hypertension
Papilloedema

Retinal neovascularization
Diabetic proliferative retinopathy
Retinal vein thrombosis
Sickle cell haemoglobinopathy
SLE
Ocular ischaemic syndrome (due to carotid occlusive disease)
Eales disease (peripheral retinal vasculitis)

Retinitis pigmentosa
Abetalipoproteinaemia
Laurence–Moon–Biedl
Refsum's disease
Friedreich's ataxia and other hereditary ataxias
Familial neuropathies
Neuronal lipidoses (ceroid lipofuscinosis)

Rheumatoid factor, + ve
Sjögren's syndrome (95 %)
Rheumatoid arthritis (70 %)
SLE
Scleroderma
Mixed connective tissue disease
Mixed cryoglobulinaemia
Polymyositis/dermatomyositis
Infection/inflammatory diseases, e.g. TB, infectious mononucleosis, subacute bacterial endocarditis, chronic hepatitis
Healthy individuals (∼5 %)

Rigors
Cholangitis
Pyelonephritis
Pneumococcal pneumonia
Malaria
Localized sepsis (abscesses)

Roth's spots
Infective endocarditis
Leukaemia
Anaemia
Vasculitis: PAN, SLE

Rubeosis iridis
Proliferative retinopathy (diabetes mellitus, sickle cell disease, retinal vein thrombosis)
Carotid artery disease, including carotid–cavernous fistula
Chronic intraocular inflammation/tumour
Chronic retinal detachment

Saddle nose deformity
Trauma
Congenital syphilis
Wegener's granulomatosis
Relapsing polychondritis
Lepromatous leprosy

Scleromalacia perforans
Rheumatoid arthritis
Ankylosing spondylitis
Vasculitis (Wegener's granulomatosis, polyarteritis nodosa)
Gout
Herpes zoster

Scotoma, central
Optic nerve disease
Retinal disease affecting the macula

Seizures
Adults
Vascular: infarction, haemorrhage, cortical venous thrombosis, vascular malformation
Trauma: head injury
Tumours
Toxic: alcohol, drugs, lead, carbon monoxide
Metabolic: hypoxia, hypoglycaemia, electrolyte disturbances ($\uparrow$ or $\downarrow$ Na^+, K^+, Ca^{2+}, Mg^{2+}), renal/hepatic failure, endocrine disorders (hypopituitarism, myxoedema, hypo/hyper-parathyroidism, Addison's disease, insulinoma), vitamin deficiency
Infection: meningitis, encephalitis, abscess, TB, cysticercosis, HIV
Inflammation: MS, vasculitis, SLE, sarcoidosis
Degenerative disorders: Alzheimer's disease, prion disease
Very raised BP

Children
Congenital anomaly
Tuberous sclerosis
Metabolic storage diseases

Sensory disturbance, distribution
Hemisensory loss (arm, trunk, leg) + ipsilateral facial sensory loss:
   Contralateral thalamic lesion
Hemisensory + contralateral facial sensory loss:
   Contralateral brainstem (ipsilateral to the facial sensory loss)
Bilateral lower limbs and trunk (below a dermatomal sensory level):
   ↓Pin prick/temperature sensation: bilateral spinothalamic tracts
   ↓Joint position/vibration sensation: bilateral dorsal columns
Hemisensory loss (leg and trunk below a dermatomal sensory level):
   ↓Pin prick/temperature sensation: contralateral spinothalamic tracts
   ↓Joint position/vibration sensation: ipsilateral dorsal columns
Upper arms and trunk ('suspended sensory loss' for pin prick and temperature):
   Central spinal cord (e.g. syringomyelia)

Glove-and-stocking:
  Peripheral neuropathy
  Cervical myelopathy
Dermatomal
Peripheral nerve

Sensory disturbance, timing of onset
Transient
Epilepsy
Migraine
TIA, stroke
CNS demyelination
Peripheral nerve or root entrapment
Psychogenic

Persistent
Brain: space-occupying lesions (tumour, subdural haematoma, abscess)
Spinal cord: cervical spondylosis, demyelination
Nerve root: spondylitic radiculopathy
Peripheral nerve: peripheral neuropathy e.g. diabetes mellitus (*See* Polyneuropathy)

SGOT
See Liver function tests

SGPT
See Liver function tests

Short 4th/5th finger
Turner's syndrome
Pseudohypoparathyroidism
Dactylitis residua (sickle cell disease)

Shortness of breath
See under Breathlessness

Shoulder pain
Overuse injuries, subluxation, fracture
Adhesive capsulitis (frozen shoulder)
Rotator cuff tendinitis
Subacromial bursitis
Rotator cuff tear
Bicipital tendinitis
Arthritis (septic, osteoarthritis, rheumatoid arthritis, gout/pseudogout)
Acute calcific tendinitis
Avascular necrosis
Referred pain:
Myocardial ischaemia (left shoulder pain)
Cervical disc herniation/spinal stenosis, nerve entrapment (long thoracic or suprascapular
    nerve)
Diaphragmatic irritation (e.g. subphrenic abscess), hepatic capsule distension, pulmonary
    tumour/infection/abscess

Skin necrosis

Warfarin, protein C/S deficiency, DIC (e.g. meningococcal septicaemia)
Vasculitis (*Primary:* Wegener's granulomatosis, cryoglobulinaemia; *Secondary:* SLE, rheumatoid arthritis)
Peripheral vascular disease
Emboli: cholesterol, subacute bacterial endocarditis
Pyoderma gangrenosum
Panniculitis (e.g. idiopathic, pancreatitis)
Calciphylaxis (small-vessel vasculitis causing skin necrosis associated with end-stage renal failure, $\uparrow Ca^{2+}$ and phosphate)

Sore throat

Pharyngitis (viral)
Streptococcal tonsillitis
Infectious mononucleosis
Gonococcal pharyngitis
Diphtheria

With pharyngeal ulcers

Herpes simplex
Herpangina
Vincent's angina (fusospirochetal infection)
Candidiasis

Spastic paraparesis

Cord compression (cervical spondylosis, disc prolapse, secondary tumour in spine, spinal cord tumour)
Multiple sclerosis
Motor neurone disease
Trauma, birth injury (cerebral palsy)
Syringomyelia

Others

Vascular: anterior spinal artery thrombosis, venous sinus thrombosis, multiple cerebral infarctions
Infection: tranverse myelitis (post-infectious, e.g. Mycoplasma), HIV, HTLV-1 (tropical spastic paraparesis), syphilis
Tumours: parasigittal meningioma
Toxic/metabolic: B_{12} deficiency (subacute combined degeneration)
Congenital: hereditary spastic paraparesis, Friedreich's ataxia

Spherocytosis

Hereditary spherocytosis
Autoimmune haemolytic anaemia
Septicaemia

Splenomegaly
Massive

Chronic myeloid leukaemia, myelofibrosis
Tropical infections: malaria, leishmaniasis, schistosomiasis, tropical splenomegaly
Gaucher's disease

Moderate

Haematological (haemolytic anaemia, lymphoma, leukaemia, myeloproliferative disorders*)
Portal hypertension (*See* Portal hypertension)

---

*Chronic myeloid leukaemia, myelofibrosis, polycythaemia rubra vera, essential thrombocythaemia.

Infection: infective endocarditis, infectious mononucleosis, tuberculosis, brucellosis
Inflammatory/connective tissue diseases: rheumatoid arthritis, SLE, sarcoidosis, amyloidosis

Splinter haemorrhages
Trauma, e.g. gardening
Infective endocarditis
Vasculitis
Psoriasis
Mitral stenosis

Sputum (purulent)
Upper respiratory source (acute sinusitis, rhinitis, bronchitis)
Infection: pneumonia, TB, lung abscess
Bronchiectasis
Bronchopleural fistula
See also Haemoptysis

ST segment
Depression
Myocardial ischaemia
Myocardial infarction (posterior)
Drugs (digoxin, quinidine)
Ventricular hypertrophy

Elevation
Myocardial infarction (acute)
Pericarditis
Prinzmetal angina
Left ventricular aneurysm
Brugada syndrome (downsloping ST elevation; may be caused by mutations in the cardiac
   sodium channel gene *SCN5A*, associated with sudden cardiac death)
High take-off

Stature
Short stature
CGPD (constitutional growth and puberty delay), familial
Syndromic: Turner's syndrome, achondroplasia, Prader–Willi
Psychosocial factors: child abuse, anorexia nervosa, emotional deprivation
Endocrine factors:
   ↓ Growth hormone: Hypopituitarism (e.g. pituitary tumour)
   Mutations: Pit1, PROP1, GHRH receptor
   Cushing's syndrome and excess exogenous corticosteroids
   Biologically inactive GH
   GH resistance (GH-receptor mutation)
   Low levels of IGF1 (Laron dwarfism)
   ↓ Thyroid hormones (hypothyroidism)
Nutritional factors
Systemic illness:
   Gastrointestinal: malabsorption (coeliac disease, milk protein intolerance, inflammatory
      bowel disease)
   Cardiovascular: congenital cyanotic heart disease
   Respiratory: cystic fibrosis
   Renal: chronic renal failure

Stature (Continued)
Tall stature
Familial
Syndromic (disproportionate):
   Klinefelter's syndrome
   Marfan's syndrome
   Homocystinuria
Endocrine:
   Excess GH (gigantism)
   Excess thyroid hormones (thyrotoxicosis)
   Excess sex steroids/precocious puberty (e.g. early phases of CAH, adrenal tumours)

Steatorrhoea
Small bowel disease/resection
Bacterial overgrowth (e.g. scleroderma, diverticulosis, autonomic neuropathy), coeliac disease, Crohn's disease, ileocaecal TB, parasite infection (e.g. giardiasis, strongyloidiasis), intestinal lymphoma, radiation enteritis, Whipple's disease, tropical sprue

Pancreatic insufficiency
Chronic pancreatitis, pancreatic cancer, cystic fibrosis

Biliary insufficiency
Biliary obstruction, primary biliary cirrhosis

Striae
Cushing's syndrome
Systemic steroids
Physiological: pregnancy (lower abdomen, breasts), adolescence (thighs, lumbosacral areas), weightlifters (shoulders)

Stridor
Partial obstruction of upper airways
Intraluminal:
   Foreign body, tumour
Intramural:
   Infection: epiglottitis, croup in children, respiratory papillomata (HPV warts on the larynx), retropharyngeal abscess
   Laryngeal oedema (anaphylaxis, smoke inhalation)
   Laryngeal carcinoma
   Cricoarytenoid rheumatoid arthritis
   Tracheal stenosis (following surgery/intubation/tracheostomy)
Extramural:
   Goitre
   Lymphadenopathy

Sweating
↑ Sweating: See Hyperhidrosis
See also Night sweats

T waves
Tall
Hyperkalaemia
Acute MI
Normal variant

Small
Hypokalaemia
Pericardial effusion
Hypothyroidism

Inverted
V_1—V_3/V_4
Normal variant (children and black people)
Right bundle branch block
Pulmonary embolism

V_2—V_5
Non-Q wave MI
Hypertrophic cardiomyopathy
Subarachnoid haemorrhage, Lithium

V_4—V_6 and lateral
Left ventricular hypertrophy
Myocardial ischaemia
Associated with LBBB

Tachycardia
Sinus tachycardia
Fever, exercise, anxiety, anaemia, drugs (caffeine, salbutamol, anticholinergics, catecholamines, nicotine), pregnancy
Hypotension (e.g. hypovolaemia, septicaemia)
Cardiac: MI, congestive cardiac failure, constrictive pericarditis
Pulmonary: pulmonary embolism, asthma, chronic lung disease
Endocrine: hyperthyroidism, phaeochromocytomas, hypoglycaemia

Supraventricular tachycardia
Idiopathic, Wolff–Parkinson–White syndrome

Atrial fibrillation/flutter
Idiopathic, thyrotoxicosis, alcohol abuse, pulmonary: embolism/infection/cancer, pericarditis, cardiomyopathy, ischaemic heart disease, rheumatic heart disease, mitral stenosis

Ventricular tachycardia
Idiopathic, ischaemic heart disease/MI, hypertensive heart disease, cardiomyopathy, myocarditis, long QT syndrome, drugs

Tachypnoea
See Respiratory rate

Target cells
Splenectomy
Haemoglobinopathies (sickle cell anaemia, thalassaemia, haemoglobin C disease)
Iron deficiency
Liver disease
Lecithin cholesterol acyltransferase (LCAT) deficiency

Teardrop cells
Thalassaemia
Bone marrow fibrosis

Telangiectasia
Normal variant
Connective tissue diseases: scleroderma, SLE, dermatomyositis
Genetic: hereditary haemorrhagic telangiectasia, ataxia telangiectasia
Chronic liver disease (esp. alcoholic cirrhosis)
Carcinoid syndrome
Pregnancy
Topical steroids (long-term)
Rosacea
Radiation dermatitis

Tenesmus
Space-occupying lesions in rectal wall/lumen, e.g. rectal carcinoma
Irritable bowel syndrome

Testicular atrophy
See Hypogonadism, male

Testicular pain and swelling
Testicular torsion
Epidydimo-orchitis
TB, sarcoid
Leukaemia
Polyarteritis nodosa, Henoch–Schönlein
Renal vein thrombosis

Testosterone, ↓
See Hypogonadism

Thrombin time, ↑
DIC (↓ fibrinogen)
Heparin

Thrombocytopaenia
See Platelets

Thrombocytosis
See Platelets

Thyroid-binding globulin (TBG)
↑ **levels**
Genetic

Pregnancy
Drugs (oestrogen, opiates, phenothiazines)
Acute viral hepatitis, acute intermittent porphyria

↓ levels
Genetic
Malnutrition
Chronic liver disease
Nephrotic syndrome
Drugs (e.g. androgens, corticosteroids)
Acromegaly

Thyroid function tests
Normal T4, T3 and TSH: Euthyroid
Normal T4 and T3, ↓ TSH: sub-clinical hyperthyroidism, same causes as overt hyperthyroidism
Normal T4 and T3, ↑ TSH: sub-clinical hypothyroidism, same causes as overt hypothyroidism
↓ T4 and T3, ↑ TSH: primary hypothyroidism (See Hypothyroidism)
↓ T4 and T3, ↓ or normal TSH: secondary hypothyroidism (See Hypopituitarism), sick euthyroid
    syndrome (systemic illness, esp. hospitalized patients)
↑ T4 and T3, ↓ TSH: primary thyrotoxicosis (See Thyrotoxicosis)
↑ T4 and T3, normal or ↑ TSH: secondary hyperthyroidism (pituitary TSHoma), resistance to
    thyroid hormone
↑ T4 and T3, normal TSH: ↑ serum thyroxine-binding globulin
Familial dysalbuminaemic hyperthyroxinaemia
Anti-T4 antibodies

Thyrotoxicosis
Graves' disease
Toxic multinodular goitre
Toxic adenoma
Thyroiditis (subacute/viral, post-partum)
Gestational thyrotoxicosis (↑ hCG)

Rarer causes
Secondary hyperthyroidism (TSH)
Follicular carcinoma of thyroid
Choreocarcinoma
Struma ovarii
Drugs: amiodarone, surreptitious thyroxine consumption (thyroiditis factitia)
TSH-receptor mutations, McCune–Albright syndrome

Tingling in hands and feet
See Paraesthesia

Tinnitus
Local
Presbycusis
Ménière's disease
Noise-induced
Ototoxic drugs, e.g. aminoglycosides, loop diuretics
Otosclerosis
Aneursms/AV malformations
Tumours: acoustic neuroma, glomus jugulare tumour, carotid body tumour

Tinnitus (continued)
Temporomandibular joint problems
Insects, e.g. maggots

General
Fever
CVS: hypertension, heart failure
Haematological: ↑ viscosity, anaemia
CNS: multiple sclerosis
Drugs: aspirin, alcohol, quinine

Tongue
Sore tongue
Ulcers: infection (herpes simplex), inflammatory (Behçet's disease), malignancy
Glossitis (iron/folate/vitamin B/riboflavin deficiency, candidiasis) See Glossitis
Sore physiologically normal tongue
Psychogenic

Swelling (See Macroglossia)

Ulceration
Aphthous ulcer
Dental trauma
Tumour
Syphilis

Tracheal deviation
Collapse
Tension pneumothorax
Large pleural effusion

Transfer factor
See Lung function tests

Tremor
Essential tremor: (postural tremor of hands/head, e.g. when holding a glass/writing, positive
family history, ↓ with alcohol or β-blockers)
Physiological tremor: (made worse by hyperthyroidism, anxiety, alcohol, drugs, e.g. β-agonist
bronchodilators, valproate, lithium, antidepressants)
Tremor at rest: Parkinson's disease and other akinetic–rigid syndromes
Action tremor: cerebellar sign (See Cerebellar signs)

Troponin, ↑
Myocardial infarction
May also be elevated in: unstable angina, chronic renal failure

Tumour markers, ↑
α-Fetoprotein: hepatoma, germ-cell tumour, pregnancy, hepatitis, cirrhosis, open neural
tube defects
CA 125: ovarian cancer, other malignancies (breast, endometrial, lung, pancreas). Benign
conditions (endometriosis, fibroids, pelvic inflammatory disease, peritonitis, cirrhosis)
CA 15–3: breast cancer, benign breast disease
CA 19–9: pancreatic cancer, colorectal cancer, cholestasis

Tumour markers, ↑ (continued)

CEA: colorectal cancer, medullary thyroid carcinoma, cirrhosis, pancreatitis, smoking

HCG: pregnancy, germ cell tumours, hydatidiform mole, choriocarcinoma

PLAP: seminoma, smoking, pregnancy, ovarian carcinoma

PSA: prostate cancer, benign prostatic hyperplasia, prostatitis, digital rectal examination, (PSA also ↑ with age and size of the gland)

Tunnel vision

Retinitis pigmentosa (*See* Retinitis pigmentosa)

Chronic glaucoma

Chronic papilloedema

U wave
Normal
Hypokalaemia
Hypercalcaemia
Hyperthyroidism

Ulcers: mouth, genital, leg
Mouth
Trauma, aphthous ulcers
Gastrointestinal diseases: Crohn's disease, coeliac disease
Infection: herpes simplex, acute ulcerative stomatitis (Vincent's angina), candidiasis TB, syphilis (rare)
Exclude: leukaemia, agranulocytosis
Inflammatory: Behçet's disease, reactive arthritis, SLE
Skin diseases: pemphigus, pemphigoid, erythema multiforme, lichen planus
Malignancy: squamous cell carcinoma
Other: Strachan's syndrome

Genital
Infection:
  Painful: herpes simplex, *Haemophilus ducreyi* (chancroid)
  Painless: Syphilis (*Treponema pallidum*), Lymphogranuloma venereum (*Chlamydia trachomatis*), Granuloma inguinale (*Calymmatobacterium granulomatis*)
Behçet's disease
Crohn's disease
Reiter's syndrome
Erythroplasia of Queyrat, squamous cell carcinoma
Trauma
Other genital rashes: fixed drug eruption, eczema, psoriasis, scabies

Orogenital
Infection: herpes simplex, syphilis
Inflammatory diseases: Behçet's disease, Reiter's syndrome
Skin diseases: pemphigus, erythema multiforme
GI: Crohn's disease
Other: Strachan's diseases (orogenital ulcers, sensory neuropathy, amblyopia; aetiology unknown).

Leg
Venous: superficial venous insufficiency, DVT
Arterial: atherosclerosis
Diabetic: ischaemic and neuropathic
Vasculitis: rheumatoid arthritis, primary vasculities, e.g. polyarteritis nodosa
Sickle cell anaemia
Pressure
Pyoderma gangrenosum
Malignancy

Upper motor neurone lesions
See Hemiparesis and Spastic paraparesis

Urea (↑ and ↓)
↑
Impaired glomerular filtration rate (GFR)
High protein diet, GI haemorrhage, catabolic states
Dehydration
Drugs: steroids, tetracycline

↓
Increased GFR (pregnancy)
Low-protein diet, starvation, liver failure
SIADH
Drugs: sodium valproate

Urgency
UTI
Bladder: stone, tumour, compression by pelvic mass
Prostate enlargement (Benign prostatic hyperplasia, cancer)
Genuine stress incontinence, detrusor instability, sensory urgency

Urinalysis
Urine colour
Red/brown
Haematuria
Haemoglobinuria
Myoglobinuria
Beetroot
Porphyria
Phenazopyridine

Rare
White: pyuria, phosphate crystals
Green: methylene blue, amitryptiline, propofol
Dark: obstructive jaundice, ochronosis, malignancy
Orange: rifampicin

Protein
See Proteinuria

Blood
See Haematuria

Urine glucose
See Glycosuria

Ketones
See Ketonuria

Urine leukocyte esterase
Urinary tract infection
Vaginal contaminant

Urine nitrite
Urinary tract infection
Gross haematuria

Urinalysis (continued)
Urine specific gravity

↑

Dehydration (e.g. diarrhoea, vomiting)
Diabetes mellitus
Adrenal insufficiency
Heart failure
Liver disease
X-ray contrast

↓

Diabetes insipidus
Excessive hydration
Renal failure

Urinary frequency
See Frequency

Urinary incontinence
Stress incontinence
Females: pelvic floor weakness/bladder neck descent (pregnancy, vaginal delivery, obesity, menopause)
Males: prostate surgery (external urethral sphincter damage)

Urge incontinence
Detrusor instability (idiopathic, secondary to bladder outflow obstruction, loss of supra-spinal inhibition with UMN lesions, e.g. stroke, MS, cord compression: disc lesions/spinal tumours, spinal cord/head injury)
Bladder stone, tumour, infection (cystitis)

Continuous incontinence
Chronic retention/overdistension/overflow:
  Outflow obstruction (See Urinary retention)
  Bladder atonia due to damage to S2, S3, S4 parasympathetic fibres in lower spinal cord, cauda equina or pelvis, diabetic autonomic neuropathy
  Fistula (e.g. vesicovaginal) secondary to obstructed labour, surgery, malignancy, radiotherapy

Note: Detrusor instability and chronic retention/overdistension of bladder can also cause stress incontinence.

Urinary retention, acute
Males
Prostatic hyperplasia/carcinoma
Obstruction of urethral lumen/bladder neck (stricture, stone, tumour, blood clot)
Post-operative*
Medication: e.g. anticholinergics, antidepressants, alcohol
Neurological: multiple sclerosis, spinal cord disease, e.g. injury/compression, diabetic autonomic neuropathy, herpes zoster

Females
Pelvic mass: fibroids, ovarian mass, pregnancy (and trauma of labour)
Obstruction of urethral lumen/bladder neck (stone, tumour, blood clot)
Post-operative*

---

*Post-operative: drugs/anaesthetics, immobility, constipation, pain, local oedema, neuropraxia, pre-existing bladder outflow obstruction.

Medication: e.g. anticholinergics, antidepressants, alcohol

Neurological: multiple sclerosis, spinal cord disease, e.g. injury/compression, diabetic autonomic neuropathy, herpes zoster

Urinary tract obstruction

In the lumen: stones, tumour, blood clots, sloughed renal papillae (NSAIDs, diabetes mellitus, sickle cell)

In the wall: stricture (ureteric/urethral), defective peristalsis, neuropathic bladder

Pressure from the outside: prostatic/pelvic mass, retroperitoneal fibrosis, phimosis

Urine microscopy

Bacteria

Urinary tract infection

Asymptomatic bacteriuria

Contamination

Casts

Epithelial cell casts: acute glomerulonephritis, acute tubular necrosis

Fatty casts: moderate/heavy proteinuria

Granular casts, finely granulated: concentrated urine, diuretics (loop), exercise, fever

Granular casts, densely granulated: glomerulonephritis, interstitial nephritis, diabetic nephropathy, amyloidosis

Hyaline casts: same as finely granulated granular casts

Red cell casts: glomerulonephritis, vasculitis, malignant hypertension

Waxy casts: advanced renal failure

White cell casts: pyelonephritis, proliferative glomerulonephritis

Cells

White cells: UTI (pyelonephritis, cystitis, urethritis), pyuria without bacteriuria: culture inhibited by antibacterial agent or wrong growth condition for fastidious organisms, TB, renal/bladder calculi, glomerulonephritis, interstitial nephritis, analgesic nephropathy, chemical cystitis

Red cells: *See* Haematuria

Tumour cells: Genitourinary malignancy e.g. bladder cancer, infiltration of renal parenchyma e.g. lymphoma

Crystals

Calcium oxalate (dumbbell-shaped, envelope-shaped, needle-shaped)

Calcium phosphate

Cystine (hexagonal shape)

Magnesium ammonium phosphate (coffin-lid-shaped)

Uric acid (rhombic plates, rosettes)

Uveitis

Inflammatory/Connective tissue diseases: Seronegative spondylarthropathies: (reactive arthritis, enteropathic (inflammatory bowel disease), ankylosing spondylitis, psoriatic arthritis), sarcoidosis, Behçet's desease, juvenile chronic arthritis

Infection: CMV, toxoplasmosis, post-operative infection, fungal, herpetic, TB, syphilis, *Toxocara*

Ocular disease: e.g. sympathetic ophthalmitis, intraocular tumours

Vertigo
Labyrinth:
  Acute labyrinthitis
  Benign positional vertigo
  Ménière's disease
  Secondary to middle ear disease
Vestibular nerve:
  Herpes zoster
  Acoustic neuroma
  Ototoxic drugs (e.g. aminoglycosides)
Brainstem:
  Ischaemia (vertebrobasilar circulation)/bleeding
  Multiple sclerosis, tumours
Other:
  Migraine
  Vertiginous epilepsy

Vesicles
See Bullous skin lesions

Visual loss
Sudden
Unilateral
Amaurosis fugax
Central retinal vein occlusion
Central retinal artery occlusion
Vitreous haemorrhage
Retinal detachment
Giant cell arteritis
Optic neuritis
Ischaemic optic neuropathy (non-areteritic)

Bilateral
Severe bilateral papilloedema (malignant hypertension, ↑ ↑ intracranial pressure)
Rapid progression of a lesion compressing the optic chiasm
Bilateral infarcts of occipital lobes
Bilateral optic neuritis (rare)

Gradual
Cataracts
Glaucoma
Diabetic retinopathy
Macular degeneration (age-related)
Optic nerve compression

Vomiting
Drugs, poisoning, alcohol
Abdominal pathology (gastrointestinal, hepatic, gynaecological)
Metabolic/endocrine: diabetic ketoacidosis, Addisonian crisis, hypercalcaemia, uraemia,
  pregnancy

Neurological: increased intracranial pressure (infection, space-occupying lesion, benign intracranial hypertension), acute labyrinthitis
Acute angle closure glaucoma

Wasting of small muscles of hands
T1
MND, spinal cord compression, syringomyelia, syphilis, poliomyelitis

Root involvement
Cervical spondylosis, neurofibromata

Brachial plexus involvement
Cervical rib, apical lung tumour, trauma

Peripheral nerve involvement
Rheumatoid arthritis, ulnar/median nerve palsy

Weak legs
Spastic paraparesis: *See* Spastic paraparesis
Flaccid paraparesis: *See* Flaccid paraparesis
Foot drop: *See* Foot drop

Webbed neck
Turner's syndrome
Klippel–Feil syndrome

Weight loss
Voluntary: diet, exercise

With ↑ appetite
Marked ↑ in physical activity
Malabsorption syndromes
Endocrine: hyperthyroidism, uncontrolled diabetes mellitus, phaeochromocytomas

With ↓ appetite
Chronic systemic illness:
    Infections (e.g. TB, brucellosis, subacute bacterial endocarditis, HIV)
    Malignancy
    Cardiopulmonary diseases
    Gastrointestinal disease
    Endocrine diseases, e.g. Addison's disease
Psychiatric: depression, eating disorder (e.g. anorexia nervosa)
Drugs: antidepressants, L-dopa, digoxin, metformin, NSAIDs, alcohol, opiates, amphetamine,
    cocaine

Weight gain
Pregnancy
Excessive caloric intake
Endocrine: PCOS, Cushing's syndrome, hypothyroidism, hypothalamic disease (trauma,
    tumour), acromegaly
Drugs: steroids, OCPs, androgenic steroids, antidepressants, anticonvulsants
Depression
↑ Fluid: congestive cardiac failure, renal failure, cirrhosis, excess IV fluids, lymphatic
    obstruction
Cessation of cigarette smoking

Wheeze
Anaphylaxis
Asthma, Allergic bronchopulmonary aspergillosis
COPD
Pulmonary oedema
Aspiration
Pulmonary embolism
Bronchiolitis: Infection (e.g. adenovirus, *Mycoplasma, Legionella*)
                Connective tissue diseases (e.g. rheumatoid arthritis, SLE, Scleroderma, Sjögren's, polyarteritis nodosa)
                Transplant (e.g. bone marrow, heart-lung)
                Toxic fume inhalation
                Ulcerative colitis
                Idiopathic
Carcinoid syndrome
Lung cancer
Lymphangitic carcinomatosis (e.g. secondary to stomach, breast, prostate and pancreatic cancers)
Bronchiectasis, cystic fibrosis
Parasitic infections (e.g. *Ascaris, Ancylostoma, Strongyloides, Schistosoma, Toxocara, Wuchereria*)

White cell count
Neutrophils
↑
Infection (bacterial)
Inflammation/connective tissue diseases/vasculitis
Tissue damage: trauma/surgery, burns, MI
Haemorrhage/haemolysis (acute)
Myeloproliferative disease: polycythaemia, chronic myeloid leukaemia
Medication: steroids
Malignancy: particularly disseminated solid tumours and necrotic tumours

↓
As part of a pancytopaenia (*See* Pancytopaenia)
Infection: viral (e.g. hepatitis, HIV, influenza), typhoid, TB, brucellosis, kala-azar
Drugs: e.g. sulphasalazine, sulphonamides, carbimazole, clozapine
Immune: autoimmune neutropaenia, SLE, Felty's syndrome
Benign racial: black Africans
Congenital: Kostmann's syndrome

Eosinophils
↑
Allergic diseases: asthma, urticaria, eczema, hay fever, food allergy
Drugs e.g. penicillin, sulphonamides
Parasitic infections e.g. *Strongyloides stercoralis*, hookworm, *Toxocara canis*
Addison's disease
Blistering skin disease: pemphigus, pemphigoid, erythema multiforme
Hodgkin's lymphoma
Mastocytosis

Pulmonary eosinophilia
Transpulmonary passage of larvae (Loffler's syndrome): *Ascaris lumbricoides*, *Strongyloides stercoralis,* hookworm

White cell count (continued)

Pulmonary parenchymal invasion: paragonimiasis

Haematogenous spread: trichinosis, disseminated strongyloidiasis, schistosomiasis, cutaneous and visceral larva migrans

Tropical pulmonary eosinophilia: *Wuchereria bancrofti, Brugia malayi*

Drugs: nitrofurantoin, phenytoin

Allergic bronchopulmonary aspergillosis

Coccidioidomycosis

Churg–Strauss syndrome

Eosinophilic pneumonia

Eosinophilic leukaemia

Idiopathic hypereosinophilic syndrome

Lymphocytes

↑

Infections, e.g. viral, toxoplasmosis, TB, brucellosis, pertussis

Chronic lymphocytic leukaemia, prolymphocytic leukaemia, acute lymphoblastic leukaemia, hairy cell leukaemia

Non-Hodgkin's lymphoma

Thyrotoxicosis

↓

Pancytopaenia (e.g. marrow infiltration, chemotherapy/radiation)

Infection: AIDS, legionnaires' disease

Steroids

SLE

Uraemia

Wrist drop

Radial nerve lesion: trauma (e.g. secondary to a prolonged period of abnormal posture of the upper arm)

Mononeuritis multiplex (*See* Mononeuritis multiplex)

C7 root lesion

Topic Index